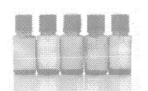

Essential Chemistry for Aromatherapy

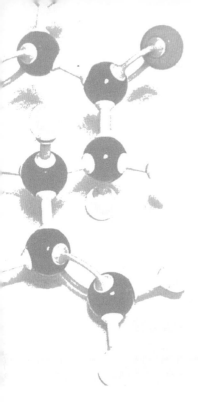

For Elsevier

Commissioning Editor: Claire Wilson
Development Editor: Kerry McGechie
Project Manager: Nancy Arnott
Designer: George Ajayi

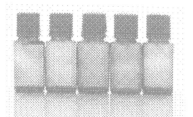

Essential Chemistry for Aromatherapy

Sue Clarke BSc (Hons) PhD

Senior Lecturer (formerly at Leigh College and Salford University) and freelance journalist, Cheshire, UK

SECOND EDITION

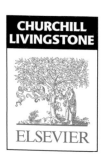

CHURCHILL
LIVINGSTONE

ELSEVIER

EDINBURGH LONDON NEW YORK OXFORD PHILADELPHIA ST LOUIS SYDNEY TORONTO 2008

CHURCHILL LIVINGSTONE
ELSEVIER

© First edition published 2002, Elsevier Ltd.
© 2008, Elsevier Limited. All rights reserved.

First edition 2002
Reprinted 2003, 2005

ISBN: 978-0-4431-0403-9

British Library Cataloguing in Publication Data
A catalogue record for this book is available from the British Library

Library of Congress Cataloging in Publication Data
A catalog record for this book is available from the Library of Congress

Notice

Knowledge and best practice in this field are constantly changing. As new research and experience broaden our knowledge, changes in practice, treatment and drug therapy may become necessary or appropriate. Readers are advised to check the most current information provided (i) on procedures featured or (ii) by the manufacturer of each product to be administered, to verify the recommended dose or formula, the method and duration of administration, and contraindications. It is the responsibility of the practitioner, relying on their own experience and knowledge of the patient, to make diagnoses, to determine dosages and the best treatment for each individual patient, and to take all appropriate safety precautions. To the fullest extent of the law, neither the Publisher nor the Author assumes any liability for any injury and/or damage to persons or property arising out or related to any use of the material contained in this book.

The Publisher

Printed in China

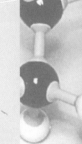

Contents

CHAPTER 1 Fundamentals of chemistry 7

CHAPTER 2 Organic chemistry 25

CHAPTER 3 Families of compounds that occur in essential oils 41

Preface

Complementary therapies, aromatherapy in particular, are increasingly popular. The demand for qualifed aromatherapists is reflected in the proliferating number of courses available. Courses relating to aromatherapy are offered in mainstream education, by private providers and as in-house training in various organizations. The standards and contents of courses vary widely, from courses running for a few hours at a weekend up to degree status. The qualifications gained, at the time of writing this text, are also very inconsistent. Currently developments are underway to establish UK national occupational standards (NOS). This is in line with the situation that now applies to other complementary practitioners such as osteopaths and chiropractors. They have to reach common standards that comply with statutory regulatory acts before they can be nationally registered. This ensures that clients can access practitioners with confidence.

The situation has been highlighted in the UK House of Lords report on CAM (Complementary and Alternative Medicine). Therapies were divided into three categories. The first category includes osteopathy, chiropractic, acupuncture, herbal medicine and homeopathy, which are described as 'professionally organized alternative therapies' and seen as the 'big five'. The second category, called 'complementary therapies', contains 12 types of therapy (including aromatherapy) that are used to complement mainstream medicine without diagnostic skills. The third category, entitled 'alternative disciplines', contains nine methodologies (including crystal therapy) that in the opinion of the CAM subcommittee favour a philosophical approach and are indifferent to the scientific principles of conventional medicine. The recommendations of this report have important implications for stimulating rigorous scientific research into CAM, and the development of better links between bodies such as the UK NHS R&D directorate, MRC (Medical Research Council), Department of Health and established research councils. Training is identified as being of paramount importance and there are calls for concerted partnership between higher educational institutions, with regulated professions acting as validating bodies to ensure that standards of training and competence are met.

A number of aromatherapy-related associations exist but unfortunately at the time of writing unification plans to produce a common register of members has not been achieved. The Aromatherapy consortium is charged with establishing a basis for a national register but does not involve unification of organisations. As the regulation and registration of complementary therapists in the UK is a voluntary self regulator it is politically controversial with perceived weaknesses. The training and regulation situation is developing, and there must be progress to ensure that aromatherapists belong to a register of fully and adequately qualified members with professional competence and standards, working to a code of conduct and practice. Aromatherapists should also be insured for both professional indemnity and public liability. Education and training are of crucial importance in achieving this goal and ensuring the meeting of common standards.

The NOS would specify a range of competencies and skills and provide underpinning knowledge within its training syllabus. A basic understanding of the concepts of science is important for an appreciation of the composition, safety and effective use of essential oils. The vast majority of students taking aromatherapy courses have little or no scientific background. Mature students, who make up a high proportion of those enrolling on these courses, often have a perception that science is difficult. For many students the scientific aspects of the course are the parts they find most daunting and incomprehensible. This book aims to explain basic background ideas and develop them into specific science applicable to aromatherapy. It should also provide a factual, accurate and easily accessible source of information for the large number of aromatherapy teachers drawn from disciplines such as beauty therapy and the social sciences.

Aromatherapy is now recognized by many people working in mainstream medicine, and qualified health professionals are increasingly taking supplementary qualifications in aromatherapy. Their medical science background will hopefully connect with the scope of the material in this book and help give credibility to the discipline.

A wide variety of aromatherapy books are available, ranging from the attractive coffee-table style to the specialized aromatology type aimed at health professionals. The most under-represented are those related to the background science. Many general aromatherapy textbooks have vague and ambiguous science sections. The small number of science texts on the market are good but assume a working knowledge of chemistry and tend to be written by chemists from the perfumery industry. The majority of students and qualified aromatherapists find these books difficult to understand, and data sheets on essential oils will refer to gas chromatography–mass spectroscopy (GC-MS), retention times, optical rotation, etc. This book aims to explain these aspects to readers with no prior knowledge of chemistry, acting as a bridge to allow them to progress to the more advanced texts. It should also enable aromatherapists to interpret and appreciate analytical data relating to the oils they use.

This book was prepared in the light of my experiences teaching an advanced science unit to qualified and practising aromatherapists. Although they had previously attended a variety of courses in both the public and the private sectors, they felt the science was inadequate and did not meet their needs. They were unable to apply what they had learned to their working situations. Their comments and experiences were addressed in preparation of this book and in subsequent teaching on an aromatology university degree module. Since publication of the first edition of this book I have taken two courses in aromatherapy. One in a Further Education College and the other with a private provider. These broadened my perspective from the student angle. My aim remains to give an objective view from someone who is outside the aromatherapy community.

SPECIAL NOTE

The material presented does not claim to be original in any way. It merely represents a selection, organization and an approach to a subject that is covered in a number of other sources. It aims to bring together those topics relevant to the science of aromatherapy, and couple these with its application to the understanding of the practice of aromatherapy. It is hoped that it will demystify the chemistry, making it more understandable and enjoyable.

The pharmaceutical and physiological properties attributed to the essential oils and their individual components are generally established in folklore or are anecdotal. The specific properties of a single compound will not necessarily always be evident when the compound is present in an essential oil; the oil may modify these properties in a number of ways. Large, statistically viable clinical trials with humans have not been carried out on the essential oils or most of their components in the way that a conventional/mainstream drug would have been evaluated. Different sources will give different points of view. *The points of view stated in this book are those of the author* and reflect the views presented in some of the established aromatherapy books in usage at the time this book went to press. However, as research and knowledge in this field is constantly being updated, the latest specialist texts should always be consulted together with information provided by manufacturers.

Sue Clarke

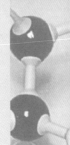

Acknowledgements

Len Cegielka, scientific copyeditor on the 1st edition, for tackling the onerous job with care and humour.

Jasbir S. Chana, Phoenix Products Ltd, A4 Bridge Road Industrial Estate, Bridge Road, Southall, Middlesex UB2 4AB. www.phoenixproducts.co.uk for advice and data supply.

Tony Clarke, Chartered Chemist, for scientific perspective, technical and IT support and infinite patience.

Dr Jane Collins Director of Research and Development (into essential oil plants), Phytobotanica UK Ltd, Lydiate, Merseyside. www.phytobotanica. com for advice, help, information, interest and supply of analytical data.

Robyn Cowan, Royal Botanical Gardens, Kew for help and advice.

Stephen Freeborn, former Director of Pharmacy, Salford Royal Hospitals NHS Trust. Now Head of Pharmacy and Medicines Management, Ascribe plc, Westhoughton, Bolton for information relating to mainstream pharmaceutical issues.

Lindsay Harper, Senior Pharmacist and Aromatherapist, **Elaine Myers** and **Joanne McEntee**, Pharmacists, and the Medicines Information Unit at Hope Hospital, Salford Royal Hospitals NHS Trust. **Alison Martin**, Pharmacist, Boots for information relating to mainstream pharmaceutical issues.

Bob Harris, Editor of the International Journal of Aromatherapy and Essential Oil Resource Consultant (EORC), Au Village, 83840 La Martre, Provence, France www.essentialorc.com for advice, help and interest.

Beverley Higham, Aromatherapist and Lecturer, Wigan and Leigh College, for initial introduction to aromatherapy.

Keren Jamieson for typing and preparing original manuscript.

Stephen Kent FRCS, Consultant ENT Surgeon, North Cheshire Hospital, for help and advice.

Geoff Lyth, Chairman of the ATC and Managing Director of Quinessence aromatherapy, Forest Court, Linden Way, Coalville, Leicestershire LE67 3JY. www.quinessence.com for advice, help, information, interest and supply of analytical data.

Valerie McCowan, Course Leader and Tutor for Complementary Therapies, Warrington Collegiate, Cheshire, for her inspired teaching of aromatherapy to me as a mature student and for advice and help.

Dr William Morden, Chartered Chemist, Director of Essential Analyses, Elm Cottage, Old Road, Whaley Bridge, High Peak SK23 7HS. www.essentialanalyses.co.uk for help, advice, information and supply of data.

Inta Ozols, formerly Publishing Manager and **Jane Dingwall**, Project Manager at Harcourt Health Sciences (now Elsevier) for support, encouragement and understanding to guide me through the 1st edition. **Karen Morley** and **Claire Wilson**, Commissioning Editors, and **Kerry McGechie**, Development Editor, **Nancy Arnott**, Project Manager **George Ajayi**, Designer Health Professions, Elsevier for similar help to get to the 2nd edition.

Len (and Shirley) Price, Pioneers of aromatherapy and aromatology. International lecturers and authors for help, advice, information and data.

Jennifer Rhind, Aromatologist and Lecturer, Napier University, Edinburgh, for review of original manuscript from an experienced practitioner's and educator's eye.

Jane Riley, Medical Herbalist, Liverpool and **Timothy Whittaker** (now retired) formerly Chief Chemist of Potters Herbal Products, Wigan for information relating to herbal products.

Alan Sanders formerly Spectroscopy Central Ltd, Maple House, Padgate Business Centre, Green Lane, Padgate, Warrington, Cheshire WA1 4JN. Now at Smiths Detection International UK, Genesis Centre, Science Park South, Birchwood, Warrington, Cheshire WA3 7BH.

James and Phillip Spiring, Spiring Enterprises Limited, Beke Hall, West Sussex RH14 9HF for help, interest, advice, molecular modelling and photography. All the photographs of molymod® molecular models were kindly provided by James C. Spiring of Spiring Enterprises Limited, Billinghurst, the inventors and sole manufacturers of the molymod® molecular model system. www.molymod.com

Robert Tisserand, for help, support and advice.

Jenny Warden, formerly Director of Traceability, Hoole Bridge, Chester, for help, interest, advice and supply of data (Traceability is no longer trading).

Charles and Justin Wells, Essentially Oils and Analytical Intelligence Limited, 10 Mount Farm, Junction Road, Churchill, Chipping Norton OX7 6NP. www.essentiallyoils.com for help, interest, information, advice and supply of data.

The many students over the years who taught me so much.

Introduction

Advances in medical science have vastly improved our health and life expectancy. Likewise, scientific developments have given us a better quality of life, improved living conditions and a range of choices that were not possible a hundred years ago. Unfortunately, the material gains have not always compensated for the increasing psychological pressures and expectations experienced in living in today's stressful and materialistic society.

The search for answers that are spiritual rather than scientific is also significant. The rise of alternative or complementary therapies reflects this need, as more people question conventional medicine. The value of a holistic approach to health and well-being, linking the mind and body with the lifestyle of an individual, is now widely recognized. Although conventional medicine has limits resulting from financial, political and bureaucratic constraints, it should be the first line of investigation and reference for health problems, and for many conditions it should offer appropriate and effective treatment. The development of a range of complementary therapies, working alongside and supplementing mainstream medicine, is more favoured now. In many circumstances it would be cruel and immoral to offer false hopes of a cure by use of an alternative therapy only, but a better partnership between conventional and complementary medicine can ensure a more effective and beneficial approach for all concerned. Complementary practitioners usually have more time to fully explore the needs of a patient, with the opportunity to follow up allied to fewer constraints. There is an argument for a more widespread use of aromatherapy in the treatment of psychologically rooted conditions and many minor ailments. These could include burns, bites, sore throats, and tired and aching muscles and joints; aromatherapy can also function as an aid to relaxation in many stressful situations. In this way, easily accessible and inexpensive remedies could be made available, with the advantage of taking some of the pressure off GPs.

In many cases the approach and techniques of the complementary therapies have a scientific basis. This is particularly true for aromatherapy using essential oils extracted from plants. Aromatherapy is scientific in terms of the biochemical and physiological functioning of the body and works in conjunction with the more esoteric and spiritual needs of the individual. It is naive and dangerous to dismiss science as bad and separate from our use of natural materials. A dictionary definition of science is 'the systematic study of the nature and behaviour of the material and physical universe, based on observation, experiment and measurement'. Scientific findings are 'a body of knowledge organized in a systematic manner'. To be credible and effective, both conventional and complementary medicine must adopt a scientific approach delivered with care and insight.

Among the complementary therapies, aromatherapy has an impressive history. It dates back as far as 2800 BC in ancient Egypt and was widespread in the Mediterranean region, with the earliest known distillation for extraction of essential oil from plant material being recorded by Herodotus in about 425 BC. During the Middle Ages the properties of aromatic plants were utilized to combat infectious diseases such as the plague; more recently, the Frenchman Gattefosse (often called the father of aromatherapy) used them to effect in the treatment of wounds of soldiers in the First World War. The art of distillation was developed to form the basis of alchemy, which has further developed into more technical chemistry. The use of herbal preparations and plant extracts is well established; the 'active' agents have been isolated and incorporated into many current pharmaceutical preparations. In aromatherapy training and practice in Britain, essential oils are administered to clients via inhalation, topical application and skin massages, and in baths. Interest in such techniques is stimulating research into the properties and actions of these oils and the development of aromatology. Aromatology additionally consists in administering oils internally by mouth, injections, pessaries and suppositories. Countries in which aromatology is practised, such as France, have practitioners who are also medically qualified. Specialized training courses are becoming increasingly popular in the UK. For reasons of safety it is not appropriate for aromatherapists to use essential oils internally on clients.

Science also has a significant history; many famous scientists were also renowned philosophers and spiritual leaders. Science has built up a vast body of knowledge that is still developing. Chemistry is just one branch of what is referred to as the physical sciences, concerned with the composition, properties and reactions of substances. A knowledge of chemistry is fundamental since all matter, whether natural or synthetic, is made up of substances or 'chemicals'. It is wrong to assume that because something is natural it must be safe and without side-effects. Many natural substances cause severe health problems: for example, the bacteria and their toxins that cause food poisoning, and pollen grains and associated allergies like hay fever. The incorrect use of 'natural' remedies is causing an increased incidence of patients reporting to their doctors with problems attributed to them. By understanding the properties of the substances that may cause us harm, we can either avoid them or deal with them in an appropriate way.

The essential oils used in aromatherapy are a potent mix of chemicals, with a vast range of properties and reactions, and should be handled with caution. A useful working definition of aromatherapy is *the use of essential oils in a controlled manner*. In order to ensure safe and effective use of these oils, the aromatherapist must be trained and have an understanding of the materials being applied. As with all things, there are risks and benefits, which must be evaluated.

This book looks at those aspects of chemistry that are relevant to essential oils. It starts with elements and simple atomic structures and builds up to molecules with basic types of bonding. Molecular diagrams and models are used to reinforce the understanding of these structures. The aromatherapy oils are mixtures of substances that come under the branch of organic chemistry. The principles of organic chemistry are developed in the context of the specialized molecules of the oils, which are based on natural products derived from the group of compounds called terpenes. Structures are explained in terms of their molecular properties and functional groups. The different chemical groups found are often an indication of the properties and therapeutic uses of the oils containing them, and explain the existence of chemotypes. The unique balance of properties imparted to many whole and pure essential oils is explored in concepts such as synergy.

The quality and composition of essential oils are of paramount importance to the aromatherapist when choosing oils. We all expect to see products such as foods and cosmetics properly labelled, giving names and amounts of ingredients along with instructions for use and associated possible hazards. This is not yet the situation with aromatherapy oils, but it is likely to develop. It will be a considerable task as essential oils may contain up to three hundred different compounds, albeit many in minuscule amounts, and criteria would have to be set to decide a convention for such labelling. Good working practices, as currently advised, are outlined in this area.

Analysis of the composition and purity of aromatherapy products relies on a number of well-established scientific techniques. The principles and application of those most commonly employed, such as GC (gas–liquid chromatography), MS (mass spectrometry) and optical rotation, are explained. The importance of the human senses in the physiological analysis and appreciation of essential oils is also outlined.

The composition of essential oils in terms of their chemical components is further evaluated by looking at a number that are popularly employed in aromatherapy. Their composition is described, and chemotypes are identified and defined using analytical data to back up the attributed properties. Analysis is important for checking the purity of an oil and this is further developed by considering methods of extraction, processing and handling that are implicated in the composition of the product. The types of products obtained from plants are distinguished along with the most commonly encountered adulteration problems. Chemical principles and a common-sense approach are adopted in sections on handling, storage and basic first aid.

Safety is always a vital consideration when using any type of chemical. There are a host of legislative issues that must be taken into account, which are designed to offer protection to both client and aromatherapist. These include COSHH (Control of Substances Hazardous to Health) and The Safety of Medicines and an increasing number of EC regulations, but the situation is constantly changing and the book summarizes the main ones currently under review. There is no guarantee that the details provided will still be accurate at any given time in the future, so the associated professional bodies must be consulted.

The therapeutic applications of aromatherapy oils and their constituent compounds are listed. However, a full consideration of these is not appropriate to this book. The properties of such oils are well documented in more specialized texts. Essential oils have been used along with other plant-based medicines over many centuries. Experience and knowledge of their effects and benefits were gathered and have been passed on from generation to generation. Generally they were found to be beneficial and safe with few reported side-effects. The amounts of the active compounds in natural products such as herbal remedies are generally lower than would be found in the formulation of a modern drug. Also, oils have a mixture of components, which balances effects in a synergistic manner. The amounts, dosage and uptake of any substance in the body should always be taken into consideration. The essential oils in the aromatherapist's dispensary are of high concentration, far exceeding that in the living plant, so correct dosage and dilutions must be carefully observed.

There will always be arguments against the use of therapies involving herbal preparations and essential oils on the grounds that they have not been subjected to rigorous scientific evaluation. Much evidence is said to be anecdotal and subjective. This again was identified in the House of Lords CAM (Complementary and Alternative Medicine) report. The holistic approach adopted within aromatherapy means that the unique circumstances of the individual client and the oils chosen for use make an objective scientific comparison impossible. The extensive resources, financial backup and situation within healthcare provision of the drug companies allow them to carry out research and clinical trials. To get a new drug onto the market takes many millions of pounds and years of work with a suitable group of patients. This would be beyond the reach of the aromatherapy suppliers, and the current medical establishment has a vested interest to resist such a development. There are, however, an increasing number of scientific papers and data being published to support the therapeutic use of essential oils. It is always interesting to note the importance of the placebo effect: this is the positive therapeutic effect claimed by a patient after receiving an inactive substance, called a placebo, that they believed to be an active drug. The placebo is an inactive substance administered to a patient usually to compare its effects with those of a real drug. It is sometimes thought to be a psychological benefit to patients by making them believe they are receiving treatment. The source of much relief to a problem can come from within the individual and is triggered or released by an appropriate stimulus. The stimulus may be a chemical, a touch or even a smile or laughter. The role of a number of chemicals produced by the brain, called endorphins, is accepted. The endorphins act in a similar way to the substance morphine, which is a very powerful opiate drug used as an analgesic, or pain reliever. In addition to their analgesic properties, the endorphins are thought to be involved in controlling the body's response to stress, in determining mood and possibly in regulating the release of a number of hormones. Acupuncture is thought to stimulate the release of endorphins to provide pain relief and, indeed, many techniques used in aromatherapy are likely to induce their release and contribute to the 'feel-good factor'.

The book sets out to make the scientific aspects of aromatherapy understandable and relevant by use of situations and examples found in the practice of aromatherapy. Data from oil suppliers, which are theoretically available to aromatherapists, are used to illustrate ideas and examples. Although these data can be obtained, this is not usually a financially viable option to the average aromatherapist. A basic analysis will often cost more than the oil. This, again, is a situation that may change in the course of time with ever-increasing legislation.

As stated in the Preface, *this book does not contain any original or new ideas.* It aims to collate the information already available from a variety of sources. These sources are listed and should be useful for further reading. This should reinforce the content of training courses and supplement ideas and concepts taught in them with other sources of information. The basic topics covered in this book should act as a stepping stone and stimulus for the reader to consult the more specialized and advanced texts.

Aromatherapy has nothing to fear from scientific knowledge and examination. Such scrutiny should help to further its applications and credibility in a wider spectrum of both practitioners and clients. It is hoped that this book will provide a better understanding of and partnership between the spiritual and scientific aspects to speed up the progress of aromatherapy.

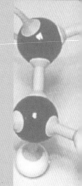

Chapter 1

Fundamentals of chemistry

A knowledge of the materials we are using will help us to understand their structure and properties. This in turn will allow us to use them more effectively and safely. In order to do this we need to apply some fundamental scientific concepts drawn mainly from chemistry.

 ## AROMAFACT

Many people feel that if something contains 'chemicals' it must be bad. There is no escaping the fact that every substance we encounter is made up of chemicals. Your favourite organically grown lavender oil is composed of a mixture of up to 300 different chemicals. To say that it is bad because it contains chemicals is nonsense. However, an understanding of these chemicals and their properties is fundamental, and this is what chemistry is about.

The science that gives us the knowledge and understanding of chemistry can enhance the use of essential oils, and is important for safe handling and practical applications, especially when linked with the experience and intuition of the aromatherapist.

Essential oils have properties that reflect their chemical composition and the range and amounts of constituents are used for evaluation of qualities such as criteria for purity, in determining extraction methods and in defining aspects such as chemotypes.

ORGANIZATION OF MATTER

The British scientist John Dalton put forward an atomic theory of matter at the beginning of the nineteenth century. This remains a sound basis for understanding the world around us and the actions and reactions of its chemical components. Dalton proposed that all substances are made of matter, which occupies space and has mass, and his theory deals with the nature of this matter.

The main points of the theory are as follow:

- All substances are made up of small particles known as *atoms*.
- An element is a substance that cannot be broken down into other substances.
- All atoms of the same element are identical in mass,[1] size and shape and differ from those of other elements.
- Atoms are indivisible and cannot be broken into smaller parts.
- Atoms can combine together in simple whole number proportions to form *molecules*.

Phases

Matter exists in three *phases* or states:

- solid
- liquid
- gas.

This can be easily explained with reference to water as an example. As a solid it is ice. Ice melts to liquid water. The liquid can then be boiled to form gaseous vapour (steam). Definite temperatures are associated with these changes (Fig. 1.1). Each substance has its own specific temperatures at which these changes of phase take place.

Properties such as boiling points are important as criteria for purity: pure water boils at 100 °C and freezes at 0 °C under the normal ambient atmospheric

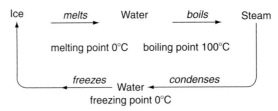

Figure 1.1   Changes of phase of water.

---

[1] *Mass* in scientific terms is a precisely defined concept that measures a body's resistance to being accelerated but it is also equivalent in practical terms to the 'amount of matter' in the body. Things of the same mass have the same *weight* when in the same situation – in normal life, here at the surface of the Earth. This is why we can use the weight of a body as commonly understood to compare the masses of bodies. In technical senses the two concepts need to be distinguished, but for our purposes the terms can be used synonymously and will be used interchangeably. Which term is used in a particular context will depend largely upon conventional usage. Thus while we speak of the mass of an atom, the term molecular weight is frequently used.

pressure. If a substance such as salt is added, the boiling point becomes higher and the freezing point becomes lower. This is useful in cold weather: salt put down on steps and roads prevents ice forming until the temperature is very much lower than the freezing point of pure water. We can also separate mixtures of liquids by *distillation*, which relies on the different boiling points of the components.

AROMAFACT

The most widespread extraction method for essential oils is steam distillation. This utilizes the volatility (the different boiling points) of the components of a mixture to allow them to be separated from other plant materials.

The arrangement and movement of the particles in matter account for its properties in the various phases. In a gas, the particles move freely and at great speed and collide frequently with one another with considerable energy; as a result, a gas completely fills the space available in any container. In a solid, there is no free movement of particles, which occupy fixed positions (although they vibrate around these positions); as a result, solids have definite shape and size. Liquids occupy an intermediate position: the particles are relatively free to move, so that a liquid flows to adopt the shape of its container, but they are attracted to each other sufficiently to keep them together and prevent the particles filling the whole space, as with a gas. The arrangements and motions of particles in the three phases of matter are shown in Figure 1.2. The movement of the particles gives them a property called *kinetic energy*; the more rapid the motion, the greater the kinetic energy. Heating increases the kinetic energy of molecules, changing them from solids to liquids, and then from liquids to gases.

State	Shape	Particle arrangement	Relative distance between particles	Diagrammatic representation	Movement of particles	Diffusion	State
Gas	No definite shape, fills container	Random	Large		Rapid	Rapid	Gas
Liquid	Takes shape of container	Fairly regular	Small		Rapid	Slow	Liquid
Solid	Has definite shape and size	Regular pattern	None (virtually touching)		Almost none (vibration about fixed position)	Very slow	Solid

Figure 1.2   The arrangements and motions of particles in the three phases of matter.

AROMAFACT

The movement of gas particles is essential in aromatherapy. A substance must be constantly losing particles into the gas or vapour phase, which can enter the air and then the nose and be detected as an odour. *Volatility* is the property of a substance to evaporate (disperse as vapour). If a few drops of pure, concentrated essential oil are put out in a room on a dish, their presence will soon be detectable at any point in that room. Oil vapour molecules mix and collide with air molecules, gradually spreading evenly through a room (by the process of *diffusion*).

The process of mixing of gas particles is called *diffusion*: molecules move from an area of high concentration (such as liquid oil in a dish) to an area of low concentration such as the air in the room. We smell food as it is heated up and cooked due to molecules of gas forming, escaping and diffusing into the air. Diffusion also takes place in liquids as molecules of one substance intermingle and spread out among those of another. Diffusion is important for movement of substances in the body.

AROMAFACT

A *volatile* substance is one that readily evaporates. Essential oils are volatile, with the top notes having the lowest boiling points and coming off most readily.

Physical changes

Changes of phase such as melting and boiling, evaporation and condensation, the dissolving of solids in a liquid or diffusion of gases are called physical changes. No new substances are formed in these processes, although the properties of the new phases or mixtures may be different.

Chemical changes

Chemical changes result in the formation of *new substances* when the composition of the original substance is changed; for example, when a metal reacts with the oxygen of the air it forms a new substance called an oxide (as when iron goes rusty). Essential oils can also react with oxygen, which alters their chemical composition and properties. Other chemical reactions can be initiated by light and are called *photochemical* reactions (*photo* means light). The photochemical process of photosynthesis is essential to green plants for the manufacture of food using light as an energy source. Heat will usually speed up chemical reactions, by increasing the kinetic energy of atoms or molecules so that they collide and interact more frequently. Living systems contain complex protein molecules called enzymes which act as catalysts to either speed up or slow down the rates of the chemical reactions occurring in the cells.

AROMAFACT

It is generally accepted that storage conditions for essential oils are important. The aromatherapist should keep oils in sealed bottles made of dark glass to protect them from the air and light, which can cause deterioration through chemical reaction. Keeping the bottles cool will slow any remaining reactions that could affect the oil's composition.

Elements

The simplest substances are the *elements*. They cannot be broken down into simpler constituents by chemical reactions. Ninety-two elements exist in nature; although some additional ones can be created experimentally by the techniques of nuclear physics, they exist only for very short periods of time before decaying radioactively. The elements can be arranged in basic groupings based on their properties: a fundamental division is into *metals* (e.g. iron, copper, gold, sodium) and *nonmetals* (e.g. carbon, oxygen, hydrogen, sulfur).

AROMAFACT

As an aromatherapist you will encounter very few elements in their pure form as constituents of essential oils. However, the numbers of ways in which elements can join up chemically to form compounds is astonishing.

For convenience, each element is given a *chemical symbol* that acts as a chemical shorthand in talking and writing about it and its reactions. The symbol always comprises one or two letters; the first letter is a capital, which may correspond to the initial letter of the element's name: Mg = magnesium, Ca = calcium, C = carbon, O = oxygen, H = hydrogen, S = sulphur, He = helium. Some chemical symbols are less obvious because they are derived from Latin names for the elements: Pb = lead (*plumbum*), Fe = iron (*ferrum*), Na = sodium (*natrium*), K = potassium (*kalium*).

Atoms

The *structure* of the atom is very important and gives the element its properties. An atom is arranged as a central *nucleus* surrounded by outer *electrons*. The nucleus is very small but very dense, being responsible for nearly all the mass (weight) of the atom. It is made up of two particles: *protons*, which carry a positive electric charge (+1) and are given a relative (arbitrary) mass unit of 1; and *neutrons*, which have no electric charge but have the same relative mass as the proton (a relative mass unit of 1). The nucleus is only 1/100000 of the diameter of the whole atom.

Most of the *volume* of the atom as a whole accounts for hardly any of the total mass of the atom. It contains negatively charged particles called *electrons*, each of which has only 1/2000 the mass of a proton or neutron. Each electron has a negative electric charge of minus one (−1).

The differences between elements are due to the differing numbers of these subatomic particles (the protons, neutrons and electrons) in their atoms. Bigger, heavier atoms are built up from more subatomic particles than smaller ones.

Atoms are electrically neutral (they have no *overall* electric charge) and the number of protons (with positive charge) is equal to the number of electrons (with negative charge).

The arrangement as well as the number of the electrons is important as this determines the chemical properties of the elements and the reactions they undergo. The electrons are found in *shells* (or *orbitals* in the language of atomic physics and chemistry) in the volume around the nucleus.

Although atoms are very small (about one hundred millionth of a centimetre in diameter), scientists have been able to learn a great deal about their structure and how it affects the behaviour of the elements. To explain the arrangement of the electrons, the idea of them in layers (shells or orbitals) surrounding the nucleus is useful. What is called the *electronic configuration* of an atom shows the number of electrons in each shell surrounding the nucleus. Shells are numbered sequentially starting at the centre and working outwards, and for each shell there is a maximum number of electrons that it can contain:

Shell 1	holds up to	2 electrons
Shell 2	holds up to	8 electrons
Shell 3	holds up to	18 electrons

The individual shells are made up of a number of *subshells* in which the electrons have different spatial arrangements (the 'shapes' of the orbitals differ). The number of subshells available in a given shell is equal to the shell number. So shell 1 comprises only one subshell (its type is designated s). Shell 2 is made up of two subshells (an s type subshell of the same shape as the 1s subshell and a second type designated p type; this is the 2p subshell). Shell 3 comprises three subshells, an s type (3s), a p type (3p), and type designated d, the 3d subshell. An s subshell can hold two electrons, so that shell 1 can hold two electrons in total. A p type subshell can hold six electrons, so shell 2 can hold eight electrons (two in the s subshell and six in the p subshell). The pattern repeats in shell 3, with now the d subshell able to hold 10 electrons. Thus shell 3 can contain two s electrons, six p electrons and ten d electrons, making a maximum of 18 electrons in shell 3. However, in the atoms we will be considering, only the 3s and 3p subshells will be involved as there are not enough electrons to start filling the d shell. Thus, for our purposes, we can consider shell 3 to contain up to 8 electrons.

Atoms are characterized by their *atomic number*, which corresponds to the number of protons in the nucleus (and to the number of electrons outside it, since these are balanced for electrical neutrality), and by their *mass number*, which corresponds to the number of protons plus the number of neutrons in the nucleus and gives the relative mass (weight) of the atom, since the electrons contribute hardly anything to the total mass of an atom. All atoms of a given element have the same atomic number and atomic mass. When the information is useful, the atomic mass can be added to the chemical symbol, written as a small superscript to the left of the symbol. Similarly, the atomic number can be added as a small subscript to the left of the symbol.

We can illustrate these concepts by applying them to three of the elements previously mentioned: helium, carbon and sodium.

Helium   Helium has an atomic number of 2 and a mass number of 4; this means it has 2 protons, 2 neutrons and 2 electrons. The electronic configuration (the arrangement of electrons in the shells) is 2 in the first shell, which is the maximum number possible for this shell. It can be represented as

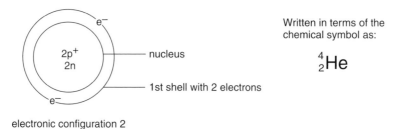

Written in terms of the chemical symbol as:

$$_2^4He$$

electronic configuration 2

where p^+ = proton, n = neutron and e^- = electron (the superscript indicates the electric charge of the particle, + positive or − negative; this can be omitted).

Carbon   Carbon has an atomic number of 6 and a mass number of 12; this means it has 6 protons, 6 neutrons and 6 electrons. The electronic configuration is 2 filling the first shell with 4 in the second shell. It can be represented as

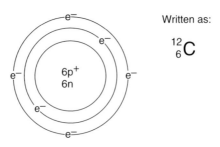

Written as:

$$^{12}_{6}C$$

electronic configuration 2.4

Sodium   Sodium has as an atomic number of 11 and a mass number of 23; this means it has 11 protons, 12 neutrons and 11 electrons. The electronic configuration is 2 filling the first shell, 8 filling the second shell with 1 in the third shell. It can be represented as

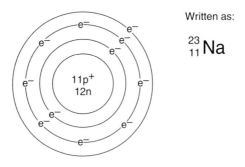

Written as:

$$^{23}_{11}Na$$

electronic configuration 2.8.1

The periodic table

A very useful arrangement of atoms in order of their atomic numbers is the periodic table of the elements. The number of electrons in an atom of an element and their configuration are related to the position of that element in the periodic table. The periodic table has vertical columns called *groups* and horizontal rows called *periods*. Only the first three periods are represented in Table 1.1.

Table 1.1   The first three rows of the periodic table of the elements, from hydrogen (H) to argon (Ar)

	Groups							
Group	1	2	3	4	5	6	7	0 or 18
Period 1	H (1)							He (2)
Period 2	Li (3)	Be (4)	B (5)	C (6)	N (7)	O (8)	F (9)	Ne (10)
Period 3	Na (11)	Mg (12)	Al (13)	Si (14)	P (15)	S (16)	Cl (17)	Ar (18)

The atomic number is shown in brackets next to each element. Going across a period, each atom has one more proton, and therefore one more electron, than its predecessor. In the first period there is one shell of electrons, from hydrogen (one electron) up to helium, which has two electrons. In the second period there are two shells of electrons, from lithium up to neon, which has eight electrons in its outer shell (shell 2) (plus two in the inner shell for a total of 10). In the third period there are three shells of electrons in the atoms, from sodium up to argon with eight electrons in its outermost shell (shell 3).

There are eight groups in the first three periods of the periodic table, numbered 1 to 7 and 18 or 0 (remember that shell 3 can hold up to 18 electrons, although in the atoms depicted only the 3s and 3p subshells are being filled, with up to 8 electrons). The group number for groups 1 to 7 corresponds to the number of *outer shell* electrons in the atomic structure. For example, hydrogen and sodium have 1 outer electron and are found in group 1; carbon and silicon have 4 outer electrons and are found in group 4; chlorine and fluorine have 7 outer electrons and are found in group 7. Helium is unusual as it has two electrons in total and its outer (only) shell is *full*. It appears in group 0 (or 18), which represents atoms with filled shells like neon and argon with 8 electrons in their outermost shells (shells 2 and 3 respectively). The possession of filled outer shells gives very stable (unreactive) elements called the *inert gases* or *noble gases* or *rare gases*.

A complete periodic table of all the elements is shown in the Glossary. In period 4, the 3d subshell is being filled up, with up to 10 more electrons, which shows why the rare gases have group number 18.

Molecules

A *molecule* is defined as the smallest unit of a substance that retains the properties of that substance or the smallest particle of matter that can exist in a free state. A molecule can comprise just one element, like the oxygen molecule (O_2), which consists of two oxygen atoms joined together, or different elements as in carbon dioxide (CO_2), made up of one carbon atom joined to two oxygen atoms.

Some elements have atoms that exist as free individual atoms, such as helium or the other inert gases. In other elements the atoms join together to form molecules. Hydrogen, oxygen and nitrogen molecules are made up of two atoms, and their molecules are written as H_2, O_2 and N_2. The way atoms link together is very specific and is due to their outer electrons forming chemical bonds.

COMPOUNDS

Compounds are substances whose molecules are made up of two or more different elements that have become chemically bonded or joined together:

- Water is a compound of the elements hydrogen and oxygen.
- Carbon dioxide is a compound of the elements carbon and oxygen.

- Table salt is a compound of the elements sodium and chlorine.
- Alcohols are compounds of the elements carbon, hydrogen and oxygen.
- Terpenes of essential oils are compounds of the elements carbon and hydrogen.

When atoms of elements join together they use only their outer electrons. As we know, the numbers of electrons are characteristic of each element's atom, and when they form bonds atoms link in fixed whole numbers to give a molecule represented by a *molecular formula*.

- Water is two H atoms linked with one O atom to give H_2O.
- Carbon dioxide is one C atom linked with two O atoms to give CO_2.
- Common salt is one Na atom linked with one Cl atom to give NaCl.
- Ethanol is two C atoms linked to six H atoms and one O atom to give C_2H_6O (which is usually written as C_2H_5OH).

AROMAFACT

The basic unit for many aromatherapy compounds is the terpene called *isoprene*. It is made up of five carbon atoms and eight hydrogen atoms. Its molecular formula is C_5H_8.

If we know the molecular formula of a compound it tells us about the size of the molecule, and a *molecular weight* (or molecular mass) can be calculated from the weights (masses) of the individual component atoms.

The chemical bonding between any atoms is due to their outer electrons and these are sometimes referred to as *valence* electrons. *Valency* is the combining power of atoms. The inert gases are known to be very stable and do not readily form chemical bonds. This is due to their outer shells of electrons being full or complete. Atoms of other elements approximate this stability by losing, gaining or sharing electrons until they have filled outer shell arrangements like those of the inert gases.

TYPES OF CHEMICAL BONDING

Electrovalent bonds

This type of bonding gives rise to *electrovalent* or *ionic compounds*. Such compounds are formed by loss or gain of electrons from the participating atoms. Atoms are normally neutrally charged, with numbers of protons (+) equal to numbers of electrons (−). If electrons are either gained or lost, an atom or group of atoms with a net overall charge due to the imbalance of + and − charges is formed; this is called an *ion*. This loss or gain of electrons is typically found between a metal and a nonmetal. If electrons are gained, the atom becomes a *negative ion* (−); if electrons are lost, a *positive ion* (+) is formed.

If we look at the structure of the atoms and their positions in the periodic table, metals are on the left-hand side in groups 1, 2 and 3, e.g.:

- Na in group 1: one outer electron
- Mg in group 2: two outer electrons
- Al in group 3: three outer electrons.

Metals can *lose* these outer electrons and form *positive ions*; the charge is due to the higher number of protons (+) that remain relative to the number of electrons. The number of electrons lost is equal to the group number in the periodic table and the resultant ion has a stable electronic configuration like that of an inert gas. The net charge on the ion is written to the right of the chemical symbol as a small superscript.

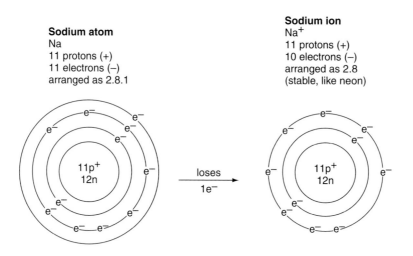

Sodium atom
Na
11 protons (+)
11 electrons (−)
arranged as 2.8.1

loses
$1e^-$

Sodium ion
Na^+
11 protons (+)
10 electrons (−)
arranged as 2.8
(stable, like neon)

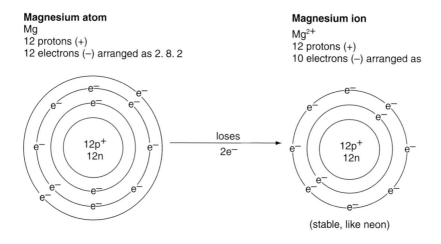

Magnesium atom
Mg
12 protons (+)
12 electrons (−) arranged as 2. 8. 2

loses
$2e^-$

Magnesium ion
Mg^{2+}
12 protons (+)
10 electrons (−) arranged as

(stable, like neon)

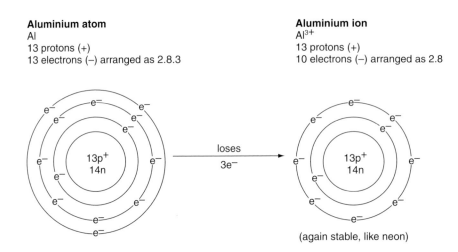

Aluminium atom
Al
13 protons (+)
13 electrons (−) arranged as 2.8.3

Aluminium ion
Al^{3+}
13 protons (+)
10 electrons (−) arranged as 2.8

loses
$3e^-$

(again stable, like neon)

Metals are described as *electropositive elements*, and the positive ions they form are called *cations*.

Nonmetals gain electrons to achieve stability. They are found in groups 4 to 7 of the periodic table. Carbon in group 4 is a unique element and will be dealt with later. Nonmetals in groups 5, 6 and 7 gain electrons to fill their shells to the maximum permissible extent, and the number they gain is 8 minus the group number. For example, oxygen is in group 6 and gains 2 electrons $(8 - 6 = 2)$ to form a negative ion, termed the oxide ion.

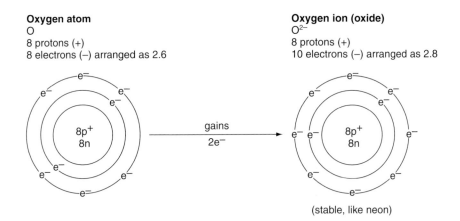

Oxygen atom
O
8 protons (+)
8 electrons (−) arranged as 2.6

Oxygen ion (oxide)
O^{2-}
8 protons (+)
10 electrons (−) arranged as 2.8

gains
$2e^-$

(stable, like neon)

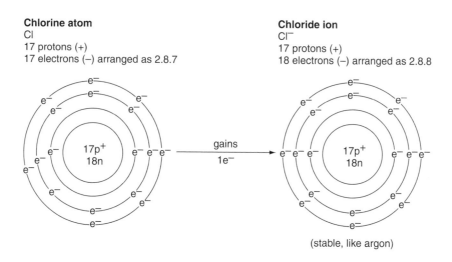

Chlorine atom
Cl
17 protons (+)
17 electrons (−) arranged as 2.8.7

Chloride ion
Cl⁻
17 protons (+)
18 electrons (−) arranged as 2.8.8

gains
1e⁻

(stable, like argon)

Nonmetals are described as electronegative elements and the negative ions they form are called anions.

Electrovalent bonds are formed between oppositely charged ions, and typically a metal donates electrons to a nonmetal. For example, sodium chloride (common salt, an important constituent of the body's fluids) is written as Na^+Cl^-. For sodium chloride only one electron is involved in the transfer and the molecular formula is written as NaCl. However, if sodium forms an ionic compound with oxygen, an oxygen atom needs two electrons to form an ion, so it will need to have two sodium atoms donating electrons:

2 Na atoms (2.8.1)   →   2 Na⁺ ions (2.8)
                  loss of 2 electrons

1 O atom (2.6)   →   1 O²⁻ ion (2.8)
             picks up the 2 electrons

The formula for sodium oxide is Na_2O.

In the same way, if calcium reacted with chlorine, the calcium atom donates two electrons, 2e⁻, but a chlorine atom accepts one; to balance this, one calcium atom reacts with two chlorine atoms to give calcium chloride, $CaCl_2$.

Ionic compounds are usually arranged as crystalline giant lattice structures of regularly repeating ions. The electrovalent bonding gives ionic compounds this property, and most ionic compounds are hard, high melting point (m.p.) solids that conduct electricity when molten or in solution (hence they are called *electrolytes* in body fluids).

AROMAFACT

Ionic compounds are not found in the chemistry of the essential oil compounds. However, they are very important in the functioning of the human body. Because they conduct electricity they are often called *electrolytes*. For this reason body fluids such as blood plasma and urine are often analysed for electrolytes as their levels can be a useful diagnostic tool.

Covalent bonding

This type of bonding gives rise to *covalent compounds*. In covalent compounds the stability of atoms is achieved by sharing rather than outright loss or gain of electrons. This sharing typically occurs between two nonmetals and is very important for the structures of essential oils and their properties. Again the position of the element in the periodic table is significant. Nonmetals are found on the right-hand side of the periodic table. To form a covalent bond, an atom must be able to put an electron or electrons into a bond and needs a space in its outer shell for the other (sharing) atom's electrons to go. Covalent bonding can occur between atoms of the same elements, e.g. in the gases hydrogen (H_2) and oxygen O_2.

The two atoms touch and the outer electron shells overlap. Each outer electron shell contributes an electron and the new pair occupies the area of overlap; the electrons are attracted to both nuclei and a bond is formed.

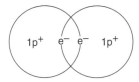

H_2, hydrogen molecule
(in the molecule a helium electron
arrangement is achieved)

There are a number of ways covalent bonds can be represented to indicate the sharing of electrons involved, but for most molecules we encounter a single pair of electrons in a covalent bond and the bond is represented simply with a single joining line, H–H. This represents a *single bond* with *one pair* of electrons.

In oxygen, with atoms with 6 outer electrons, stability is achieved by imitating the stable neon atom with 8 outer electrons. This is done by each oxygen atom using 2 electrons from its outer shell, making a total of 4 in the bond. This can be written as:

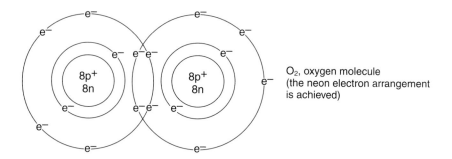

O₂, oxygen molecule
(the neon electron arrangement
is achieved)

This is shown most commonly with two joining lines, O=O. This represents a *double bond* with *two pairs* of electrons. The bonds are formed only by the outer or valence electrons.

Covalent bonds are commonly formed between atoms of different elements to form compounds. For example, methane (natural gas) is the simplest hydrocarbon (a compound made up only of carbon and hydrogen). In the following diagram only the outer or valence electrons are shown. The carbon atom has 4 outer electrons, and shares with 4 hydrogen atoms, each sharing its one electron:

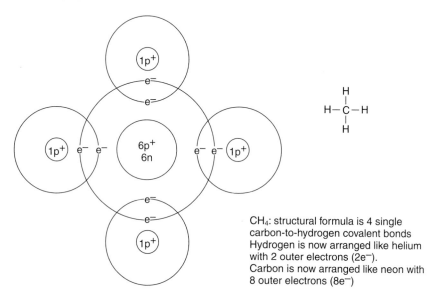

CH_4: structural formula is 4 single
carbon-to-hydrogen covalent bonds
Hydrogen is now arranged like helium
with 2 outer electrons ($2e^-$).
Carbon is now arranged like neon with
8 outer electrons ($8e^-$)

In a similar way, a triple bond involves sharing of *three* pairs of electrons and is indicated by three lines: e.g. between the carbon atoms in ethyne, H–C≡C–H.

Covalent compounds are typically gases, volatile liquids or low melting point solids. They are usually insoluble in water but dissolve easily in organic solvents such as ether, hexane and alcohol.

There are other types of bonding, but they are beyond the scope of this book.

AROMAFACT

The compounds found in essential oils and their carrier oils are all covalently bonded and their properties reflect this.

An understanding of the combining power of atoms (their valency) can explain the molecular formula and the arrangement of atoms in a compound. Knowing the molecular formula we can also determine the size of the molecule and its *molecular weight*. This is defined as the weight of one molecule and is calculated by adding together the atomic masses (weights) of its components. For our purposes the molecular weight will be the number of times the molecule is heavier than an atom of hydrogen, the simplest atom, because hydrogen has a relative atomic mass of one (1). Carbon has a relative atomic mass of 12 and the relative atomic mass of oxygen is 16. The calculation of molecular weights is illustrated in Table 1.2.

The molecular weights for water, carbon dioxide, methane and isoprene are 18, 44, 16 and 68, respectively.

AROMAFACT

Molecular weight is significant in essential oils as it can determine their extraction method, physical properties such as boiling point, and biological properties such as absorption into the body.

The numerical value of the molecular weight expressed in grams (e.g. 16 g in the case of methane) is often used to represent the quantity of a substance. The *gram molecular weight* comprises the same number of molecules of any substance (18 g of water, 44 g of carbon dioxide or 68 g of isoprene contain the same number of molecules of the respective compounds). This number

Table 1.2   Calculating molecular weights

Compound	Formula		Molecular weight
Water	H_2O	$2 \times H (=1) + 1 \times O (=16) = 2 + 16 =$	18
Carbon dioxide	CO_2	$1 \times C (=12) + 2 \times O (=16) = 12 + 32 =$	44
Methane	CH_4	$1 \times C (=12) + 4 \times H (=1) = 12 + 4 =$	16
Isoprene	C_5H_8	$5 \times C (=12) + 8 \times H (=1) = 60 + 8 =$	68

of molecules is named one *mole*; the weight of one mole of any substance is the numerical value of its molecular weight in grams. In chemistry, so-called *molar* solutions are used: a one-molar solution of a substance contains the gram molecular weight (one mole) of that substance made up to *one litre of solution*. Dilutions are not usually quoted in this way in aromatherapy, but you should be aware of the convention in case you encounter it in technical literature.

MIXTURES

So far we have considered pure substances of atoms that can join up with bonds to form molecules, which can contain atoms of the same element (e.g. H_2 or O_2) or atoms of different elements in compounds (e.g. H_2O, CO_2, CH_4).

Many substances exist as *mixtures*. A mixture is made up of two or more substances that are not chemically bonded together: e.g. sand and salt; brine, which is salt and water and other impurities; or a saline solution, which is made up of water with sodium chloride salt dissolved in it. The amounts of the substances can vary in a mixture, unlike a compound which has the same fixed proportions of atoms in every molecule and therefore in the bulk substance.

AROMAFACT

An essential oil is a mixture, often containing hundreds of compounds, and reflects the characteristics of a mixture. With very few exceptions, these individual compounds are covalently bonded volatile liquids that contribute their individual properties to the oil. An individual component may be harmful on its own but, when diluted and with other ingredients, it may have an additive and beneficial effect; this is an example of *synergy*. As with all mixtures, the composition of oils may vary and thus the overall characteristics of an oil may vary. For example, an oil can occur as different *chemotypes*, in which oils from different individuals from the same species of plant have different proportions of chemicals owing to the different environments the plants were grown in. The composition may also vary depending on the plant species and subspecies and such variations are genetically determined. This is explained in detail in Chapter 7. Individual components or groups of components in a mixture can be separated by physical methods such as dissolving or distilling. The removal of particular useful compounds from essential oils is done on a large scale in the cosmetics, pharmaceutical and food industries, exploiting physical properties such as boiling point or solubility. This has a minimal effect on the chemical properties of the compound removed. An aromatherapy–grade oil should have no components removed, added or enhanced: this would constitute *adulteration*. Adding the blue compound chamazulene to Moroccan chamomile to make it look like the more expensive German chamomile would be such an adulteration.

In the following chapters we will apply what we have learnt concerning physical and chemical changes, molecules and bonding to explore the structures of the molecules that form the essential oils. The structure of the molecules in a compound and the constituent compounds in a chemical have a big impact on its properties and these will also be reflected in the essential oils containing them.

AROMAFACT

Essential oils are mixtures of different chemical compounds and the composition will vary according to factors such as source, age, storage conditions and chemotypes of those compounds. Mixtures have properties that reflect all of their components, so by looking at the different compounds in an oil we can see how they not only have effects on different physiological systems in the body but can also complement each other. The fact that they are mixtures allows us to identify their components and analyze them with techniques such as chromatography.

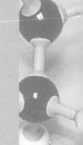

Chapter 2

Organic chemistry

IMPORTANT CONCEPTS IN ORGANIC CHEMISTRY

Essential oil chemistry is a part of organic chemistry, which covers a vast range of compounds. Early ideas suggested that organic compounds were all obtained from either plant or animal sources, i.e. that they were natural products, and arose only through 'vital forces' inherent in living cells. This definition is no longer true as a result of modern laboratory synthetic methods. The modern definition of organic chemistry is that it is the *chemistry of covalently bonded carbon compounds*.

AROMAFACT

There is a very dangerous misconception that if a substance is natural it is not harmful, and can be used therapeutically without the fear of any side-effects. Natural products often contain very powerful and toxic compounds and some form a basis for mainstream drugs. Essential oils are very complex mixtures of organic compounds, many of which should be used with great care. Their roles in the plant body are often protective and defensive, e.g. to repel invading organisms. Essential oils contain compounds with varying physiological effects and toxicity. In a genuine aromatherapy-grade essential oil, the more toxic components are often balanced by others that act as 'quenchers'. There is a phenomenon called *synergy* whereby the components making up the oil can cooperate to produce their healing effect. A knowledge of the oil components is needed for their safe use and this is why it is vital to use high-grade essential oils in a controlled way

The important points in organic chemistry are outlined below.

1. Carbon and only very few other elements are involved

The number of organic compounds *far* exceeds that of inorganic compounds, but very few other elements are involved along with the ubiquitous carbon.

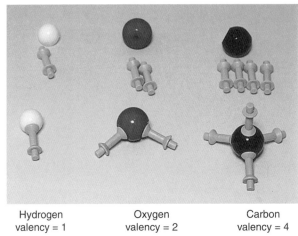

Hydrogen	Oxygen	Carbon
valency = 1	valency = 2	valency = 4

Figure 2.1   Atoms most commonly encountered in organic chemistry: carbon (black), hydrogen (white) and oxygen (grey). In colour the models are carbon (black), hydrogen (white) and oxygen (red). Their valencies are represented by the number of 'sticks', which are shown attached to the atoms in the spatial configurations that chemical bonds to these atoms occupy (e.g. pointing to the vertices of a tetrahedron in the case of carbon); the directionality of the bonds produces the shapes of different molecules. These are the basic kinds of atom that build up by covalent bonding to form the organic molecules found in essential oils. Courtesy Spiring Enterprises Ltd.

Most of them are other nonmetals, most commonly carbon (C) and hydrogen (H), which are always present; oxygen (O), nitrogen (N), sulfur (S) and phosphorus (P), which are commonly found; and chlorine (Cl), bromine (Br), iodine (I) and fluorine (F), which are present in other compounds (see Fig. 2.1).

2. The bonding is mainly covalent

Most organic compounds are low melting point solids, liquids or gases that are insoluble in water but soluble in organic (sometimes referred to as nonpolar) solvents such as ether, benzene and hydrocarbons. They do not conduct electricity. This is in contrast to ionic or electrovalent compounds with their bonding by electrostatic forces, which usually result in solids that are soluble in inorganic (sometimes referred to as polar) solvents such as water and that will conduct electricity when molten or in solution.

AROMAFACT

Essential oils are most commonly applied to the skin diluted and dissolved in another oil called a carrier for use in a massage. Water is not an appropriate or efficient carrier for massages, although some components may be water soluble. Adding essential oils to a bath will bring the oil into contact with the skin and the hot water will help the oil to evaporate so that the volatile molecules enter the nasal passages by inhalation.

3. Large molecules are common

Compounds are encountered with molecular formulae such as $C_{20}H_{40}$, with 20 carbon (C) atoms and 40 hydrogen (H) atoms. Many important biological compounds are what are called *macromolecules* and are very large. They are *polymers* made up of many repeating units. For example, cellulose (plant cell wall material) is made up of many linked glucose units and has a molecular weight of 150 000–1 000 000. Insulin (a protein) is made up of 51 amino acid residues and has a molecular weight of about 5700.

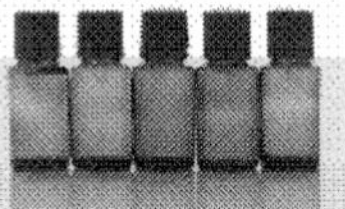

AROMAFACT

Most essential oils are liquids with constituents that exhibit a range of molecular sizes. Monoterpenes have molecular formulae $C_{10}H_{16}$, while sesquiterpenes have the formula $C_{15}H_{24}$. Although quite large molecules are present in essential oils, the oils do not contain any macromolecules.

4. Structures are based on carbon's valency of 4

The carbon atom has 4 outer electrons, which are usually shared in covalent bonds that point to the vertices of a tetrahedron (a triangular pyramid).

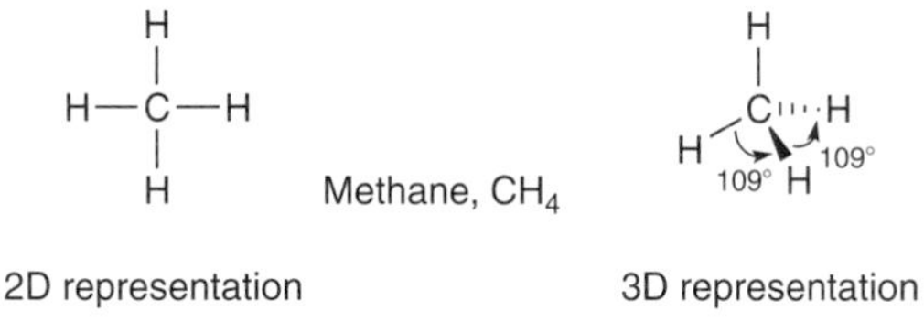

Methane, CH_4

2D representation   3D representation

In representing molecules it is common to use a two-dimensional representation with the chemical bonds drawn in the plane of the page, as shown above for methane. However, it is sometimes important to show the three-dimensional tetrahedral arrangement of single bonds around the carbon atom. To do this a 'wedge' convention is used. In the 3D representation of methane above, bonds drawn as plain lines are lying in the plane of the page; the black wedge indicates that that bond points out of the plane of the page and the broken wedge indicates that the bond points below the page. The angle between each pair of bonds is about 109°.

5. Carbon atoms have the ability to bond to other carbon atoms in extended structures

Organic compounds can be found with many forms of 'carbon skeleton'.

Straight chains

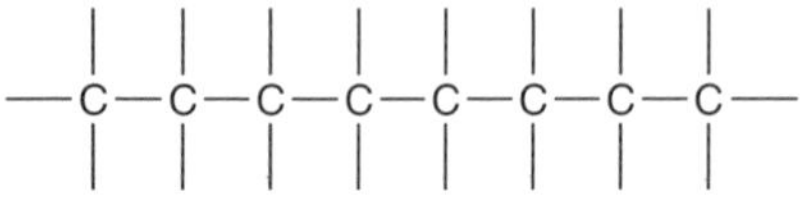

Branched chains

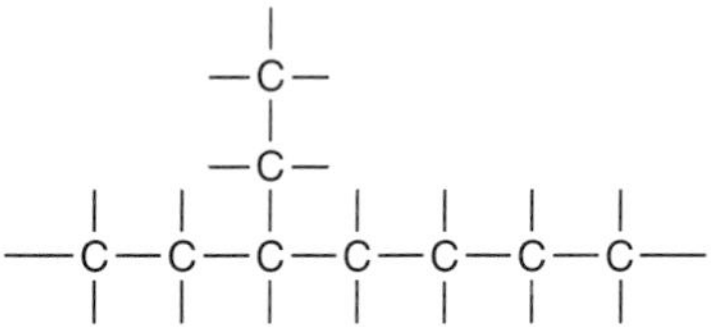

Rings – most commonly with 5 or 6 carbons

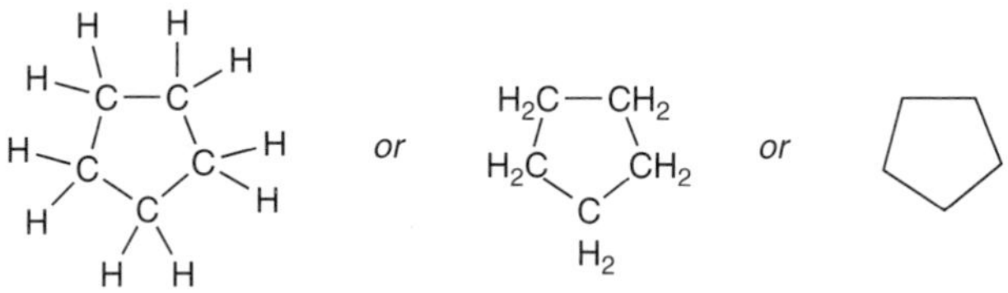

Cyclopentane, C_5H_{10} Skeletal formula

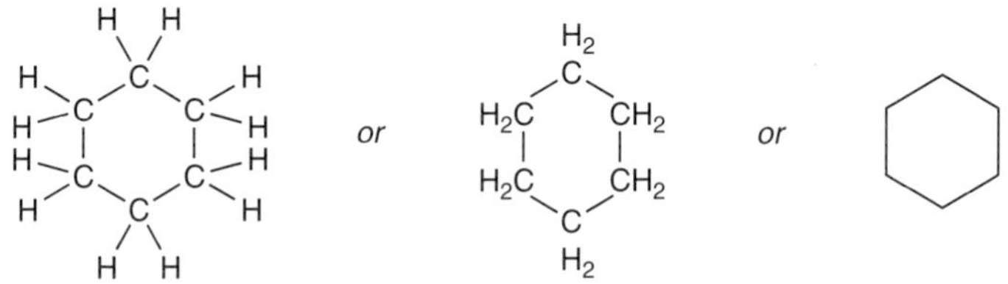

Cyclohexane, C_6H_{12} Skeletal formula

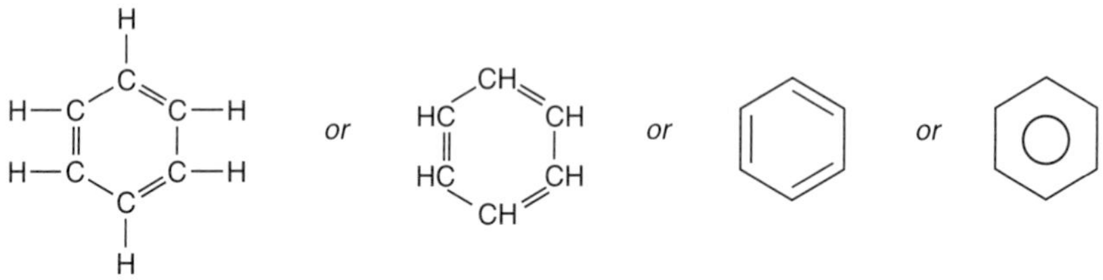

Benzene, C_6H_6

A combination of rings and chains

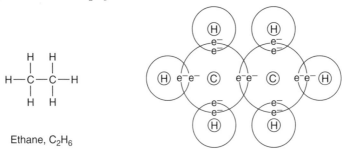

Methylbenzene, also called toluene (presence of methyl group is implied by single bond in the far right form)

6. Multiple bonding is common

Carbon can form multiple bonds (double or triple bonds; see Ch. 1) between its atoms when forming compounds. This can be shown in some simple hydro-carbons (see Fig. 2.2). In covalent bonds, the sharing of a pair of electrons comprising one electron from each atom involved in the bond is called a *single bond* and is represented by a single line. The bond is formed by two electrons; for example, in ethane, C_2H_6:

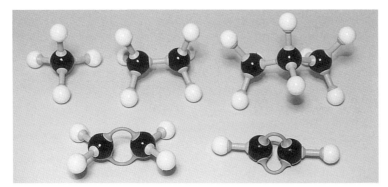

Figure 2.2   Simple hydrocarbons, showing bonding. *Top row, left to right*: methane, CH_4; ethane, C_2H_6; propane, C_3H_8 (all *alkanes*). *Bottom row, left to right*: ethene, C_2H_4 (an *alkene*, with a C-to-C double bond); ethyne, C_2H_2 (an *alkyne*, with a C-to-C triple bond). Courtesy Spiring Enterprises Ltd.

(In this and the following diagrams, only the *outer* electrons, taking part in the bonding, are shown; and for simplicity the nucleus of each atom is represented only by the element's symbol.)

For a *double bond*, each carbon contributes 2 electrons, so that two pairs partake in the bonding; for example in ethene, C_2H_4:

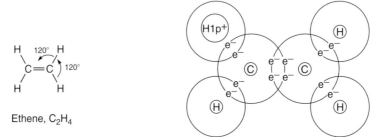

Ethene, C_2H_4

A double bond (4 electrons; two pairs) is represented as =. The angle between bonds to the carbon atoms involved in a double bond is 120° and all the bonds lie in the same plane. The ethene molecule is 'flat' in contrast to the tetrahedral arrangement of single bonds.

As there are fewer hydrogen atoms in ethene (four) than the maximum possible number in the single-bonded ethane (six), it is said to be *unsaturated*.

For *triple bonds*, each carbon contributes 3 electrons, so that three pairs partake in the bonding; for example in ethyne, C_2H_2:

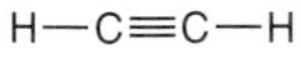

H—C≡C—H

Ethyne, C_2H_2

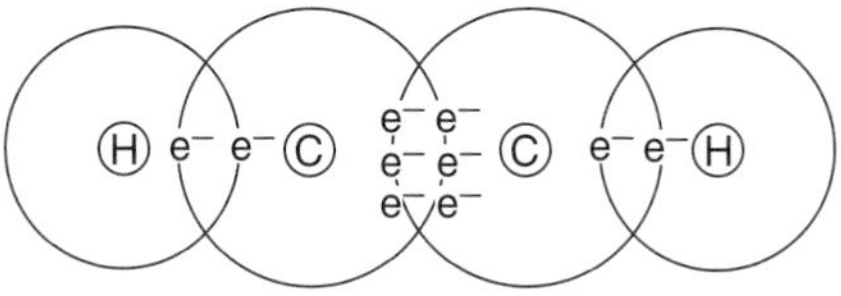

When carbon atoms form triple bonds, all the bonds to those atoms lie in a straight line – i.e. the angle between the single and triple bonds is 180°.

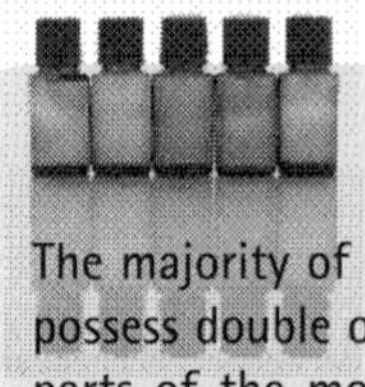

AROMAFACT

The majority of essential oils have compounds that are *unsaturated* (i.e. they possess double or triple bonds). These multiple bonds tend to be very reactive parts of the molecule that can often combine with oxygen if an oil is not stored correctly.

In nature, many compounds are *polyunsaturated*, that is they have more than one double or triple bond. They are found in vegetable oils and some vitamins, where they are thought to be beneficial in the diet for a variety of reasons.

7. Isomerism is common

Many compounds have the same molecular formula as other compounds and so contain the same number of atoms of the same elements, but the atoms are arranged differently. This is called *isomerism*. It can be illustrated using some examples.

Functional isomers

Take the molecular formula C_2H_6O. This can represent the two compounds

Dimethyl ether
(an ether)

Ethanol
(an alcohol)

Dimethyl ether and ethanol are said to be *isomers*: they are different compounds with different functional groups (the –O– ether group and the –OH alcohol group) (see Fig. 2.3).

Geometric isomers

In α- (alpha-) and β- (beta-) pinenes it is the position of the double bond that differs, and this makes them isomers. They are made up of the same

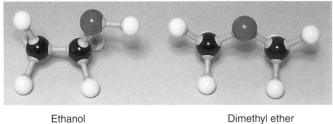

Ethanol
CH_3CH_2OH

Dimethyl ether
CH_3OCH_3

Figure 2.3 Functional group isomers. Both compounds have the same molecular formula, C_2H_6O, but different functional groups. Courtesy Spiring Enterprises Ltd.

atoms in their molecular formula $C_{10}H_{16}$ and the same number and types of bonds, but here they are arranged differently in space, and this is a type of *stereoisomerism* (from the Greek *stereos*, meaning 'solid', i.e. involving three-dimensional shape). When a molecule is unsaturated, the double bond does not readily permit rotation about its axis, thus fixing the different groups into their positions in space. When identical groups are on the same side of the double bond, the isomer is called the *cis* isomer, and when identical groups are on the opposite sides of the double bond, the isomer is called the *trans* isomer.

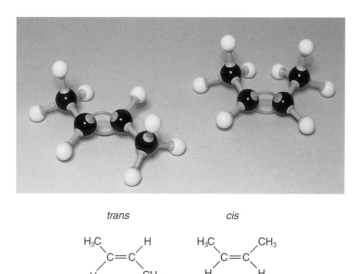

The *cis*/*trans* relationship is also used more generally, when the attached groups are not identical but are located on opposite sides of the same double bond in different isomers; in this sense it describes the overall 'shape' of the carbon skeleton of otherwise identical isomers (see Fig. 2.4).

Figure 2.4 Geometric isomers. Butene, with groups $-CH_3$ (methyl) and $-H$ (hydrogen) arranged differently (*cis* and *trans* arrangements) on the carbon skeleton with a 'fixed' double bond. Courtesy Spring Enterprises Ltd.

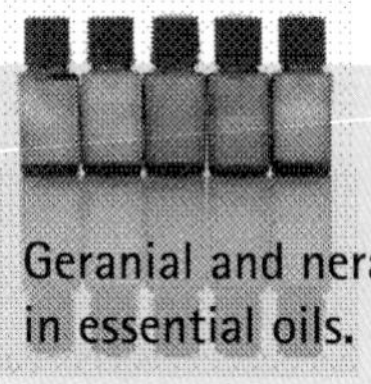

AROMAFACT

Geranial and neral are examples of *cis/trans* isomeric alcohol molecules found in essential oils.

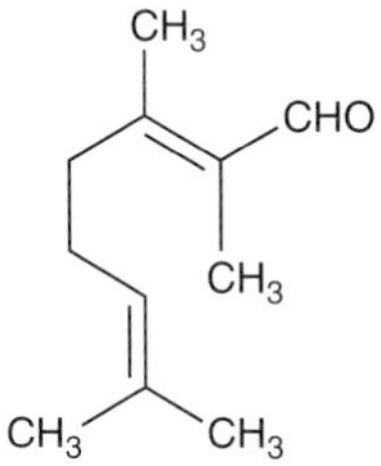

Geranial
(*trans*)

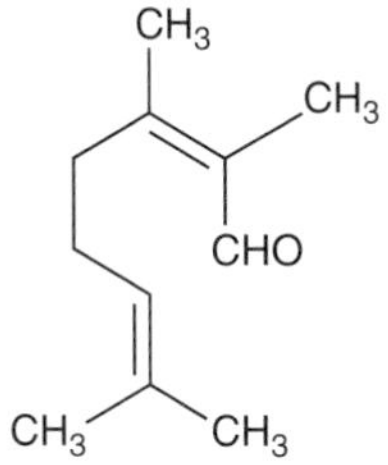

Neral
(*cis*)

Geranial is also called α-citral and neral is called β-citral. The general name citral is quoted as a constituent of many essential oils such as lemongrass. 'Citral' is actually a mixture of these *cis* and *trans* isomers. The methyl group, CH_3, is always joined by a C–C bond to the molecule although, for simplicity, the bond often appears to go to the H atom or the middle of the group.

Optical isomers

Optical isomers are also an example of *stereoisomerism*, with different arrangements of atoms in space. The important property of optical isomerism relies on the *chirality* (from the Greek word for hand) or 'handedness' of a molecule, i.e. whether it is right-handed or left-handed. The resulting isomers are called optical isomers and one form of the molecule is the mirror image of the other. The property of chirality in a molecule gives rise to structures that are mirror images that *cannot be superimposed*, just as the left and right hands cannot be superimposed. For this to happen (for the molecule to be *chiral*), there must be an *asymmetric carbon atom* present: that is, one with four different atoms or groups attached to the four tetrahedrally arranged bonds.

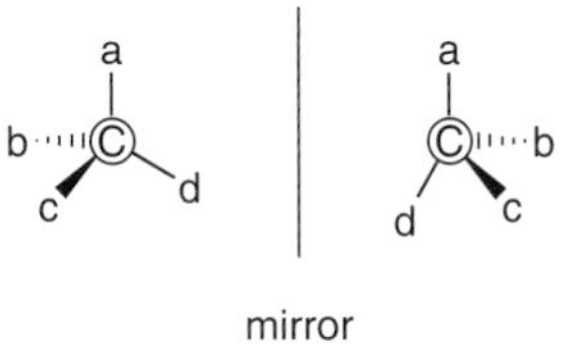

mirror

The two isomers formed are called the *d*- and *l*-isomers: they have the same physical properties such as boiling points but they differ in their effect on a special type of light called *plane-polarized light*, which vibrates in a particular plane rather than randomly. The isomers can be distinguished using this plane-polarized light because they will cause the plane of vibration to rotate by the same amount but in opposite directions for each isomer. If the rotation produced is clockwise it is termed *dextrorotatory* and the isomer is designated the *d*-form; if the rotation produced is anticlockwise it is termed *laevorotatory* and the isomer is designated the *l*-form. The property of being able to affect the plane-polarized light in this way is called *optical activity*. Naturally occurring optically active compounds usually consist of one isomer only. Those synthesized in the laboratory usually contain equal amounts of the *d*- and *l*-forms and are called *racemic modifications* (or racemic mixtures or racemates), which are optically inactive (the two rotations cancel out) (see Fig. 2.5).

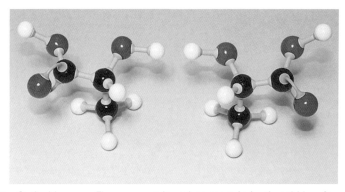

Figure 2.5   Optical isomers. The asymmetric carbon atom in lactic acid has four different groups attached: –CH$_3$, –H, –OH and –COOH. The two molecules are mirror images of one another and are *chiral* – they differ in the same way that left and right hands differ. Courtesy Spiring Enterprises Ltd.

AROMAFACT

The amount by which a given optical isomer rotates the plane–polarized light is a characteristic signature of that compound or substance. When measured under a set of standard conditions this quantity is termed the specific rotation, alpha, and written in square brackets [α]. It can be used as a measure of the purity or authenticity of an essential oil in analysis and quality control procedures. This is discussed further in Chapter 5.

Almost all essential oils show optical isomerism and this gives them differing biological properties, including their odours. This illustrates the significance of optically active isomers in living systems. Human cells detect changes by receptor sites that respond to specific stimuli, including chemicals. There is a difference in the way a chiral molecule and its optical isomer interact with a chiral receptor site. This is analogous to the difference between a right hand and a left hand fitting into a right glove.

AROMAFACT

Examples of essential oil compounds showing these different odours include *d*-limonene, which has a dull citrus odour while *l*-limonene has a turpentine odour; similarly, *d*-linalool has a floral, woody (lavender-like) odour, while *l*-linalool has a floral (petitgrain-like) odour.

The *d*- and *l*-carvones are optical isomers that exist in different oils: *d*-carvones are found in caraway oil, whereas *l*-carvones are found in spearmint oil.

REPRESENTING ORGANIC MOLECULES

There are a number of ways of drawing and writing the structures and formulae of molecules. It could be as simple as its molecular formula, for example methylbenzene is C_7H_8, or it can be done in a way that gives some indication of structure: $C_6H_5CH_3$, indicating an unsaturated aromatic ring (C_6H_5) with a methyl (CH_3) chain. The concept of the aromatic ring is explained below in the example of benzene.

A fuller representation of arrangement and bonding can be drawn diagrammatically:

or

This is rather unwieldy and is not the representation most often employed. Using certain conventions it can be simplified:

or

In such representations the convention is to assume a carbon atom at each apex of the ring and that the carbon valency of 4 is made up by the appropriate number of hydrogen atoms, which are not shown explicitly. A similar convention is used to simplify the writing of the structure of noncyclic compounds as well, as illustrated in some of the examples below.

Butane   Molecular formula C_4H_{10}; a straight-chain hydrocarbon; saturated, single bonds.

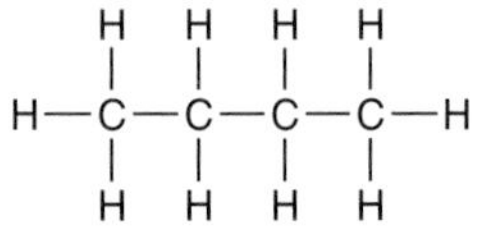

$$H-\overset{\overset{\displaystyle H}{|}}{\underset{\underset{\displaystyle H}{|}}{C}}-\overset{\overset{\displaystyle H}{|}}{\underset{\underset{\displaystyle H}{|}}{C}}-\overset{\overset{\displaystyle H}{|}}{\underset{\underset{\displaystyle H}{|}}{C}}-\overset{\overset{\displaystyle H}{|}}{\underset{\underset{\displaystyle H}{|}}{C}}-H$$

$$CH_3CH_2CH_2CH_3$$

Ethanol   Molecular formula C_2H_6O; an alcohol.

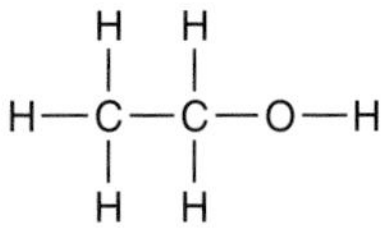

$$H-\overset{\overset{\displaystyle H}{|}}{\underset{\underset{\displaystyle H}{|}}{C}}-\overset{\overset{\displaystyle H}{|}}{\underset{\underset{\displaystyle H}{|}}{C}}-O-H$$

$$C_2H_5OH \quad \text{or} \quad CH_3CH_2OH$$

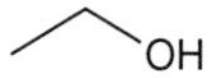

Cyclohexane   Molecular formula C_6H_{12}; cyclic saturated ring structure with single bonds.

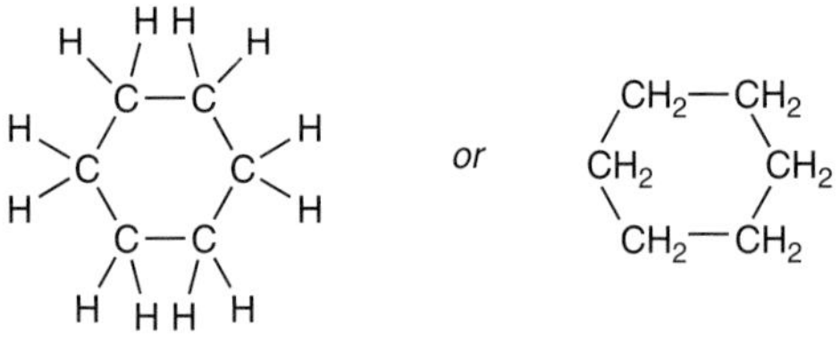

The shorthand form shows all single bonds in a 6-sided carbon skeleton ring:

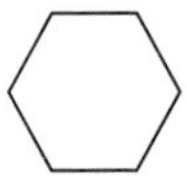

Benzene   A special case is C_6H_6. This is a cyclic unsaturated 6-sided carbon skeleton ring with alternate single and double bonds. It is often represented as

The hexagonal ring structure of benzene with its alternating single and double bonds always presented a problem. If you transpose all the single and double bonds, you end up with the identical structure: what decides between which atoms there are double bonds and between which single bonds? Also, benzene did not show the typical properties of an unsaturated double-bonded compound, suggesting that its bonds were somehow different. When the bond lengths were measured using X-ray analysis, it was found that all the bonds had the same length rather than there being two different values normally associated with single bonds and double bonds. The reactions of benzene also differed from those of a normal double-bonded structure.

This was originally explained describing the structure as a 'hybrid' of the two possible structures. The two forms are known as *canonical forms* and the 'blended' structure was called a *resonance hybrid*.

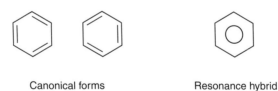

Canonical forms   Resonance hybrid

Effectively, the structure was assumed to have six '$1\frac{1}{2}$-bonds'.

Modern chemical theory elegantly solves the problem by showing the formation of a *molecular orbital* extending over the whole ring, within which six of the electrons contributing to the bonding in benzene – one from each carbon atom – are able to move freely around the ring. These electrons circulate freely and are not attached to any one particular carbon atom or pair of carbon atoms. The electrons are said to be *delocalized*, that is they are spread out, which theory predicts to result in a more stable (lower-energy) molecular configuration.

Thus the central circle in the 'resonance hybrid' representation actually captures the physical reality of the bonding in benzene.

This delocalized ring structure is called *aromatic*. Structures possessing this feature are frequently associated with substances with distinct aromas and the concept of *aromaticity* derives from this fact. While in colloquial terms 'aromatic' is commonly applied to describe strongly fragrant compounds, in chemical technical terminology it refers purely to the possession of this type of chemical structure, irrespective of the fragrance (which in practice may not be at all what we mean colloquially by aromatic).

FUNCTIONAL GROUPS

Compounds made up of only hydrogen and carbon are called *hydrocarbons*. They make up only a small number of the total organic compounds.

When looking at an organic molecule we find that only certain parts and bonds take part in the chemical reactions. Usually the carbon chain or skeleton remains unchanged. The atom or group of atoms that defines the chemical reactivity of a particular class of organic compounds and determines its properties is called the *functional group*. Commonly occurring functional groups are alkenes (hydrocarbons with double bonds), alcohols, aldehydes, ketones, carboxylic acids and esters.

AROMAFACT

The functional group names can be used in characterizing and describing the odours of many perfumes and some of the essential oils. Aldehydic smelling oils are due to compounds with functional groups called aldehydes, and sweet and fruity smelling oils are due to compounds with functional groups called esters.

A large amount of organic chemistry is concerned with the reactions and transformations of one functional group to another. An understanding of the functional group explains the particular set of properties associated with compounds within a series or 'family'.

HOMOLOGOUS SERIES

These are useful arrangements of compounds into 'families' and are very common in organic chemistry and biochemistry. Members of homologous series have a number of characteristics in common.

1. They all have the same *general* formula.
2. They have similar properties, both physical and chemical, i.e. they have the same functional group.

This can be simply illustrated with the *alkanes*, which are saturated noncyclic hydrocarbons. They all have the same general formula, C_nH_{2n+2}, where n is the number of carbon atoms (1 or 2 or 3 or …).

- Methane has 1 carbon atom: $C_1H_{2+2} = CH_4$.
- Ethane has 2 carbon atoms: $C_2H_{4+2} = C_2H_6$ (or CH_3CH_3).
- Propane has 3 carbon atoms: $C_3H_{6+2} = C_3H_8$ (or $CH_3CH_2CH_3$).
- Butane has 4 carbon atoms: $C_4H_{8+2} = C_4H_{10}$ (or $CH_3CH_2CH_2CH_3$).

The systematic names of the higher members of the homologous series of alkanes indicate the number of carbon atoms present in the chain (*pentane* has 5, *hexane* has 6, ... *decane* has 10, and so on), but the names of the first few members are based on chemical history [methyl (1), ethyl (2), propyl (3) and butyl (4)] and one just has to learn what these represent.

Major homologous series found in organic chemistry are summarized in Table 2.1.

Table 2.1 Homologous series of compounds

Compound	Formula	Melting point (°C)	Boiling point (°C)
Alkanes			
Methane	CH_4	−182	−161
Ethane	CH_3CH_3	−183	−88
Propane	$CH_3CH_2CH_3$	−188	−42
Butane	$CH_3(CH_2)_2CH_3$	−138	−0.5
Pentane	$CH_3(CH_2)_3CH_3$	−130	36
Hexane	$CH_3(CH_2)_4CH_3$	−95	69
Decane	$CH_3(CH_2)_8CH_3$	−30	174
Eicosane	$CH_3(CH_2)_{18}CH_3$	37	344
Cycloalkanes			
Cyclopentane		−94	49
Cyclohexane		7	81
Alkenes			
Ethene	$CH_2=CH_2$	−169	−104
Propene	$CH_2=CH-CH_3$	−185	−48
Cyclohexene		−103	83
Arenes			
Benzene		6	80
Methylbenzene (toluene)		81	218
Alcohols			
Methanol	CH_3OH	−98	65
Ethanol	CH_3CH_2OH	−114	78
Propanol	$CH_3CH_2CH_2OH$	−126	97
Butanol	$CH_3CH_2CH_2CH_2OH$	−89	118
Methylpropanol	$(CH_3)_3COH$	−26	82
Cyclohexanol		25	161

continued

Table 2.1 Homologous series of compounds / Cont'd

Compound	Formula	Melting point (°C)	Boiling point (°C)
Aldehydes			
Methanal (formaldehyde)	HCHO	−92	−21
Ethanal (acetaldehyde)	CH_3CHO	−121	20
Propanal	CH_3CH_2CHO	−81	49
Ketones			
Propanone	CH_3COCH_3	−95	56
Butanone	$CH_3CH_2COCH_3$	−86	80
Carboxylic acids			
Methanoic (formic) acid	HCO_2H	9	101
Ethanoic (acetic) acid	CH_3CO_2H	17	118
Propanoic acid	$CH_3CH_2CO_2H$	−21	141
Esters			
Ethyl ethanoate (acetate)	$CH_3CO_2CH_2CH_3$	−84	77
Ethyl propanoate	$CH_3CH_2CO_2CH_2CH_3$	−74	99
Methyl ethanoate	$CH_3CO_2CH_3$	−98	57
Methyl propanoate	$CH_3CH_2CO_2CH_3$	−87	80

Chapter 3

Families of compounds that occur in essential oils

The chemistry of essential oils is organic and vast. To avoid confusion a formal system was developed: the *IUPAC* (International Union of Pure and Applied Chemistry) system. This names compounds based on the arrangement of the component atoms into functional groups, e.g. alcohols contain –OH.

AROMAFACT

For aromatherapy compounds the older established or 'historical' names (sometimes called 'trivial' names) are commonly used. This book will use both as appropriate, e.g.:
- Isoprene is systematically named 2–methylbuta–1,3–diene.
- Menthol is systematically named 2–isopropyl–5–methylcyclohexanol.

There are two main types of component in essential oils: hydrocarbons (carbon and hydrogen only) and oxygenated hydrocarbons, which also contain oxygen. These are subdivided into groups based on their structures (Table 3.1). In this chapter, the general physicochemical and therapeutic properties associated with each group are given but it must be emphasized that not *all* members will have every property; for example acetic acid (vinegar) and the polyacids in dietary fat are all of the form X–COOH but differ drastically. Interactions with other groups in the molecule and in the oil can also affect properties.

AROMAFACT

It is the oxygenated constituents that have a significant impact and, along with sesquiterpenes, determine and characterize the odours of almost all essential oils.

Table 3.1   Two major classes of compounds found in essential oils

Hydrocarbons	Oxygenated compounds
• Also called aliphatic hydrocarbons • Names end in *-ene* as they are *unsaturated* (have double bonds) **Terpenes** based on the isoprene unit (5 carbon atoms) *Monoterpenes*: 2 isoprene units (up to 10 carbon atoms) *Sesquiterpenes*: 3 isoprene units (up to 15 carbon atoms) *Diterpenes*: 4 isoprene units (up to 20 carbon atoms)	• If they are derived from terpenes they are called *terpenoids* Alcohols Phenols Aldehydes Ketones Esters Lactones

THE TERPENES

The terpenes are a large group of naturally occurring hydrocarbons (made up of carbon and hydrogen only) found in essential oils. They are based on the *isoprene unit* with the molecular formula C_5H_8 (Fig. 3.1). Isoprene is a chain structure described as *aliphatic* or *acyclic*, which means a compound with its carbon atoms in chains not closed rings:

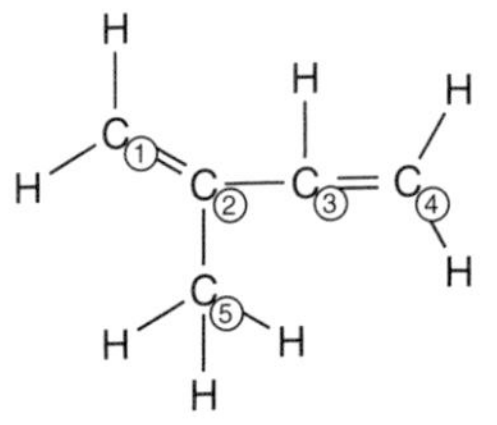

The *systematic* or *IUPAC* name is 2-methylbuta-1,3-diene. This means that the longest chain of carbon atoms is 4 (like butane), giving the 'buta' part of the name; it is an alkene ('ene' represents an alkene) with two ('di') double bonds starting on carbon atoms 1 and 3, giving the name buta-1, 3-diene, and the methyl group is attached to the carbon atom 2 ('2-methyl'). (When no ambiguity can arise, the name may also be written 2-methyl-1, 3-butadiene.) From this point forward these more systematic names will be used.

For most practical purposes it is called by the 'trivial' name of isoprene and has been known for a long time as it forms the basis of another important natural product – rubber.

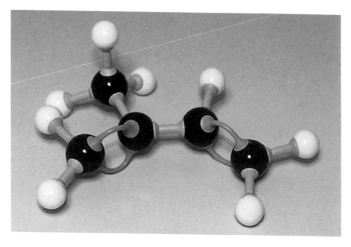

C_5H_8

Figure 3.1   Isoprene (C_5H_8): The monomer, or single unit, that builds up into the terpenes. Courtesy Spiring Enterprises Ltd.

AROMAFACT

BEWARE: there are various representations of isoprene to be found in general aromatherapy books, often showing the arrangement of the carbon skeleton as

$$C-C-C-C \quad \text{with } C \text{ above}$$ or

These are inaccurate since they do not show the important position of the double bonds. Probably the most useful shortened form is

The isoprene unit acts as *monomer* or single unit that builds up in repeating units to make the groups of terpenes found in the essential oils. Their names usually end in -ene.

There are several groups of terpene hydrocarbon based on the number of isoprene units incorporated.

Monoterpenes

Monoterpenes are made up of two isoprene units, joined head to head. They have a molecular formula of $C_{10}H_{16}$ (Fig. 3.2).

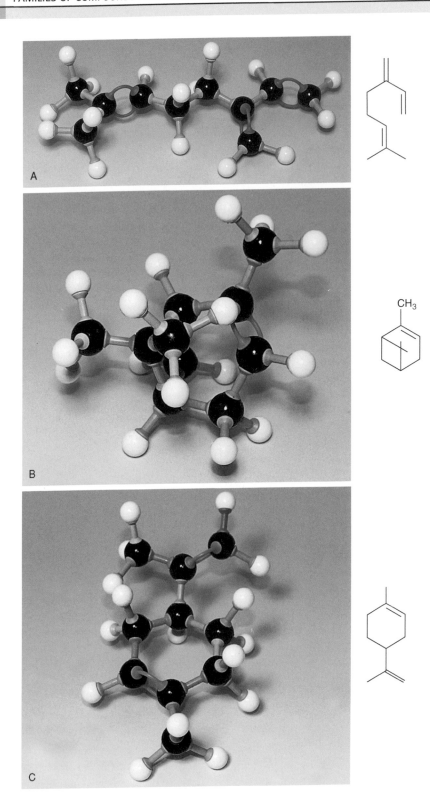

Figure 3.2   Monoterpenes (C₁₀H₁₆). (A) Myrcene, an acyclic monoterpene. (B) α-Pinene, a dicyclic structure. (C) d-Limonene, a monocyclic structure. Courtesy Spiring Enterprises Ltd.

Myrcene

Double bond disappears from isoprene as new single bond of monoterpene is formed

New bond formed here

Myrcene is an example of a monoterpene and is found in essential oils of bay, verbena, pine and juniper, and in many others.

AROMAFACT

Different acyclic monoterpenes are made up of two isoprene units, but the positions of the three double bonds vary.

Ocimene   Found in essential oil of basil.

Ocimene

One new bond formed, so three double bonds remain.

Myrcene and ocimene are not arranged in ring structures: they are *acyclic*. However, many monoterpenes link up to form rings or *cyclic* structures, for example in limonene.

d–Limonene   Found in essential citrus oils, pine leaves and peppermint.

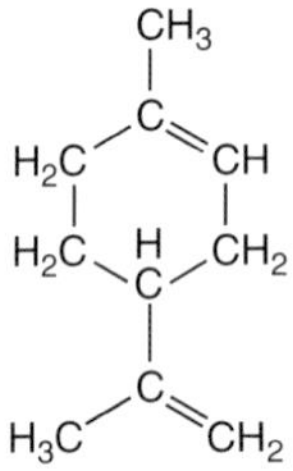

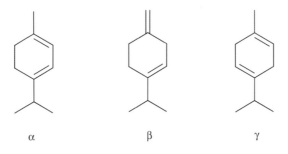

$C_{10}H_{16}$ 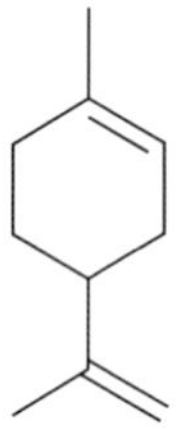   d–Limonene

Two new bonds are formed, so two double bonds remain.

Terpinolene   Found in essential oils of eucalyptus, tea tree and turpentine.

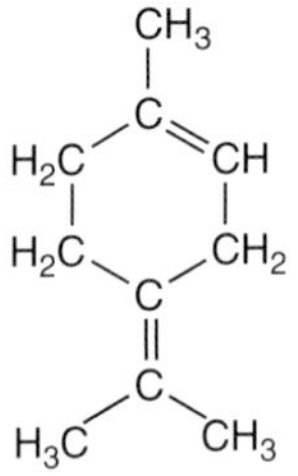

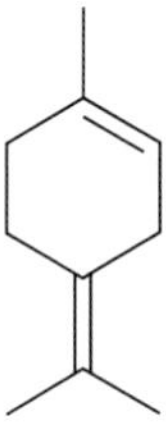

Terpinolene

Terpinene   Found in essential oils of tea tree and juniper.

α   β   γ

Terpinene

α- (alpha-), β- (beta-) and γ- (gamma-) terpinene are isomers, with the position of the double bond varying.

Other cyclic monoterpenes, e.g. pinenes, form 'bridged' structures, but the molecular formula is still $C_{10}H_{16}$.

Pinenes   Found in essential oils of juniper, pine and cajeput.

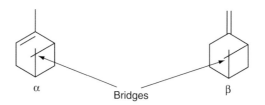

α   β

Bridges

AROMAFACT

Pinene is thought to be the most abundant hydrocarbon in nature.

Properties of monoterpenes

Physical and chemical properties
1. Colourless, mobile liquids
2. Highly volatile, low boiling points, evaporate very quickly
3. Weak, uninteresting odours
4. Fairly reactive, prone to oxidation (reaction with oxygen) even under cool conditions.

AROMAFACT

CAUTION: The oxidation products of monoterpenes are thought to be irritants.

Therapeutic properties
1. Antiseptic
2. Bactericidal, antiviral
3. May be
   - analgesic
   - expectorant
   - decongestant
   - stimulant.

Box 3.1 Monoterpenes found in essential oils

- Camphene
- Menthene
- Pinene
- Carene
- Myrcene

- Sabinene
- Cymene
- Ocimene
- Terpinene
- Dipentene

- Phellandrene
- Thujene
- Limonene

Sesquiterpenes

Sesqui means half as much again, so sesquiterpenes have a molecular formula one and a half times a monoterpene: they are made up of three isoprene units. The molecular formula is $C_{15}H_{24}$ (Fig. 3.3).

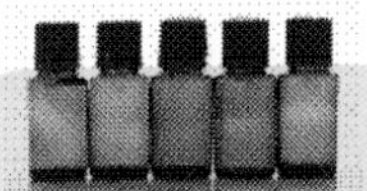

AROMAFACT

Sesquiterpenes make up the largest group of terpenes in the plant world. They are of particular significance in aromatherapy.

Farnesene   A branched chain hydrocarbon found in oils of citronella, German chamomile, yarrow, rose and cassie absolute.

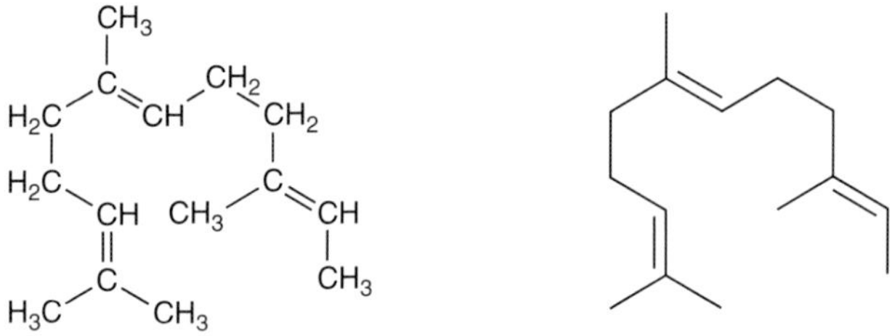

Farnesene

15 carbons, 24 hydrogens: $C_{15}H_{24}$

Bisabolene   A cyclic structure (with a carbon ring in the molecule) found in myrrh oil and German chamomile.

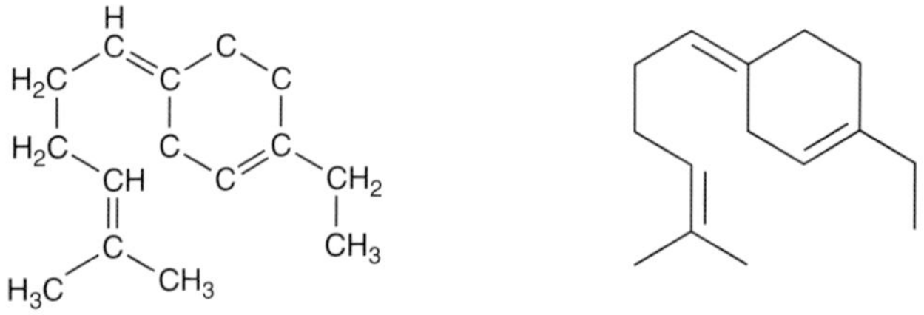

Bisabolene

Caryophyllene   Cyclic and has a strong woody, spicy odour, found in oil cloves, lavender, sweet thyme and ylang ylang.

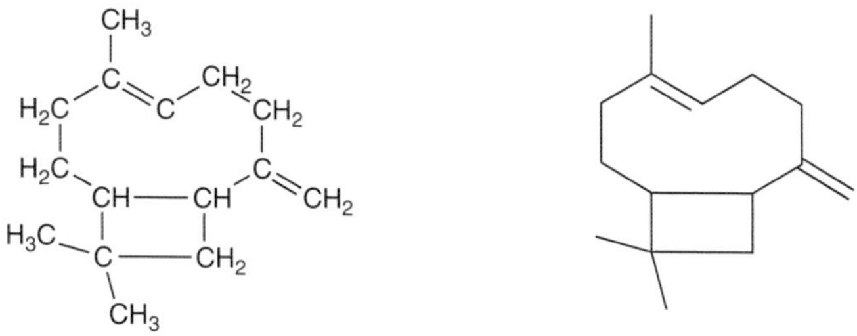

Caryophyllene

Chamazulene   A bicyclic unsaturated hydrocarbon with the molecular formula $C_{14}H_{16}$. It does not belong to the sequiterpenes but is historically included with them. It is an azulene which are compounds derived from sequiterpenes. Chamazulene is formed by the breakdown of matricine during the steam distillation process.

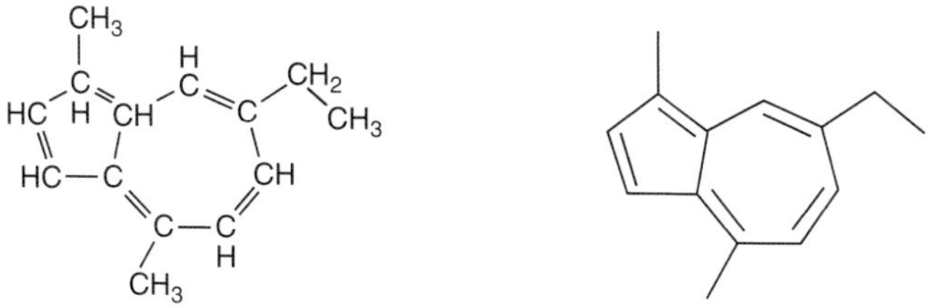

Chamazulene

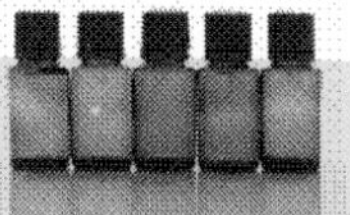

AROMAFACT

Chamazulene has been the subject of extensive research. It is considered to have anti–allergy and anti–inflammatory properties and to be beneficial to cells. It gives German chamomile its characteristic blue colour.

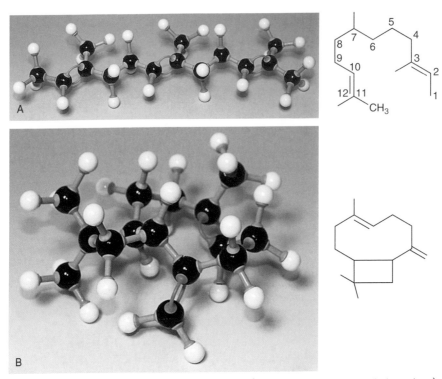

Figure 3.3 Sesquiterpenes ($C_{15}H_{24}$). (A) Farnesene (3,7,11-trimethyl-2,6,10-dodecatriene) (acyclic). (B) Caryophyllene (bicyclic). Courtesy Spiring Enterprises Ltd.

Properties of sesquiterpenes

Physical and chemical properties
1. Greater molecular weight than monoterpenes, so less volatile with higher boiling points
2. Still prone to oxidation but more slowly by atmospheric oxygen
3. Strong odours.

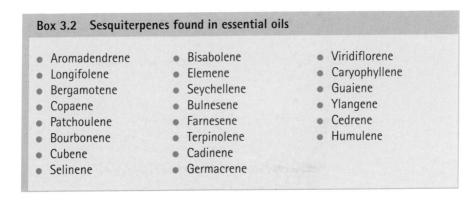

Box 3.2   Sesquiterpenes found in essential oils

• Aromadendrene	• Bisabolene	• Viridiflorene
• Longifolene	• Elemene	• Caryophyllene
• Bergamotene	• Seychellene	• Guaiene
• Copaene	• Bulnesene	• Ylangene
• Patchoulene	• Farnesene	• Cedrene
• Bourbonene	• Terpinolene	• Humulene
• Cubene	• Cadinene	
• Selinene	• Germacrene	

AROMAFACT

Only a few sesquiterpenes and their derivatives are volatile – these are notably the azulenes such as chamazulene, bisabolol and farnesene.

Therapeutic properties   Different sesquiterpenes have been described as being:

- antiseptic
- antibacterial
- anti-inflammatory
- calming and slightly hypotensive
- some may be analgesic and antispasmodic.

AROMAFACT

The sesquiterpenes and their derivatives are of particular interest owing to their important pharmacological activity.

Diterpenes

Diterpenes are made up of two monoterpene units (four isoprenes): $2 \times C_{10}H_{16} =$ *molecular formula*, $C_{20}H_{32}$.

Diterpenes are not so common in essential oils as their higher molecular weight and boiling point prevents them coming over in the extraction process of steam distillation. They are most likely to occur in resins.

Camphorene   Cyclic compound, found in the high boiling fraction of camphor oil, boiling point (b.p.) 177–178 °C.

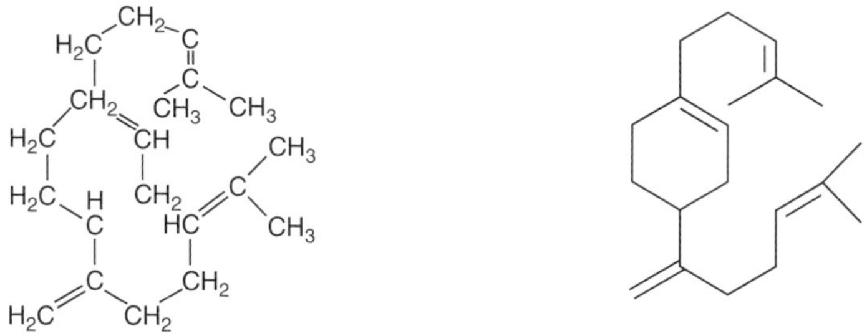

Camphorene

Properties of diterpenes   The molecular structure of the diterpene camphorene is given in Figure 3.4.

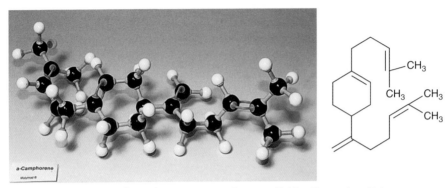

Figure 3.4 Diterpenes $(C_{20}H_{32})$. Camphorene. Courtesy Spiring Enterprises Ltd.

Physical and chemical properties Diterpenes are similar to sesquiterpenes but the larger molecules and molecular weights give them higher boiling points and lower oxidation rates.

Therapeutic properties Certain diterpenes have been described as:

- antifungal and antiviral
- possibly expectorant and purgative
- possibly having a balancing effect on the endocrine system.

Important biological compounds that are derivatives of diterpenes include gibberellic acid, which is a plant growth hormone.

Triterpenes

Six isoprene units combine to give a molecular formula $C_{30}H_{48}$ for the triterpenes. Their derivatives – the triterpenoids – include sterols (found in all plant and animal cells), steroids (many hormones) and saponins (important plant products).

Tetra- or quadraterpenes

Eight isoprene units combine to give a molecular formula $C_{40}H_{56}$ for the tetra- or quadraterpenes. Their derivatives include the carotenoids, which are important starting materials for vitamin A, fat-soluble vitamins D, E and K, cholesterol and sex hormones.

AROMAFACT

Note that tri- and tetraterpenoids are not hydrocarbons but are derived from them. They are not found in essential oils but form starting materials for a range of important natural products.

Polyterpenes

Polyterpenes are compounds comprising several hundred isoprene units and give rise to natural rubber. *Poly* means 'many', so that rubber is made up of many repeating isoprene units. The name for a compound made up of many such repeating units is a *polymer*. There are many both naturally occurring and synthetically produced polymers of importance with many applications.

The vast majority of these compounds are produced in plants but are obviously outside the scope of aromatherapy.

AROMAFACT

SUMMARY: In essential oils, most constituents are terpenes and terpenoid molecules. The method of extraction can influence the terpene content. In citrus oils extracted by expression (squeezing or pressing the plant material), the terpenes present are similar to those found in the living plant tissue; for example, orange, lemon, mandarin and grapefruit essential oils may be made up of up to 90% of the monoterpene limonene. When extraction is by steam distillation the action of the hot water and steam on thermolabile (heat-sensitive) molecules present in the plant is responsible for the formation of the bulk of the terpene content. Solvent extraction often produces absolutes that are very low in terpenes or do not contain them at all, when compared to a distillation of the same material, for example as found in lavender and rose products.

OXYGENATED COMPOUNDS

Compounds of this type are named after the hydrocarbon or terpene plus the functional group:

- A monoterpenol, or monoterpene alcohol, is a monoterpene with an alcohol functional group.
- A monoterpenone, or monoterpene ketone, is a monoterpene with a ketone functional group.
- A monoterpenal, or monoterpene aldehyde, is a monoterpene with an aldehyde functional group.

This will become clearer as we proceed through a number of examples.

Alcohols

AROMAFACT

Alcohols are considered the most therapeutically beneficial of essential oil components, with low toxicity and pleasant fragrances. When employed correctly essential oils rich in alcohols present minimal risk and are generally safe for use on children and the elderly.

The alcohol functional group is –OH and the name ends in -ol; for example, geraniol and linalool (found in geranium and lavender, respectively). If the alcohol functional group is attached to a monoterpene, the compounds are called monoterpenols (Fig. 3.5).

Monoterpenols

Monoterpenols, e.g. geraniol, linalool and citronellol, are acyclic.

Geraniol

trans-2,7-Dimethylocta-2,6-dien-1-ol

Found in oils of rose, geranium, citronella, palmarosa

Warm, floral and sweet odour

Linalool (sometimes called linalol)

3,7-Dimethylocta-1,6-dien-3-ol

Found in oils of ho, rosewood and coriander

Light, floral, spicy, woody with slight citrus odour

Citronellol

3,7-Dimethylocta-6-en-1-ol

Found in oils of rose, geranium, citronella, eucalyptus and citriodora

Fresh, light floral odour like roses

Terpineol

1-Methyl-4-isopropylcyclohex-1-en-8-ol

A major component of pine oils, and present in small amounts in many other essential oils such as eucalyptus and cajeput

Delicate, sweet, floral and lilac odour

AROMAFACT

There is some concern about sensitisation with essential oils high in linalool, geraniol and citronellol. However, pure linalool is not a sensitiser. It is the oxidation products such as hydroperoxides that have been shown to have sensitising properties. Due to the oxidation hazard the correct storage and handling of essential oils containing these alcohols is important. (see Chapter 8)

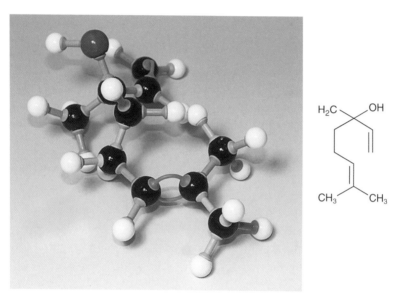

Figure 3.5   Alcohols. Linalool (3,7-dimethyl-1,6-octadien-3-ol; $C_{10}H_{18}O$), a monoterpene alcohol. Courtesy Spiring Enterprises Ltd.

Box 3.3   Monoterpene alcohols found in essential oils

- Borneol
- Isopulegol
- Nerol
- Citronellol

- Lavandulol
- Terpineol
- Fenchyl alcohol
- Linalool

- Terpin-4-ol
- Geraniol
- Myrtenol

Therapeutic properties   Monoterpenols are considered to be:

- anti-infective – antiviral, antibacterial (bactericidal)
- immune system stimulants
- good general tonic and balancing
- uplifting
- warming.

AROMAFACT

The type of chemical constituent is quoted when explaining the influence of *chemotype*. This occurs when plants have the same botanical species and name but have significantly different chemical constituents in their oils, which then exhibit different therapeutic properties. Different types of alcohols are found in essential oils of thyme grown in different situations. For *Thymus vulgaris* the position, altitude and other environmental factors cause the formation of essential oils with differing types of alcohols.

- Thyme at top of mountain: high in linalool, better quality safe oil from stronger plants.
- Thyme at very bottom of mountain: oil contains significant amount of phenol.
- Thyme near bottom of mountain: higher in geraniol, intermediate composition.

Phenol is not actually an alcohol, although the molecular structure is similar. The difference between alcohols and phenols should be recognized. Phenols need to be used with caution in aromatherapy.

Sesquiterpenols

A sesquiterpenol is a sesquiterpene with an attached alcohol group. A few important examples are found in essential oils.

α- (alpha-) Bisabolol   Found in German chamomile; it is thought to have anti-inflammatory effects.

α-Bisabolol

α- (alpha-) Santalol   Found in sandalwood oil in high amounts. Sometimes used for urinary tract infections, but may act via immune system.

α-Santalol

Farnesol   Found in rose essential oil. It is bacteriostatic and non-irritant; sometimes used in the formulation of deodorants.

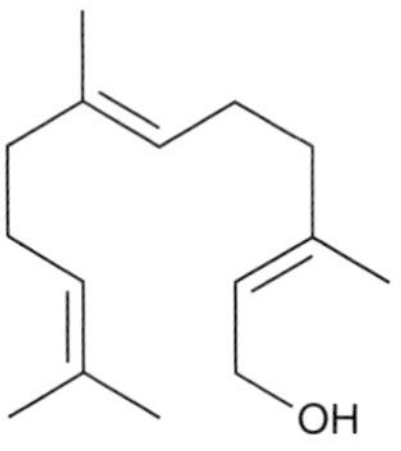

Farnesol

Sesquiterpenols are found in appreciable amounts in oils of ginger, carrot, valerian, patchouli and vetiver. The pharmacological effects are quite varied and general properties assigned to them include anti-inflammatory, stimulant to liver and glands, and tonic.

Box 3.4   Sesquiterpene alcohols found in essential oils

- Atlantol
- Caryophyllene alcohol
- Nerolidol
- Bisabolol

- Elemol
- Patchoulol
- Cadinoll
- Eudesmol
- Santalol

- Cedrol
- Farnesol
- Viridiflorol

Diterpenols

A diterpenol is formed from a diterpene and an alcohol group. As diterpenols have higher molecular weights and boiling points they do not vaporize or come through in essential oil distillation extraction. They have structural similarities to human steroid hormones and may have a balancing effect on the endocrine system. An example is sclareol, found in Clary sage essential oil, with a molecular mass just small enough to vaporize and be extracted by steam distillation.

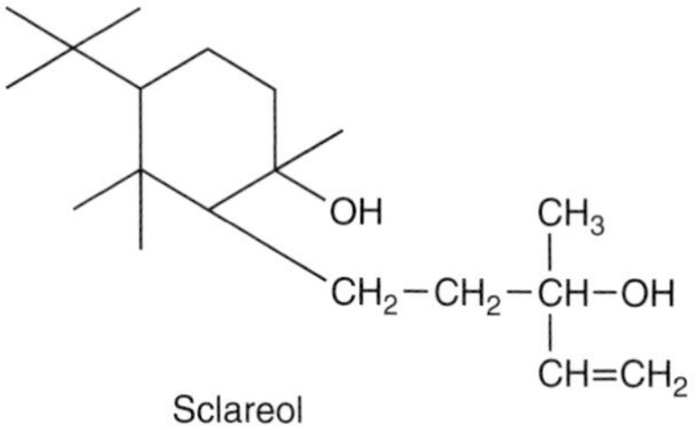

Sclareol

Also present in essential oils are *non-terpene-derived aliphatic alcohols* such as decanol, hexanol, heptanol, octanol and nonanol, and *aromatic alcohols* such as benzyl alcohol and phenylethyl alcohol.

Phenols

Phenols appear superficially similar to alcohols, possessing an –OH group, but in practice they are very different. The names of phenols also end in -ol, e.g. carvacrol.

In phenols the –OH group is attached to an *aromatic ring* or *phenyl ring*:

Benzene: 6-membered carbon ring
(see p. 37)

The parent compound *phenol* is

Phenol is a very potent chemical; in solution it is known as carbolic acid and was used as an early antiseptic. It does not occur in nature as carbolic acid. As it is harmful to living cells it is no longer used, but may be used for cleaning surfaces and equipment.

In aromatherapy the family of phenols are called substituted phenols, as one or more of the five remaining available hydrogen atoms of the ring is replaced by another group of atoms. Examples are carvacrol, thymol and eugenol (Fig. 3.6).

Carvacrol (5–isopropyl–2–methylphenol)   Found in essential oils of thyme, sage and oregano. Phenolic, spicy odour.

Carvacrol

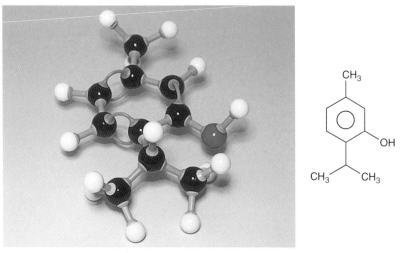

Figure 3.6   Phenols. Thymol ($C_{10}H_{14}O$). Courtesy Spiring Enterprises Ltd.

Thymol (2–isopropyl–5–methylphenol)   Found in essential oils of thyme and oregano. Strong medicated, herbaceous odour.

Thymol

Eugenol (4–allyl–2–methoxyphenol)   Eugenol is not actually derived from a terpene molecule (as opposed to carvacrol and thymol) but it is a phenol and is found in essential oils of clove, cinnamon leaf, pimento, ylang ylang and rose. It has a spicy, pungent odour typical of clove.

Eugenol

Properties of phenols
Physical and chemical properties
1. Slightly acidic
2. Very reactive, similar to but much stronger actions than alcohols.

Therapeutic properties   A number of therapeutic actions are attributed to the phenols:

- antiseptic, anti-infectious, bactericidal
- stimulant to immune system – can activate healing
- stimulant to nervous system – effective in some depressive illnesses.

AROMAFACT

CAUTION: Essential oils high in phenols must be handled with great care. They can be toxic to the liver and irritant to the skin and mucous membranes.

Essential oils high in phenols that are skin irritants include cinnamon, clove, aniseed oil, basil, tarragon, red thyme and origanum.

Thyme and origanum are widely used in the pharmaceutical field, mainly due to the germicidal and antiseptic properties of phenolic components.

Box 3.5   Phenols found in essential oils

- Carvacrol
- Eugenol
- Cresol
- Thymol

Phenolic ethers

A number of phenols appear in essential oils as phenolic ethers. The hydrogen atom of the –OH group is replaced by an alkyl or aryl group. An *alkyl* group is a saturated or unsaturated hydrocarbon chain structure; *aryl* groups are joined to the compound by a carbon atom of an aromatic ring. The names of compounds in this class end in -ole.

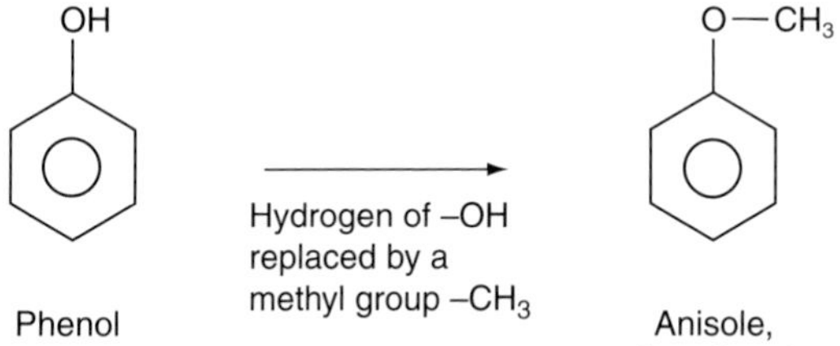

OH

Phenol

Hydrogen of –OH replaced by a methyl group –CH_3

O—CH_3

Anisole, a phenolic ether

Other examples include anethole, safrole and estragole.

Anethole

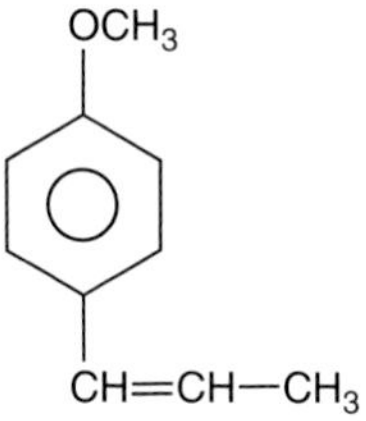

OCH$_3$

CH=CH—CH$_3$

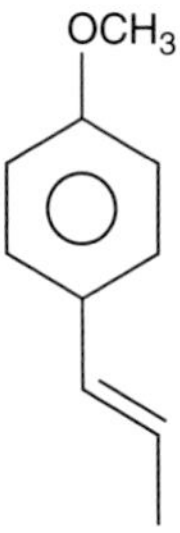

OCH$_3$

Anethole

Anethole is found in essential oils of anise and fennel. It exists as *cis* and *trans* forms, with the *cis* being more toxic. (Recall that *cis* and *trans* forms of a molecule are isomers that differ in the arrangement of groups attached to double bonds; see Ch. 2.)

Safrole

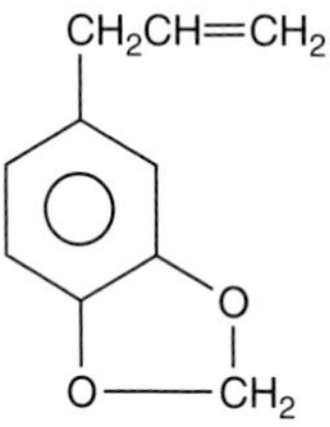

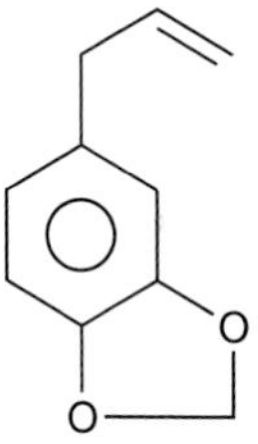

CH$_2$CH=CH$_2$

O—CH$_2$

Safrole

Safrole is found in oils of camphor and saffras. It has been used medicinally as a counterirritant and for parasitic infections. It is also a listed carcinogen and cannot be used as a fragrance ingredient.

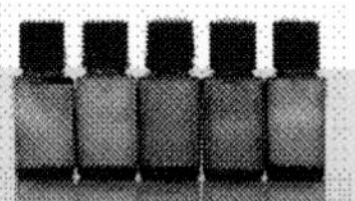

AROMAFACT

The IFRA recommendation is that essential oils containing safrole should not be used at a level such that the total concentration exceeds 0.01% in consumer products. Essential oils with a high safrole content include Brown camphor oil (80%) and Sassafras (85–95%). Even the East Indian nutmeg oil has up to 3.3% and this needs considering when formulating blends.

Methyl chavicol (also called estragole)

Estragole

Box 3.6   Phenol ethers found in essential oils

- Anethole
- Myrtenyl methylether
- Estragole (methyl chavicol)

- Myristin
- Methyl eugenol
- Safrole

Estragole is found in essential oils of basil, fennel, chervil, ravensara and tarragon. Although it is not restricted by any regulatory agencies, there is evidence of potential carcinogenic properties in high doses. (see Fig. 3.7)

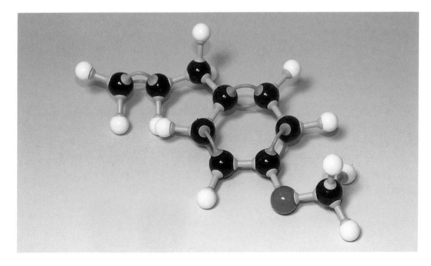

Figure 3.7   Phenolic ether. Methyl chavicol (estragole) ($C_{10}H_{12}O$). Courtesy of Spiring Enterprises Ltd.

AROMAFACT

Phenolic ethers have similar properties to the phenols but are generally more powerful; several are neurotoxic if present in large amounts in an oil. This would indicate 'short term use only in low concentration'.

Aldehydes

The aldehyde functional group is

$$-\overset{\overset{\displaystyle O}{\displaystyle \|}}{\underset{\underset{\displaystyle H}{}}{C}}$$

and aldehyde names end in -al (e.g. citral, citronellal) or aldehyde (e.g. cinnamic aldehyde).

Citronellal (3,7-dimethyl-6-octenal)   Found in essential oils of citronella, eucalyptus citrioda and melissa. Citrus, strong smell very characteristic of citronella. (Fig. 3.8)

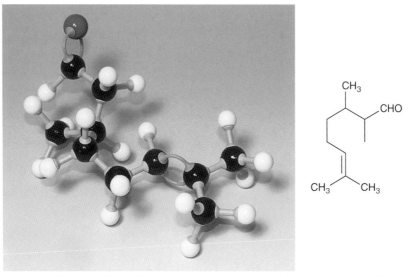

Figure 3.8   Aldehydes. Citronellal ($C_{10}H_{18}O$), monoterpene aldehyde. Courtesy Spiring Enterprises Ltd.

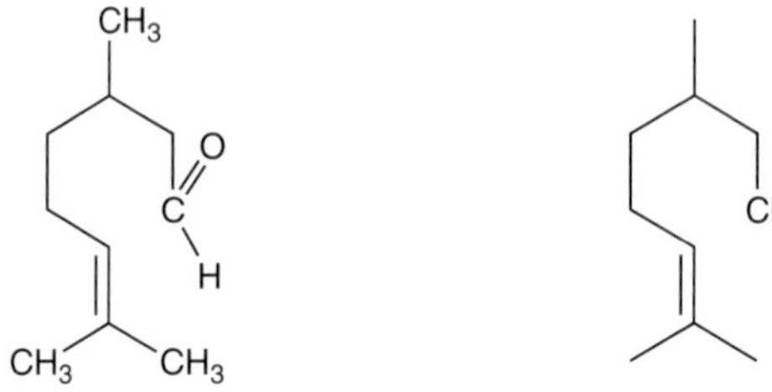

Citronellal

Cinnamic aldehyde (3–phenylprop–2–enal)   This is not a terpene derivative but is an example of an aldehyde. Found in essential oils of cinnamon bark, cassia (Chinese cinnamon). Warm, spicy and balsamic.

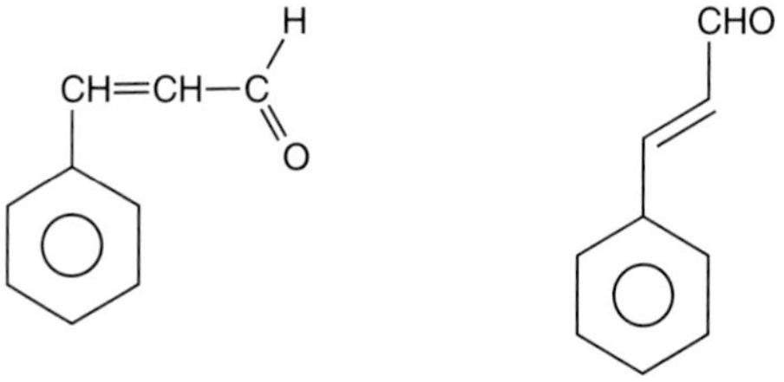

Cinnamic aldehyde

Geranial (α–citral; trans–3,7–dimethyl–2,6–octadienal)   Found in essential oils of lemongrass, lemon, lime, melissa and verbena. Light, sharp, fresh lemon odour.

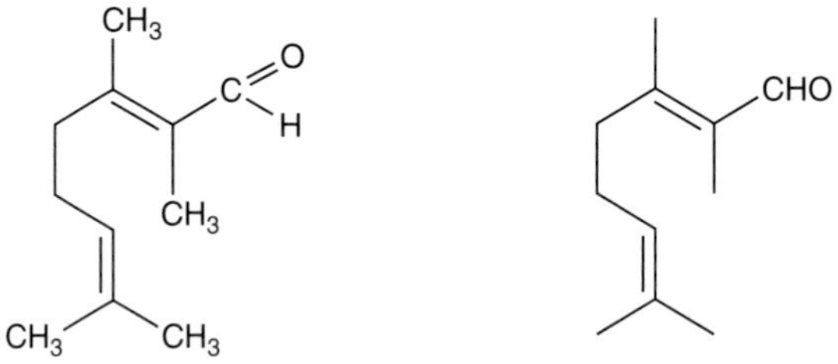

Geranial

Beta-citral (the *cis* form) is called neral and is not as fresh smelling as the α form.

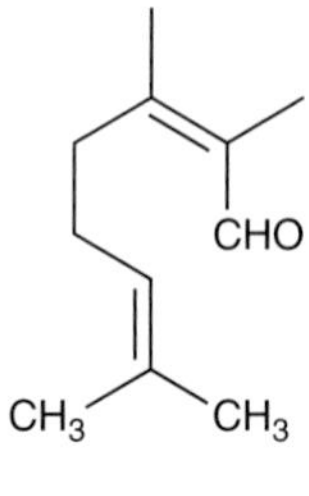

Neral

AROMAFACT

Aldehydes have very powerful aromas and widespread use in the perfumery industry. Chanel No. 5 is described as having an aldehydic smell. The aldehydes used in perfumery are not the terpene derivatives but are usually synthetic fatty aldehydes.

Careful storage of essential oils high in aldehydes is crucial. Over a period of time, or in poor conditions, the oxidation of the aldehydes to acids will render them useless for aromatherapy.

Aldehydes are very reactive molecules and oxidize (combine with oxygen) to form organic acids called carboxylic acids. This may cause them to be skin irritants and skin sensitizers if not stored correctly.

AROMAFACT

CAUTION: A sensitizer substance may cause a rash on initial use, which then reappears whenever that substance is applied. This needs to be noted, as the same aldehyde may be present in another oil and will have the same effect. For example cinnamic aldehyde has a recommended level of not more than 0.05% for skin contact (see page 259).

Properties of aldehydes   Aldehydes are often described as having properties intermediate between alcohols and ketones. Therapeutically, certain aldehydes have been described as:

- anti-infectious (but not as consistent as alcohols)
- tonic
- vasodilators, hypotensive
- calming to the nervous system
- temperature reducing (antipyretic).

Box 3.7   Aldehydes found in essential oils

- Acetaldehyde
- Cuminaldehyde
- Piperonal
- Anisaldehyde
- Decanal
- Phellandral
- Benzaldehyde

- Geranial
- Sinensal
- Caproic aldehyde
- Myrtenal
- Teresantal
- Cinnamaldehyde
- Neral

- Valeranal
- Citral
- Nonanal
- Citronellal
- Perillaldehyde

AROMAFACT

Citral as a pure isolated compound is a very powerful irritant, however, when present in the whole oil of lemon (where it makes up about 5%), its possible hazards appear to be reduced by the presence of the other 95% of constituents, most of which are terpenes. It is important to remember that citral rich oils like lemongrass may act as skin irritants and sensitisers in some people.

This is an example of the terpenes acting as quenchers. Quenching occurs when certain constituents of an oil may cause a reduction (not a complete negation) in side effects caused by other constituents. This concept has been scientifically challenged but in aromatherapy mixing an oil containing citral with one containing equal amounts of d-limonene has been shown to reduce the irritant and sensitising properties of the citral. This is reinforced by the IFRA (International Fragrance Association) guidelines that say citral should be used as a fragrance ingredient in conjunction with substances preventing sensitisation, as for example 25% d-limonene, or mixed citrus terpenes, or a-pinene. This recommendation is based on results showing sensitisation potential for the individual ingredient, but reduction of sensitising reactions in a number of compounds with lemongrass oil, as well as in mixtures of 80 parts citral to 20 parts d-limonene, or mixed citrus terpenes, or a-pinene. (However see page 47 there is potential danger from formation of peroxides from the oxidation of limonene and other monoterpenes.)

Ketones

Ketones contain the carbonyl group and their names end in -one.

$$\diagdown \atop \diagup C = O$$

AROMAFACT

Ketones are not very common in the majority of essential oils, and aromatic ones are particularly rare.

Carvone In the *dextro* (*d*) form carvone is found in caraway and dill essential oils. In the *laevo* (*l*) form it is the main constituent of spearmint oil (Fig. 3.9).

d-Carvone

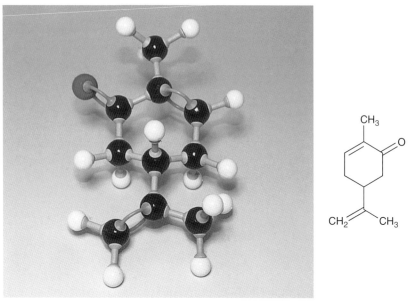

Figure 3.9 Ketones. *l*-Carvone ($C_{10}H_{14}O$), a monocyclic monoterpene ketone. Courtesy Spiring Enterprises Ltd.

AROMAFACT

Carvone is found in gripe water and seems to be harmless, showing no adverse ketone hazards.

Menthone (2-isopropyl-5-methylcyclohexanone) Found in essential oils of peppermint and *Mentha arvenis*. Minty, woody, fresh odour.

Menthone

cis-Jasmone [3-methyl-2-(2-pentenyl)-2-cyclopentenone] A constituent of jasmine absolute. Floral, warm, spicy 'celery-like' odour.

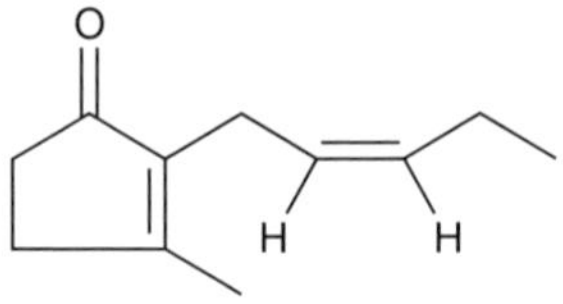

cis-Jasmone

Camphor (C$_{10}$H$_{16}$O) Found in essential oils of ho leaf, lavandin, spike lavender, rosemary and sage. An important compound used in many applications including medical preparations, but it is classified as toxic.

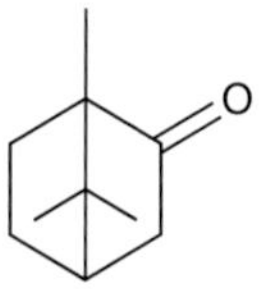

Essential oils that contain high amounts of ketones are aniseed, sage, hyssop, fennel, rosemary, caraway, pennyroyal, peppermint, spearmint and dill.

Box 3.8   Ketones found in essential oils

- Acetophenone
- Fenchone
- Menthone
- Atlantone
- Ionone
- Methylheptenone
- Camphor
- Irone
- Methoxyphenylacetone
- Carvone
- Jasmone
- Nootkatone
- Octanone
- Pulegone
- Valeranone
- Pinocamphone
- Tagetone
- Verbenone
- Pinocarvone
- Thujone
- Piperitone
- Undecan-2-one

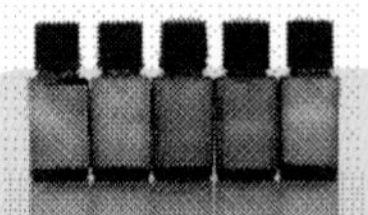

AROMAFACT

CAUTION: Ketones must be used very carefully. Not all essential oils containing ketones are necessarily hazardous but they should be well diluted up to a maximum of 2% and only used externally. They should not be used for prolonged periods.

Therapeutic properties   Therapeutic properties associated with some ketones include:

- calming and sedative
- mucolytic, some may be expectorant
- analgesic
- digestive
- encourage wound healing.

AROMAFACT

CAUTION: Ketones must be used with great care. Hyssop may provoke epileptic fits. Oils such as wormwood and thuga, which are high in the ketones thujone and pulegone, may cause miscarriage. These oils should never be used during pregnancy. In France, hyssop and sage are available only through pharmacies.

Acids

Organic acids contain the carboxyl group

$$\begin{array}{c} \overset{O}{\underset{O-H}{\overset{\|}{-C}}} \end{array} \quad \text{or} \quad -COOH$$

and their name ends in acid (Fig. 3.10). They are very rare in essential oils but are found in nature in many situations; for example:

H–COOH	Formic or methanoic acid (an aliphatic acid). Found in sweat, urine and stinging nettles.
CH$_3$–COOH	Acetic or ethanoic acid (an aliphatic acid). Found in vinegar and some aromatic waters.
CH$_2$–COOH (phenyl ring)	Phenylacetic acid (an aromatic acid). Found in neroli essential oil.

Acids are important because they react with alcohols to form esters. Many esters present in essential oils are formed as reaction products during the distillation process in extraction.

Box 3.9   Acids found in essential oils

- Anisic acid
- Palmitic acid
- Benzoic acid

- Phenylacetic acid
- Cinnamic acid
- Valerenic acid

- Citronellic acid
- Vetiveric acid

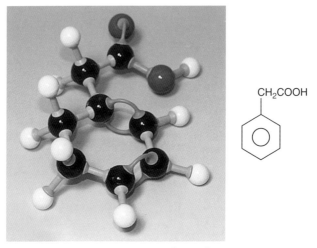

CH₂COOH

Figure 3.10   Aromatic acids. Phenylacetic acid $(C_8H_8O_2)$, not a terpene but an organic acid. Courtesy Spiring Enterprises Ltd.

Esters

AROMAFACT

Esters form the most widespread group of compounds in plant essences and fragrances.

Esters are formed by reaction of acids with alcohols:

Organic acid + Alcohol   →   Ester + Water

e.g.

COOH   COOCH₃

OH   OH

+ CH₃OH   ⟶   + H₂O

Salicyclic acid + Methanol   ⟶   Methyl salicylate   + Water
(found in oil of wintergreen)

The functional group of esters is

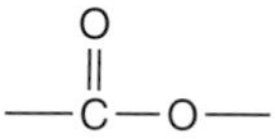

$$-\overset{\overset{\displaystyle O}{\displaystyle \|}}{C}-O-$$

and the names end in -ate or ester.

Esters are generally safe to use, with low toxicity (see exception of methyl salicylate and sabinyl acetate found in Spanish sage). Although few essential oils have esters as their main components, esters are found in greater numbers than other functional groups.

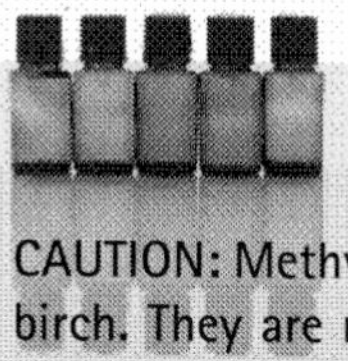

AROMAFACT

CAUTION: Methyl salicylate makes up 90% of essential oils of wintergreen and birch. They are not suitable for aromatherapy, although the pungent wintergreen is often an ingredient in sports gels for external use only.

Examples of significant esters include benzyl acetate, linalyl acetate, geranyl acetate and citronellyl formate.

Benzyl acetate Found in jasmin absolute and essential oils of ylang ylang and neroli. Floral and fruity odour (typical of jasmin). (Benzyl acetate is not a terpene derivative but is found in many essential oils.)

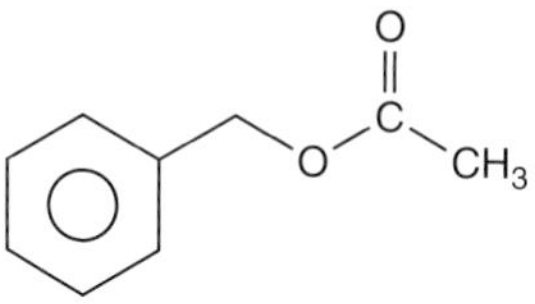

Benzyl acetate

Linalyl acetate (3,7–dimethyl–1,6–octadien–3–yl acetate) Found in essential oils of bergamot, lavender, lavandin, spike lavender, Clary sage, neroli and petitgrain. Floral, fruity, sweet and herbaceous odour.

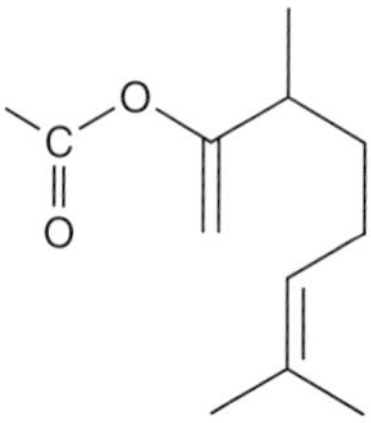

Linalyl acetate

Geranyl acetate (trans–3,7–dimethyl–2,6–octadien–1–yl acetate)   Found in many essential oils including geranium, citronella, lavender, petitgrain and sweet marjoram. Fruity, floral, fresh, rose-like odour.

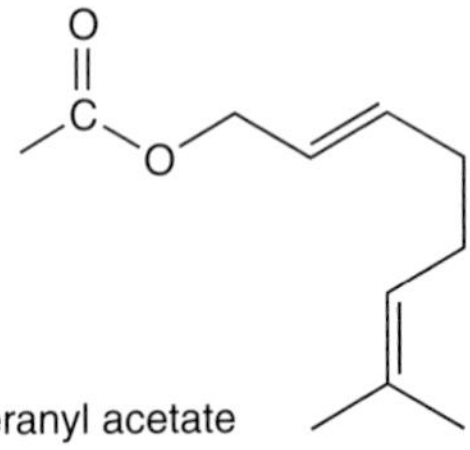

Geranyl acetate

Citronellyl formate (3,7–dimethyloct–6–en–1–yl formate)   Found in geranium oil. Fruity, floral, light rose-like odour.

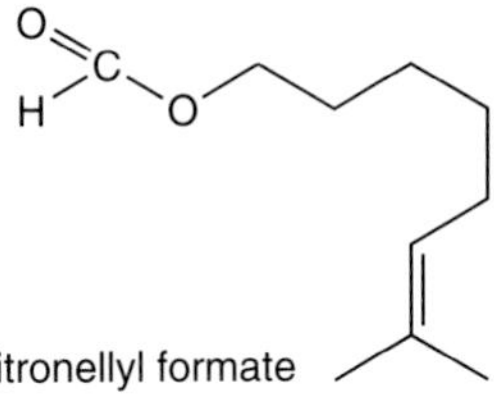

Citronellyl formate

Properties of esters   Properties commonly associated with esters include:

- gentle in action, similar to alcohols
- characteristic sweet, fruity odours
- antifungal
- anti-inflammatory
- antispasmodic
- calming and tonic to nervous system
- effective for skin rashes.

Box 3.10   Esters found in essential oils

- Benzyl acetate
- Geranyl acetate
- Methyl salicylate
- Benzyl benzoate
- Geranyl tiglate
- Neryl acetate
- Bornyl acetate
- Hexyl acetate
- Propyl angelate

- Bornyl isovalerate
- Lavandulyl acetate
- Sabinyl acetate
- Butyl angelate
- Linalyl acetate
- trans-Pinocarveol acetate
- Citronellyl acetate
- Menthyl acetate

- Citronellyl butyrate
- Methyl anthranilate
- Terpineol acetate
- Citronellyl formate
- Methyl benzoate
- Vetiverol acetate
- Eugenyl acetate
- Methyl butyrate

Lactones and coumarins

A lactone is an ester in which the functional group of the ester has become part of a ring structure with carbon atoms. Names of lactones end with -in or -one, e.g. umbelliferone.

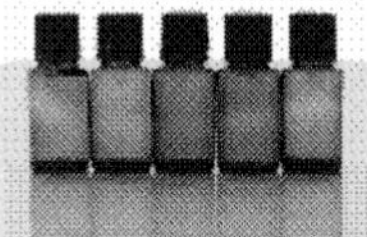

AROMAFACT

Lactones are only found in expressed oils and some absolutes, e.g. jasmine, as their molecular weights are too high for them to come over in distillation. Although they are present in low amounts in essential oils, they are wide-spread in nature.

Coumarins are a type of lactone.

Coumarin (2–hydroxycinnamic acid lactone) Found in hay and beans. Sweet, coconutty, soft odour of hay, and used in the perfumery industry.

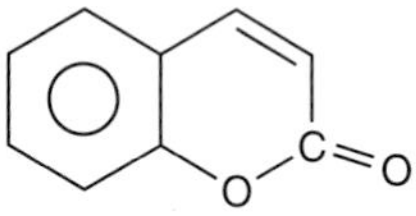

Coumarin

Umbelliferone (7–hydroxycoumarin) Found in many plants.

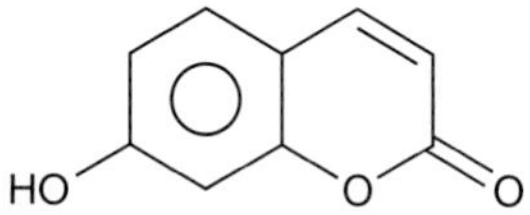

Umbelliferone

Furocoumarins, e.g. bergaptene (5–methyloxypsoralen) (Fig. 3.11) Found in essential oil of bergamot (about 0.3%) and in small amounts in orange, mandarin and lemon.

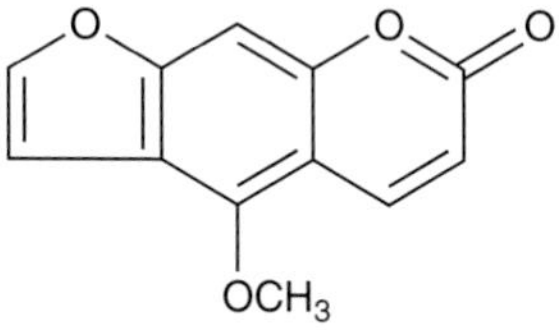

OCH_3

Bergaptene

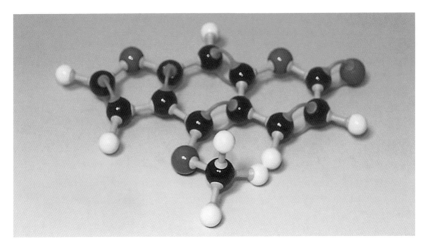

Figure 3.11 Furocoumarins. Bergaptene ($C_{12}H_8O_4$). Courtesy Spiring Enterprises Ltd.

Box 3.11   Lactones, coumarins and furocoumarins found in essential oils

Lactones
- Achilline
- Costuslactone
- Dihydronepetalactone
- Alantrolactone
- Epinepetalactone
- Nepetalactone

Coumarins
- Aesculatine
- Citropten

- Heniarin (7-methylcoumarin)
- Coumarin
- Dihydrocoumarin
- Umbelliferone (7-hydroxycoumarin)

Furocoumarins
- Bergaptene
- Bergaptol
- Psoralen

AROMAFACT

CAUTION: Bergaptene is a furocoumarin and should not be confused through its name with the terpenes. It is potentially photocarcinogenic. This means it may induce a cancer that is triggered off by the action of light with this chemical on the body cells. Cancer is due to a malfunction of the DNA or genetic material of the chromosomes that causes cells to divide in an abnormal and uncontrolled way. Bergaptene appears to interfere with the skin cells that produce melanin. Melanin is the pigment that gives the colour to skin and protects it against the harmful UV (ultraviolet) rays that can induce the cancer. Oils containing furocoumarins should never be used before sunbathing or using sunbeds.

Properties of lactones   Some lactones are:
- mucolytic and expectorant
- temperature reducing.

Coumarins   Many coumarins are skin sensitizing and phototoxic and, consequently, they should be used with caution. Properties associated with coumarins are:
- anticoagulation
- hypotensive
- uplifting *yet* sedative.

Furocoumarins
1. Caution with bergaptene – potentially carcinogenic
2. Some are antifungal and antiviral.

AROMAFACT

The recommended maximum safe level of bergaptene (from IFRA) is 0.0015%, so 100 g oil must not contain more than 0.0015 g.
  CAUTION: A typical bergamot oil may have 0.3%, i.e. 0.3 g in 100 g, so it must be diluted. The maximum safe strength of the essential oil would be 0.5 g in 100 g carrier or 1 g in 200 g carrier.
  When blending oils, check that others do not contain any photosensitizing components as their effect will be additive.

Oxides

Oxides in essential oils have an oxygen atom within a ring structure, usually made from an alcohol, and are named after the alcohol with the termination oxide, e.g. linalool oxide (Fig. 3.12). They are found in a wide range of essences, especially those of a camphoraceous nature, e.g. eucalyptus, rosemary, tea tree and cajeput.

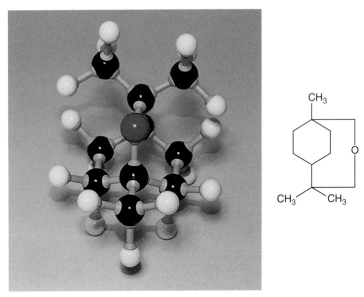

Figure 3.12   Oxides. 1,8-cineole ($C_{10}H_{18}O$). Courtesy Spiring Enterprises Ltd.

Eucalyptol (1,8-cineole; was also called cajuputol)   The most commonly encountered oxide in aromatherapy. Found in eucalyptus, cajeput and wormseed essential oils. It is a very chemically stable molecule and has a camphorlike smell.

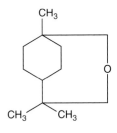

Eucalyptol

1,8-Cineole has been shown to be expectorant and to stimulate glands of the respiratory and digestive systems.

Box 3.12   Oxides found in essential oils

- Bisabolol oxide
- Cineole
- Rose oxide

- Bisabolone oxide
- Linalool oxide
- Sclareol oxide

- Caryophyllene oxide
- Pinene oxide

AROMAFACT

CAUTION: Oxides can be skin irritants and act in a similar way to phenols and should not be used in concentrations of more than 2%. (It is recommended not to use them on children.)

OTHER COMPOUNDS

Other types of compound can also be found in essential oils. They will probably be present only as trace amounts but may need to be considered when using the oil.

- *Ethers*. We have previously considered the phenolic ethers, which are quite a significant group, but there are also others, e.g. phenyl ethyl ether found in pandanus essential oil.
- *Furans*. Cyclic structures with an O atom in the ring, e.g. menthofuran found in many of the mint essential oils.
- *Sulfur-containing compounds*. These are not derived from the terpenes. They have very pungent smells, e.g. diallyl disulfide found in garlic.

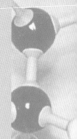

Chapter **4**

Processing, extraction and purity

EXTRACTION FROM NATURAL PRODUCTS

When considering quality and composition of an essential oil the method of extraction plays a crucial role. An essential oil is that oil extracted from plant material that is volatile at room temperature, but there are a number of other products whose nature and means of production need to be clarified – absolutes, resinoids, tinctures, floral waters, etc. (see Fig. 4.1).

The descriptions and definitions given here are only a brief summary and for further detail more specialized texts can be consulted.

Essential oils are extracted from different parts of the plant – petals, leaves, fruits, roots, barks, etc. – and this should be known when considering an oil.

The efficiency and yield of oil will depend on the method used and is usually reflected in price.

AROMAFACT

The time of year and even time of day the material is harvested can be crucial; for example, jasmine should be picked in the evening, rose in the morning before the dew goes off it. When the oil is found deep in plant tissue, the tissues need breaking up or powdering before extraction is possible; for example, cedarwood essential oil is extracted from wood chips or sawdust.

Distillation

Distillation is the most commonly used method for the extraction of essential oils. There are two techniques of distillation: *water* and *steam*.

Water distillation

The distillation apparatus, commonly called a 'still', consists of a vessel for plant material and water, a condenser to cool and condense the vapour produced and a method of collection, or 'receiver'. Material from the appropriate

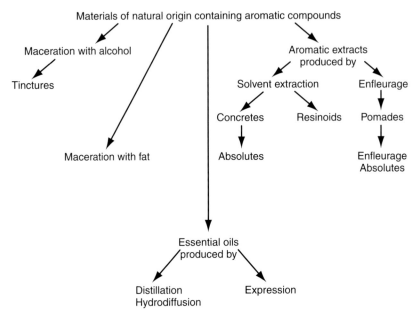

Figure 4.1   The various types of aromatic extract derived from plant materials.

part of the plant for extraction is immersed in water in the distillation vessel. This is then heated to boiling point and the steam (water vapour) carries out the volatile oils. The water safeguards some components by preventing over-heating as the temperature will not exceed 100 °C (the boiling point of water at normal pressure). However, the distillation can be a long process and the water may damage some other compounds.

AROMAFACT

Essential oils with a high percentage of esters can become *hydrolyzed* (hydrol-ysis is a chemical reaction of a substance with water) by contact with the hot water, which breaks them down to their constituent alcohols and carboxylic acids (see Ch. 3, esters). In lavender, linalyl acetate can break down into lina-lool and acetic acid, so a short distillation time is favourable.

The extraction of essential oils from plant material can be easily carried out in the chemistry laboratory using the apparatus shown in Figure 4.2.

Steam distillation

In steam distillation, steam – which is water vapour – is passed through the plant material at high pressure. Constituents that are insoluble in the water

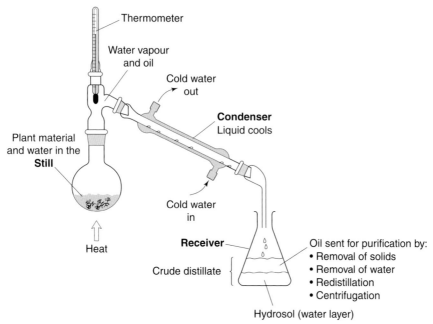

Figure 4.2 Laboratory water distillation apparatus for extraction of oils from plant materials.

but volatile enough to be driven off by the steam come over and are cooled, condensed and collected in the receiving vessel.

The resultant liquid is a mixture of immiscible oil and water, which separate out. Steam distillation is economical in processing large amounts of material, requiring little labour or complex extraction apparatus. A simple industrial steam distillation setup is shown in Figure 4.3.

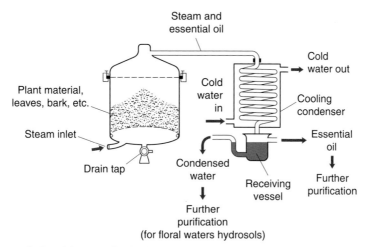

Figure 4.3 Industrial steam distillation setup.

AROMAFACT

The aqueous (water) portions left over from initial distillation are called hydrosols or floral waters, e.g. lavender, rose. They have many uses alongside essential oils and are utilized in the skin care and perfumery industries.

Steam distillation is quick, which minimizes damage to the compounds in the essential oil. The technique is good for extraction of volatile compounds from the monoterpenes (10 carbon atoms) to the diterpenes (20 carbon atoms).

 AROMAFACT

Certain compounds present in the essential oil can be changed by the steam. This can be illustrated by comparing a steam–distilled extract with that of the solvent extract. In rose extracts compounds such as phenylethyl alcohol make up a major proportion of the solvent-extracted material, but this is practically all lost in the steam distillation extract as it dissolves in the water. However, the process can be advantageous in German chamomile, where matricin is decomposed to form the characteristic blue compound chamazulene.

Essential oils extracted by water or steam distillation need further purification, especially drying to remove water. Essential oils produced by distillation are limited to compounds with a maximum molecular weight of 225–250.

Hydro-diffusion

Also called *percolation*, this is the newest method of extraction, developed in the 1990s. It is similar to steam distillation but is quicker and simpler. Steam percolates downwards through the plant material, and the extracted oil and steam are condensed in the same manner as in conventional steam distillation.

Expression

Expression is the use of a crushing, mechanically applied pressure to squeeze oils from plant material. It was originally done by hand but is now mechanized, with use of centrifugal separators. Expression is used almost exclusively for citrus fruits with oil glands in the outer rind of the fruit.

AROMAFACT

Expression is good for the top notes, e.g. in bergamot and lemon esssential oils, which are very volatile owing to being high in monoterpenes. Many of these would be lost in distillation because of the high temperatures. It is also a cheap method, using by-products from the juice industry.

Solvent extraction

Aromatic plant material is placed into organic solvents such as acetone (propanone) or hexane, which dissolve out the oils. Other solvents used are methanol, ethanol, toluene and petroleum ether. In some processes the plant material is broken up, to aid penetration of solvent into the tissues, by placing it in a rotating drum with internal blades to ensure thorough mixing. The materials that become dissolved include not only the essential oil but also natural waxes, resinous materials, chlorophyll and other pigments.

The residue obtained is repeatedly washed with fresh amounts of the same solvent to maximize yield. Solvent is then recovered in a still at reduced pressure, which lowers the solvent's boiling point and permits the use of gentle heat. The concentrated extract is not distilled but is retained in the vessel in a liquid state. When it is removed and cooled, the concentrated extract solidifies to a waxy consistency called a *concrete*, which is made up of approximately 50% odourless wax. The unwanted wax is removed by washing with alcohol, which extracts the essential oil. The alcohol mixture is then filtered and alcohol is removed by vacuum distillation. The final residue is called the *absolute*. A typical solvent extraction plant is shown in Fig. 4.4; in this system the solvent is pumped through a bed of the plant material.

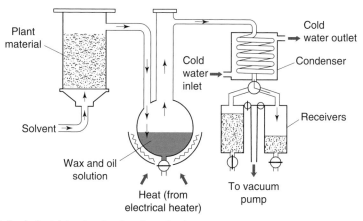

Figure 4.4   Industrial solvent extraction plant.

AROMAFACT

An absolute may not contain all the volatile oils from a plant; it will only have those that are alcohol soluble, e.g. rose absolute. Even after processing, some products may still contain some wax, e.g. orange flower.

If the residue from the initial extraction is of a resinous nature, it is called a *resinoid*, e.g. benzoin, myrrh, frankincense. Many resinoids will yield essential oils when distilled if they contain sufficiently volatile aromatic constituents.

AROMAFACT

Frankincense and myrrh can be prepared in the form of both resinoids and essential oils, whereas benzoin, which is insufficiently volatile to be distilled, is a resinoid only. Resinoids are used in the perfumery industry as fixatives that prolong the fragrance effects.

Carbon dioxide extraction

Introduced in the 1980s and now very popular, this technique uses as the solvent liquid carbon dioxide under conditions described as 'supercritical'. In the normal solvent extraction technique, an organic solvent is used that is liquid at room temperature. By application of pressure to the extraction equipment, solvents that are normally gases at room temperature can be compressed and liquefied (see 'Organization of matter' in Ch. 1). Carbon dioxide, when pressurized in this way, becomes a 'supercritical' fluid at above 33 °C. In the supercritical state it is too hot to be a conventional liquid and too pressurized to be a conventional gas. In this state it has excellent solvent properties for organic molecules. Once the extraction is complete, the pressure can be released and carbon dioxide becomes a gas again.

The process has the advantage of producing products with no solvent residues. The technology is expensive and complex, but the high-quality oils it gives should ensure its development and greater use, which will ultimately reduce its costs. The resultant extract is usually sold as an essential oil even though using the strict definition of a solvent extract it should be thought of as an absolute.

AROMAFACT

Essential oil produced by supercritical carbon dioxide extraction is more similar to that present in the living plant, i.e. more top notes, a higher proportion of esters and some larger molecules. However, the presence of fewer terpenes may be due to their lower solubility in the carbon dioxide compared with conventional organic solvents.

Enfleurage

Enfleurage is a method that is almost obsolete, producing a rather impure product. Thin layers of cold, odourless fat such as lard are coated onto glass plates called *chassis* and the plant material is spread in layers onto the top of the fat. Other chassis with fat and plant material are stacked onto each other and the essential oil is absorbed into the fat. When the fat is saturated, it is washed with hexane to dissolve the essential oil. After removal of hexane, the residue is washed with alcohol and the resultant solution is evaporated to give purer essential oil, or more strictly an absolute. The *true pomades* are products of enfleurage as they are the fragrance-saturated fat.

AROMAFACT

Enfleurage was used to extract oils from delicate petals. It is very labour intensive and can take up to three months. It was a widespread manufacturing practice in the south of France before tourism became a major economic factor.

Maceration

Maceration is the removal of substances by soaking materials in an appropriate liquid. Hot fat is used in maceration to extract essential oils from plant material. The saturated fat is then washed with alcohol to leave pure essential oil, e.g. calendula oil. Maceration is used for extraction of essential oils that cannot be extracted by distillation.

AROMAFACT

The processing will affect the composition and quality of an essential oil. The plant material used for extraction is dead, and is subjected to conditions including heat, solvents and pressure, all of which can have an effect on composition of the final product. The products formed are *products of natural origin*; they are not necessarily natural products that are present in the living plant.

TERMINOLOGY OF EXTRACTS

It is useful to clarify some of the terminology that has been encountered in production of products of natural origin.

- *Plant extracts* contain all compounds that are soluble in both the solvent used and alcohol; not all of them are necessarily volatile.
- *Distilled oils* contain only volatile compounds (these are only a limited number within a plant).
- *Expressed oils* contain compounds of all molecular sizes.
- *Macerated oils* contain compounds of all molecular sizes (not necessarily all the volatiles) that are soluble in vegetable oil.
- *Absolutes* contain compounds of all molecular sizes that are soluble in both solvent and alcohol (not necessarily all the volatiles).
- *Resinoids* contain compounds of all molecular sizes that are soluble in the solvent used (not necessarily all volatiles).
- *Concretes* are the waxy or fatty extract produced by solvent extraction of plant material with an organic solvent after the solvent has been recovered. They contain compounds of all molecular sizes and are usually solids containing natural wax, essential oil and pigments from the plant.
- *Pomades* are the product of enfleurage, whereby substances of all molecular sizes are dissolved in the extracting fat.
- *Hydrosols* (or *hydrolat* or *floral water*) comprise the water collected from distillation of plant material used to extract essential oils. They contain water-soluble plant extracts and usually contain a tiny proportion of the essential oil. Their properties are often similar to those of the corresponding essential oil, but owing to their dilute nature they are considered to be gentler.
- *Tinctures* contain compounds of all molecular sizes that are soluble in the alcohol that is used as the solvent in the maceration process.

ESSENTIAL OILS

Finally, a definition of an *essential oil* and its properties, which are fundamental to aromatherapy. There are many descriptions in use but they should refer to the totally volatile product that is extracted by physical processes from a single natural plant species and that has an odour and composition character-istic of an essential oil from that species. Most essential oils are produced by distillation and expression. This means that concretes, resinoids, gums, abso-lutes and hydrosols do not fit the category.

The term *essential* oil does not reflect its role in the plant's functioning and metabolism. Plant volatile oils function as *secondary metabolites*. (A metabolite is a compound produced by the plant's metabolism.) Primary metabolites are the compounds needed for the plant to live and include the food substances produced in photosynthesis. The secondary metabolites vary widely in chem-ical structure and serve a variety of purposes within the plant. They include protective, survival and reproductive roles. However, they are responsible for giving a plant its aroma and flavour and have significant physiological and psychological effects on animals and people.

AROMAFACT

When extracted, the essential oil produced is very concentrated, often over 100 times more than it is in the plant. It takes approximately 2000 kg of rose petals to produce 1 kg of essential oil.

There are a number of characteristic chemical and physical properties asso-ciated with essential oils. When fresh they are usually colourless, volatile, non-oily, and insoluble in water but soluble in alcohol, ether and other organic solvents and fixed (vegetable/carrier) oils. They will dissolve grease, sulfur, iodine and phosphorus. Their varying chemical compositions give them their unique and characteristic odours. Their physical characteristics include their boiling points, between 160 and 240 °C, densities of 0.759 to 1.096, and high refractive indices; and most are optically active (see Ch. 2). The measure-ment of these physical characteristics is a valuable analytical tool in determin-ing composition and purity. See Chapter 5 for further explanations of these techniques.

Using this knowledge we can appreciate that the composition of essen-tial oils will depend upon a number of factors including methods of process-ing and storage. Essential oils are also subject to adulteration which can have dangerous consequences for the aromatherapist.

THE EFFECTS OF PROCESSING AND MANIPULATION ON OIL COMPOSITION

The quality of an essential oil and its composition have been evaluated in terms of the methods used to extract it from the plant. It will be affected by types of solvent, heat, pressure and time of the processing. The oil will also reflect the *quality of the plant material* used, which depends upon its age, harvesting method, conditions of storage and any impurities present. The *method of growth* is also significant. The species, position and habitat of the plant will determine composition and chemotypes (see the examples in Chapter 7 looking at the composition of essential oils). Soil composition is vital, as the plant obtains its mineral nutrients through its roots in solution. The use of pesticides and herbicides is thought to cause a build-up of undesirable and dangerous compounds in the plant and these may then be present as tiny residues in the essential oil. Organically grown plants are usually a safer bet for producing high-quality essential oils. However, such oils are still quite rare and expensive.

Rectification and adulteration

These interventions cause changes in the composition of a pure essential oil. *Rectification* generally implies the idea of 'putting right' a composition, such as by removing water or terpenes by vacuum distillation. *Adulteration* usually implies that a substance is added to the oil; this might be accidental introduction of an impurity or might be a deliberate addition to or alteration of the composition of the oil.

The interventions can include removal, substitution, additions and mixing of oil components. An increasing number of 'reformulated' or synthetic mixtures are also produced. The term *cutting* is applied to changes to oils that make an original oil go farther; the cutting agent acts as a diluting agent.

Removal

Redistillation of an essential oil can remove terpenes (deterpenation) to make the oil more alcohol-soluble and longer-lasting. This is most commonly done in citrus oils and they are called *terpeneless* or *folded oils*.

AROMAFACT

The fragrance industry uses large quantities of deterpenated bergamot oil.

Substitution

This is when an oil is substituted with a cheaper oil, e.g. petitgrain for neroli, or lemongrass for lemon verbena.

AROMAFACT

Lavandin essential oil is often sold as lavender essential oil but is much cheaper. It is made from a hybrid plant bred from true lavender and spike lavender. The true lavender grows at high altitudes (between 600 and 2000 metres above sea level), whereas lavandin will grow easily on lower ground (between 400 and 600 metres). Lavandin can be propagated from cuttings, grows readily and yields about twice as much oil as lavender. Lavandin essential oil is used as a source of linalool for the perfume industry.

Nature identicals

These are essential oils whose components are obtained from plant sources but whose supplier has compounded an essential oil from scratch using fractions from other oils.

AROMAFACT

Fractions from essential oils of eucalyptus, rosemary and oreganum can be used to compound a commercial white thyme oil.

An essential oil may also have measured amounts of nature identical compounds added, e.g. α-pinene added to frankincense. Figure 4.5 shows a chromatographic 'fingerprint' of a genuine and a compounded frankincense oil.

Synthetics

As their name suggests, synthetics are made up entirely from chemicals produced in the laboratory from various sources including plant material. They are often cheaper and of inferior quality as they will never contain the full range of compounds found in a genuine essential oil.

AROMAFACT

Synthetic methyl salicylate may be sold as wintergreen.

The term reconstructed oil (RCO) is used to describe these laboratory-produced oils. They are not suitable for aromatherapy.

AROMAFACT

Synthetics are cheaper, and, in some cases, it may be difficult to distinguish them from the genuine essential oil. Perfumes will contain between 50% and 100% synthetic ingredients.

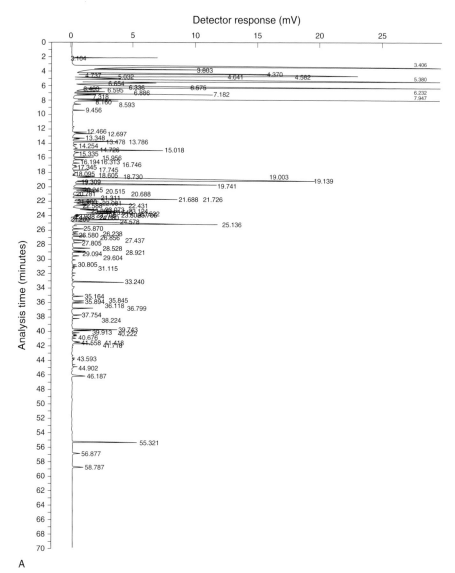

A

Figure 4.5 The use of gas chromatography (GC) to distinguish a 'fake' oil from a genuine essential oil. The size of the peaks represents the output of the detector (in this case measured in millivolts) and each peak corresponds to a different constituent separated from the original mixture. The horizontal axis represents the time during the analysis at which that constituent emerged from the GC column (over a total analysis time of 70 minutes). (A) The result of gas chromatography of a genuine frankincense. (B) This is the GC chart of a completely fake mix. It contains the common adulterant DEP (diethyl phthalate), which is represented by the very large peak at 47 minutes, and DEP amounts to up to 90% of this sample. The rest of the sample is a synthetic perfume and shows a completely different 'fingerprint' of peaks from the genuine oil. Oils adulterated with DEP are often totally synthetic and contain no genuine essential oil. The technique of GC analysis is explained in Chapter 5. The analysis was carried out by Jenny Warden of Traceability.

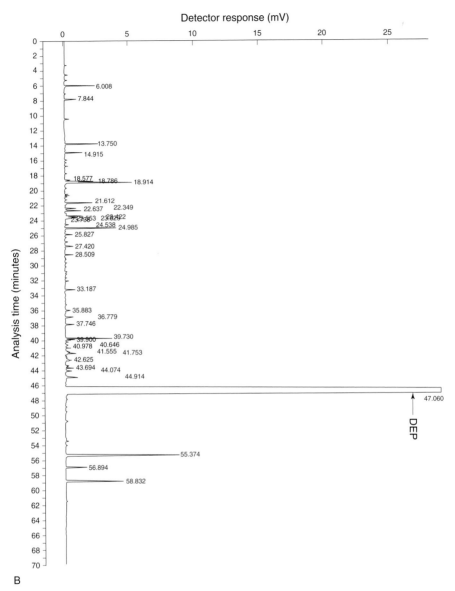

B

Figure 4.5   *Contd*

Folding

In this process, different batches of the same essential oil may be mixed together. Oils become more concentrated in some components and other components may become relatively reduced. The term 'folded oil' is also used for essential oils with a component removed in order to concentrate more desirable constituents. When terpenes are removed, the resultant oil is termed a folded or terpeneless oil. Folding may be done to extend the shelf-life of the oil, especially when terpenes are removed.

AROMAFACT

Some aromatherapists prefer to use bergamot essential oil with the compound bergaptene removed. Bergaptene is an example of a furocoumarin, not a terpene, and it is phototoxic.

Cutting

Cutting is a term used for methods of making the original oil go farther. This can be done with odourless solvents or other compounds.

Odourless solvents can be added to dilute an essential oil. Alcohol is commonly used for a wide variety of essential oils. Diethyl phthalate (DEP) is added to sandalwood, and dipropyl glycol (DPG) or phenylethyl alcohol (PEA), which is a natural component of rose otto, is often added to the essential oil.

AROMAFACT

The fixed oils that the aromatherapist uses as carrier oils are often added to concentrated essential oils. Some retail outlets sell essential oils in dilutions as low as 1% in a carrier oil. Many people think they are buying the concentrated oil; only with careful examination of the small print on the label does the dilution of the composition become apparent.

Additions

A number of substances can be added to a genuine essential oil. They include a cheaper oil, e.g. orange added to bergamot, or essential oil from a different part of the plant added to the desired oil, e.g. clove leaf or stem added to clove bud.

AROMAFACT

The German chamomile essential oil is much favoured by aromatherapists but is quite expensive. A good indication of a genuine German essential oil is its dark blue colour due to the presence of the compound chamazulene. Synthetic chamazulene is sometimes added to the cheaper Moroccan chamomile, which is then sold as German.

An essential oil used for aromatherapy should not be chemically altered in any way for it to be effective. A true oil is a very complex mixture containing hundreds of compounds that themselves may vary in terms of factors previously described – growth conditions and so on. The unidentified compounds contribute to the overall synergistic effect of the oil, as do the known substances.

The composition and purity of an essential oil sample can be determined using modern analytical techniques (see Fig. 4.5 for an example). This is expanded in more detail using actual examples of essential oils in Chapter 7.

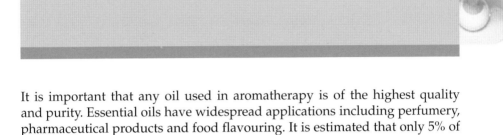

Chapter 5

Analytical techniques

It is important that any oil used in aromatherapy is of the highest quality and purity. Essential oils have widespread applications including perfumery, pharmaceutical products and food flavouring. It is estimated that only 5% of all essential oils produced are used in aromatherapy.

As previously stated, aromatherapy-quality oils must be *pure* and *natural*, with no manipulation of their composition after extraction. In conventional terms, a chemically pure substance is made up of chemically identical atoms or molecules that have a uniform structure. As essential oils are made up of a mixture of many organic compounds, subject to variation produced by factors such as the growth conditions of the original plants and the extraction processes used, there will be some variation in the composition of oils with the same name.

When analyzing oils, there are a number of techniques that are consistently used. They can give us two types of information:

- *Qualitative information*. This *identifies* the components present in a substance, that is, what it is made up of. Most essential oils have about 50 readily accessible compounds, with total number present as high as 350.
- *Quantitative information*. This shows the *amounts* of components present in a substance.

AROMAFACT

For an essential oil such as lavender, the same major components will be present; these are linalool, linalyl acetate and 1,8-cineole. This is the qualitative knowledge. The different types of lavender essential oils will contain different amounts of constituent compounds. Spike lavender, *Lavandula latifolia*, has high amounts of 1,8-cineole (25–37%), while true lavender, *Lavandula angustifolia*, has very small amounts (0–5%). *Lavandula latifolia* may contain up to 60% camphor, while *Lavandula angustifolia* has only up to about 12%. This is quantitative information. A quantitative analysis is needed to help identify different types of oil and can distinguish chemotypes.

The main technique used is *gas–liquid chromatography* (abbreviated GLC or nowadays just GC), which is especially useful when combined with mass spectroscopy (MS); the combination is often referred to as GC-MS. They can provide both quantitative and qualitative information that is very accurate and reliable when compared to known analytical measurements of oils that are stored in databases.

CHROMATOGRAPHY

Chromatography refers to a range of closely related techniques used for separating mixtures. Chromatography is used extensively in analysis of mixtures in a wide range of applications. Many different techniques have been developed to identify specific compounds in specialist applications.

AROMAFACT

Essential oils are made up of a mixture of compounds, so chromatography can be used for separating and identifying them. It can also detect any impurities, making it particularly useful as a tool for defining purity.

All chromatography relies on a *mobile phase* moving through a *stationary phase*. The components of the mixture are attracted to both phases and become distributed between them. It is the *differing* relative strength of attraction of the components for the two phases that is important. If a component is strongly attracted to the stationary phase, it will be held back, while one with a strong attraction for the mobile phase will quickly move along with it. The choice of materials in the stationary and mobile phases must be suitable to allow the components of the mixture to move at different speeds and thus be separated.

The rate at which a component moves will depend on its equilibrium concentrations in mobile and stationary phases. By the technical term equilibrium concentrations we are essentially referring to the solubilities of that component in each of the phases. The ratio of these concentrations is known as the *distribution coefficient* (symbolized D).

$$\text{Distribution coefficient (D)} = \frac{\text{Component concentration in mobile phase}}{\text{Component concentration in stationary phase}}$$

The substance must be in the same molecular form in both phases for this relationship to apply (i.e. we must be comparing the concentrations of identical forms). This D value will always be the same for a given component distributed between a particular combination of phases. This means that the separation can be reproduced to give the same result with the same substance when using the same system.

Gas–liquid chromatography (GC or GLC)

In GC the mobile phase is a *gas* and the stationary phase is a *liquid*. It is one of the most widely used techniques for separation of materials and for analysis and can give both qualitative and quantitative information about a sample.

A typical GC apparatus is shown in Figure 5.1.

- The carrier gas (1) acts as the mobile phase; it is typically a chemically inert gas (e.g. N_2, H_2, Ne) – that is one that will not react with either the stationary phase or the sample being investigated.

- The sample is injected into a sample port (2), where it vaporizes.

- The sample is carried through the *column* (3) by the carrier gas/mobile phase. The column is enclosed in a thermostatically controlled oven (4). Depending on how firmly each component of the sample 'sticks' to the stationary phase – i.e. its *affinity* for the stationary phase – the mobile phase carries it through the column more or less quickly. Components that stick least tightly to the stationary phase move fastest, while those that are held more firmly move through more slowly. The time taken for a component of a mixture to pass through the column is known as its *retention time*. The retention time of a substance depends on how its vapour is distributed between the mobile and stationary phases.

- The *detectors* (5) that are used work in different ways, but all respond to a component as it leaves the column in a stream of carrier gas. The magnitude of the response depends on the concentration of the component. A common detector is a *flame ionization detector* (FID). This passes the emerging gas

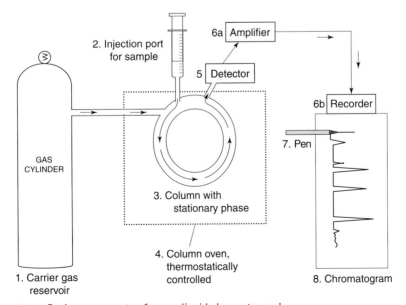

Figure 5.1   Basic components of a gas–liquid chromatograph.

through a hydrogen flame; as components arrive, they burn in the flame to produce ions. The presence of the ions causes a flow of current between two charged plates, which indicates the arrival of a component.

- The *recorder* (6b) plots the signal from the amplifier (6a) used to boost the detector signal, in this case the FID current, against time to produce the *gas chromatogram* (8), which appears as a series of peaks on a printout. Each peak represents a different component.

The gas chromatograph can be calibrated by using a series of known or standard solutions to produce a calibration graph so that the retention times of peaks from the known sample can be compared with the unknown sample. The *chromatogram* can be examined for the number of peaks produced and peaks can be identified by their *retention times*. The quantity of compound present in each peak can be found by measuring the area under the peak.

A typical GC analysis chart is shown for a geranium oil in Figure 5.2.

AROMAFACT

All reputable suppliers will be able to provide you with a GC chromatogram, to give you an indication of the major components of an essential oil.

The gas chromatograph is particularly useful when it is linked to a *mass spectrometer*. This combination is called *gas chromatography–mass spectrometry* (GC-MS).

MASS SPECTROMETRY (MS)

Mass spectroscopy is particularly useful for elucidating the components of essential oils. It can determine relative atomic masses, molecular masses (relative molecular weights) and, in the more powerful instruments, obtain molecular formulae with sufficient accuracy for unambiguous identification. Also, each substance produces a fragmentation pattern in the mass spectrometer. This can be used to distinguish between closely related molecules by comparing their fragmentation patterns. These patterns can be used to identify known substances by a 'fingerprinting' technique or to give evidence for the arrangement of the atoms in a compound. Thousands of mass spectra are stored in computer databases. These are used so that rapid and accurate comparisons can be made and samples identified.

With the development of high resolution mass spectroscopy the mass of the molecular fragment can be measured to seven significant figures. These very accurate relative atomic masses make it possible to distinguish molecules with very similar molecular mass values.

In a mass spectrometer a compound is vaporized and its molecules are bombarded with high-energy electrons. In collisions the electrons transfer

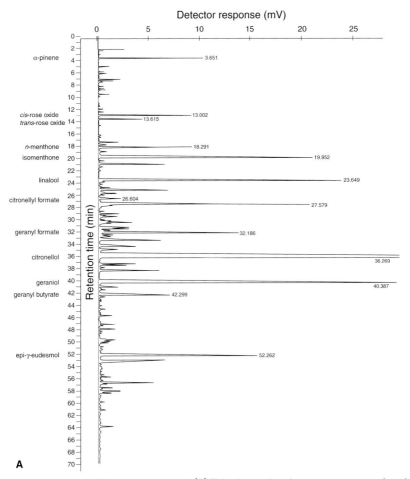

Detector response (mV)

Retention time (min)

α-pinene — 3.651

cis-rose oxide — 13.002
trans-rose oxide — 13.615

n-menthone — 18.291
isomenthone — 19.952

linalool — 23.649

citronellyl formate — 26.604 — 27.579

geranyl formate — 32.186

citronellol — 36.269

geraniol — 40.387
geranyl butyrate — 42.299

epi-γ-eudesmol — 52.262

A

Figure 5.2 Results of GC of geranium oil. (A) This shows the chromatogram, or printed chart, in an analysis that has run for 70 minutes (see the horizontal axis). (B) These are the type of data you would expect to get along with the chart. (Column 1) *Peak number* in order of retention times – the lower the number, the quicker the compound passes through the column, i.e. the faster it moves in the mobile phase. The order of the peaks represents the volatilities of the compounds: the monoterpenes come off first, sesquiterpenes and their oxygenated compounds in the middle, with the compounds of low volatility last. (Column 2) *Peak name* identifies the compound. (Column 4) *Retention time* is the time the vaporized compound takes to pass through the column. (Column 3) *Result percentages*. These figures are measures of the areas of individual peaks expressed as a percentage of the total area of all of them. This means that all the individual peak areas should add up to 100%. The figures are calculated automatically by a special computer called an integrator. In practice the relative area of each peak is not precisely proportional to the percentage of the corresponding constituent in the essential oil; this has to be worked out using an additional response factor for the substance.

Continued

```
Run mode          :  Analysis
Peak measurement  :  Peak area
Calculation type  :  Percent
```

Peak no.	Peak name	Result (%)	Retention time (min)	Time offset (min)	Area (counts)	Sep. code	Width 1/2 (s)	Status codes
1	α-Pinene	0.56	3.651	−0.000	22 299	VV	1.8	
2	cis-Rose oxide	1.23	13.002	0.000	48 909	PB	4.9	
3	trans-Rose oxide	0.50	13.615	−0.000	19 835	BB	4.2	
4	n-Menthone	1.67	18.291	−0.000	66 462	VV	6.2	
5	Isomethone	6.65	19.952	0.000	265 009	VV	13.3	
6	Linalool	5.81	23.639	0.181	231 414	PV	9.4	
7	6,9-Guaiadiene	0.48	26.604	−0.000	19 309	VV	6.5	
8	Citronellyl formate	7.55	27.579	−0.000	301 367	VV	12.8	
9	Geranyl formate	3.20	32.186	0.000	127 409	VV	8.9	
10	Citronellol	31.59	32.269	0.001	1 258 215	VV	24.9	
11	Geranoil	15.26	40.387	−0.000	607 863	BB	15.8	
12	Geranyl butyrate	1.61	42.299	−0.000	63 936	VP	7.9	
13	Epi-γ-eudesmol	5.12	52.262	0.000	203 727	VV	12.2	
	Totals	81.25		0.182	3 235 754			

Total unidentified counts: 747 156
Detected peaks: 289   Rejected peaks: 237   Identified peaks: 13

B

Figure 5.2   *Contd*
For this sample the results show identification of 13 major components out of 289, making up 81.25% of the total components. The volatile monoterpene α-pinene (peak 1) is the first off the column. The alcohols citronellol (10) and geraniol (11) are responsible for the odour characteristics of geranium, which is lifted and activated by the two rose oxides (2 and 3). The 6,9-guaiadiene (7) is a non-terpene hydrocarbon that acts as a back note but it is not a powerful odour. Component 12 is geranyl butyrate; component 13 is epi-γ-eudesmol. Chromatograms and data supplied by Jenny Warden of Traceability.

energy to the molecules: the molecules *ionize* and *positive* ions are formed (a positive ion is a molecule that has lost one or more electrons, but is otherwise unchanged). The bombarding electrons have enough energy to break the covalent bonds in the molecules, and the molecules or ions *fragment* into smaller positively charged ions.

The ions produced are then formed into a beam and accelerated in a magnetic field and deflected by another magnetic field. For ions with the same charge, the deflection in the magnetic field is *greatest* for *ions of lowest mass*. The degree of deflection also depends on the amount of charge on the ion – more highly charged ions will be deflected more than ions of the same mass with a lower charge. These two factors are taken into account by the mass spectrometer, which records the relative abundance of each type of particle in terms of its mass (m) to charge (z) ratio (m/z).

Figure 5.3 shows the typical arrangement of a mass spectrometer. Figure 5.4 shows MS charts for the two monoterpenes [α]-pinene and limonene, and the oxide 1,8-cineole.

The results of mass spectrometry are usually interpreted in terms of the relative molecular weights of fragments produced. This pattern of fragments is recorded in a *mass spectrum*.

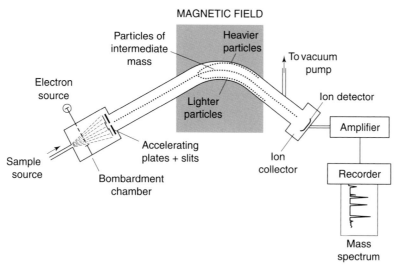

Figure 5.3 Typical layout of a mass spectrometer, showing its main components.

Infrared (IR) spectroscopy

Infrared spectroscopy is used for identifying substances, in particular to show which functional groups are present in an organic compound. It relies on the fact that bonds in organic molecules vibrate, twist and bend at fixed frequencies. When infrared radiation passes through a compound, the molecules will absorb radiation with just the right energy to make those bonds vibrate, twist or bend more rapidly. Since the energy that can be transferred from infrared (or any other electromagnetic radiation) depends on the frequency or wavelength of the radiation, the excitation of the different bonds absorbs different frequencies or wavelengths.

The energy required depends on the type of atoms and the nature of their bonds. Bonds involving light atoms vibrate more rapidly *with higher frequencies* than do bonds involving heavy atoms. Multiple bonds vibrate at higher frequencies than single bonds.

Radio waves (also electromagnetic radiation) are characterized by frequencies given in kilohertz or megahertz (as on radio tuners). Infrared radiation

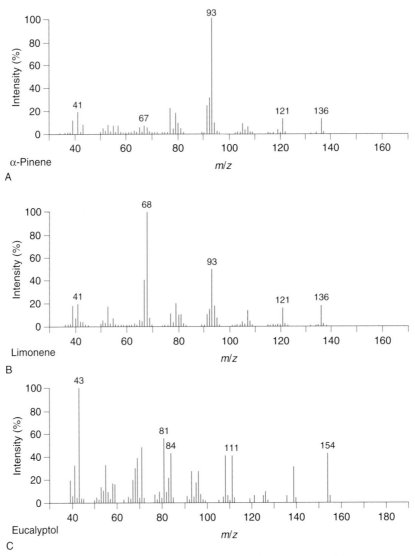

Figure 5.4   Mass spectra. The monoterpenes α-pinene (A) and limonene (B) both have the molecular formula $C_{10}H_{16}$ and their mass spectra are similar; however, the obvious differences at m/z 68 and m/z 93, coupled with accurate and reproducible retention times from GC, enable an identification for each compound. (C) The oxide eucalyptol (1,8-cineole), with molecular formula $C_{10}H_{18}$, produces this characteristic pattern when analyzed by mass spectrometry. MS data supplied by Bill Morden of Analytical Intelligence Ltd.

involves frequencies ten thousand to a million times higher, and for convenience IR is characterized by frequencies given in a unit called the *wavenumber*. This is proportional to the frequency (high wavenumber is equivalent to high frequency) and is written in the form cm^{-1} ('pronounced' *reciprocal centimetres*). The infrared region of the electromagnetic spectrum is in the range

250 to 5000 cm^{-1}. Most infrared spectrometers operate at wavenumbers 600 to 4000 cm^{-1}.

Certain bonds and functional groups absorb infrared frequencies of a characteristic wavenumber; for example:

Carbonyl group	C=O at 1680–1750 cm^{-1}
Alcohol group	C–OH at 3640 cm^{-1}
Alkane bonds	(C–C–H) in CH$_3$ at 2962 and 2872 cm^{-1}
Alkene bonds	(C=C–H) in C=CH$_2$ at 3085 and 3018 cm^{-1}

The region 1400–650 cm^{-1} is known as the 'fingerprint region' and is usually checked for identification as absorptions in this region are characteristic of a substance. This can be compared to infrared spectra of known substances for identification.

The infrared spectrum of an unknown compound can give clues to its structural arrangement. When infrared radiation of wavenumbers covering the full range of the IR region is passed through a compound, an *absorption spectrum* is obtained in which the strength of absorption is plotted against the wavenumber. For a particular compound, or substance containing a number of compounds, a characteristic pattern or 'fingerprint' is produced.

Figure 5.5 shows the typical arrangement of an IR spectrometer, the instrument used to produce IR spectra. An infrared spectrophotometer passes a beam of infrared radiation from a suitable source (1) through a liquid sample (2). The intensity of the beam of infrared that passes through the sample (i.e. is not absorbed by the sample) is compared with the intensity of a reference beam that passes through a reference sample (3) of pure solvent, for a range of wavenumbers determined by the monochromator (4). Taking the output of a detector (5), a recorder (6) plots a graph of percentage *transmission* (the light

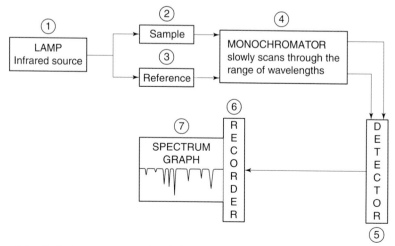

Figure 5.5   Typical arrangement of an infrared spectrometer.

passing through) against the wavenumber to produce the spectrograph (or just *spectrum*). Absorptions appear as inverted peaks or dips in the recordings of the infrared spectra (7). Figure 5.6 shows the IR spectrum of *Rosmarinus officinalis* oil.

OPTICAL ROTATION

This is a property of the arrangement in space of the atoms in a compound, i.e. their *stereochemistry*. A carbon atom with four different groups attached to it by single bonds is said to be *asymmetric*. This was previously described under isomerism in Chapter 2.

Normal light can be regarded as a transverse wave motion (vibrating at right angles to the direction of travel, like waves on water). When normal light, which has all possible directions of vibration, is passed through certain solids it becomes plane-polarized – that is, it vibrates at right angles to the direction of propagation in only one plane instead of all possible planes. This is shown in Figure 5.7.

Optically active substances are termed *dextrorotatory* (*d*-) when they rotate plane-polarized light to the right, while *laevorotatory* (*l*-) substances rotate it to the left. A mixture of *d*- and *l*-forms is called *racemic*.

Optical rotation is measured with an instrument called a *polarimeter*. It produces plane-polarized light and passes it through a sample of liquid and measures the angle through which the plane of vibration of the plane-polarized light is rotated as it passes through a sample. The angle of specific rotation is called alpha and written [α]; it will be expressed as either a positive or a negative value, depending on the direction of rotation. There is no simple connection between the handedness of a particular isomer and the sign of its optical rotation.

Figure 5.6   Infrared spectrum of *Rosmarinus officinalis* oil. The essential oil is a mixture of several major components. (i) 1,8-Cineole [I below] makes up to 60% of the essential oil. It is an oxide with a ring structure containing an oxygen atom in an ether (–C–O–C–) arrangement. This is shown in the peak in the region 980–1000 cm^{-1}, which is characteristic of a 'strained' ether grouping. (ii) The monoterpenes myrcene, α- and β-pinene and p-cymene together make up to 37% of the essential oil. The spectrum shows saturated hydrocarbon (–C–H) alkane bond vibrations in a large peak just below 3000 cm^{-1}, with fewer unsaturated (–C=C–H) alkenes in the region above this. (iii) Camphor (II below) makes up to 21% of the essential oil. It is a ketone, with a carbonyl group (–C=O). This is shown as a strong peak at 1750 cm^{-1}, which is characteristic of aliphatic ketones. Other peaks at 1100 and 1200 cm^{-1} may also be due to this group. (iv) This particular sample does not show any strong peaks for benzyl acetate, an ester, which can make up to 3% of the essential oil. Borneol, an alcohol with an –OH group, which only makes up to 2% of the total composition may be indicated in the broad absorption in the region of 3500 cm^{-1}, but this could be due to water (H–O–H). Spectrum supplied by Alan Sanders formerly of Spectroscopy Central Ltd.

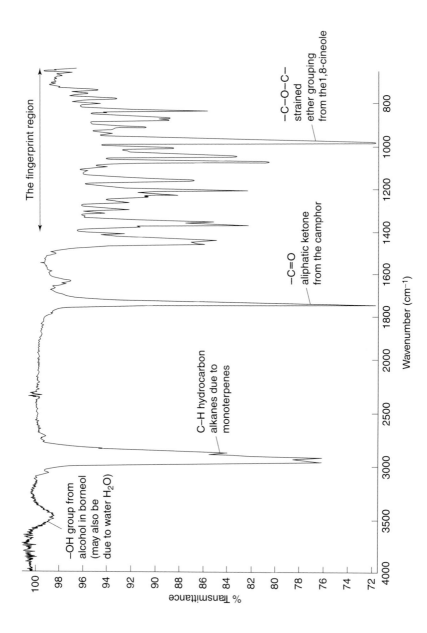

Ordinary light   Plane-polarized light

Figure 5.7 A schematic representation of 'normal' light, which vibrates at right angles to the direction of travel (which is directly towards the reader in this representation) randomly in all possible planes, and of plane-polarized light, which vibrates only in one plane.

The optical rotation of an essential oil is a summation of the optical rotations of its constituents, and is in relation to their proportions within that oil. For most oils a value within a range will be quoted owing to variations in the natural composition, e.g.:

Lavandula angustifolia	−5 to −12	(lavender)
Citrus reticulata	+65 to +75	(mandarin)
Citrus bergamia	+12 to +24	(bergamot)
Rosmarinus officinalis	−5 to −20	(rosemary)
Santalum album (East Indian)	−15 to −20	(sandalwood)

However, any deviation away from this range is a good indication that an oil is not pure.

AROMAFACT

Measurement of optical rotation is an important aid to detecting adulteration, as added compounds that might have been produced in bulk chemical synthesis will have chemicals with different optical activity from that of the natural oil.

SPECIFIC GRAVITY (SG)

The measurement of specific gravity compares the weight of a certain volume of a substance with the weight of the same volume of pure water when measured at the same temperature and pressure.

$$SG = \frac{\text{Mass of given volume of a substance}}{\text{Mass of an equal volume of pure water}}$$

It is usually measured these days by an electronic meter.

AROMAFACT

For an oil,

$$SG = \frac{\text{Weight of a certain volume of essential oil}}{\text{Weight of same volume of pure water}} \text{ (at same temperature)}$$

This measurement is usually done at 20°C. Most essential oils will be less dense than water and so have an SG less than 1:

Lavandula angustifolia	0.878–0.892 (lavender)
Citrus reticulata	0.854–0.859 (mandarin).

Some woody oils have an SG above 1, and collect beneath the distillation water during extraction:

Syzygium aromaticum	1.041–1.054 (clove bud)
Cinnamomum zeylanicum	1.000–1.040 (cinnamon bark).

Like specific optical rotation values, the specific gravity of an essential oil is specified within a range. It is quite a narrow range and any deviation from these limits can indicate impurity.

AROMAFACT

Rosewood essential oil should have an SG of 0.872–0.887. It is made up of 84–93% linalool. Linalool has an SG of 0.87. If a sample of rosewood had an SG much less than 0.872, this could be due to the addition of extra linalool, which is a cheap diluting compound.

REFRACTIVE INDEX

When light passes from the air into a liquid (or vice versa) it is *refracted*: its direction of travel is altered and a light ray is 'bent'. This can be simply illustrated by putting a pencil into a glass of water. A pencil sticking partly in and partly out of the water looks bent at the water's surface. This is because the light rays travelling from the pencil to the eye are refracted or bent where they emerge from the water.

Air and water have different densities and the velocities of light are different in each medium. When a ray goes into a denser medium, it changes direction and enters at a *smaller* angle than that at which it approached the point of incidence. This is shown in Figure 5.8. The relationship between the angle of incidence (*i*) and the angle of refraction (*r*) defined in Figure 5.8 is called the *refractive index* (RI) and is defined as follows:

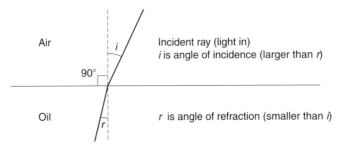

Figure 5.8   The bending (refraction) of a light ray on passing from a less dense medium (air) into a more dense medium (oil), and definitions of the angles of incidence (*i*) and refraction (*r*).

$$RI = \frac{\text{Sine of angle } i}{\text{Sine of angle } r}$$

The refractive index is always more than 1 for light passing from less dense medium (air) into a more dense one (oil).

(The *sine* of an angle is a trigonometric function. In a right-angled triangle containing a given angle, it is the ratio of the length of the side opposite that angle to the length of the hypotenuse. The hypotenuse is the side opposite the right angle. Sines of angles can be looked up in mathematical tables or can be displayed on scientific calculators using the 'sin' button.)

The refractive index is measured by an instrument called a *refractometer*. Each essential oil has a refractive index within fairly narrow limits, e.g.:

Lavendula angustifolia	1.457–1.464	(true lavender)
Citrus reticulata	1.475–1.478	(mandarin)
Syzygium aromaticum	1.528–1.537	(clove bud)

Deviation from these values can indicate adulteration, poor-quality oil or even a different substance altogether.

These physical measurements such as specific optical rotation, specific gravity and refractive index for evaluating composition and purity of an oil are widely quoted and can be read from data sheets. However, the power and value of the human nose should not be overlooked. In addition to being an important entry point for essential oils into the body, it is invaluable for making an initial examination of an oil sample. For this reason, the sense of smell and the nose and associated structures are included at this point.

THE SENSE OF SMELL

The sense of smell is called olfaction. In order to have a scent a compound must be volatile and exert a sufficient vapour pressure at room temperature. A typical scent molecule, called an odorant, usually has a molecular weight of less than 300. This includes the majority of molecules found in essential oils.

We have seen that a number of analytical machines are available to detect and tell which compounds are present in an essential oil, and we should regard our nose and associated structures as our own analytical tool.

AROMAFACT

Humans have a poor sense of smell compared with many animals. Research has also shown that there is variation between people, with women generally better at detecting smells than men. The machine closest to the human nose is the gas–liquid chromatogram, which can be sensitive enough to detect a pico-gram (10^{-12} or $1/1000\,000\,000\,000$ g) of a substance. The nose can sometimes do better than this and detect components present in amounts too small to register a peak on the GC chart recorder.

Olfaction, in common with the other senses, provides information about changes in our environment for warning, recognition and pleasure. It is closely associated with taste and it has been estimated that up to 90% of what we taste is actually smell and that smell is 10 000 times more sensitive than taste.

AROMAFACT

A person who has lost some or all of their sense of smell is described as anosmic. Like other senses smell declines with age but the odour memory (see below – Limbic system) remains when others have diminished.

Detection and mechanism of smell

The mechanism of olfaction has many theories but is not fully understood and is still the subject of research. The nose is the human organ that detects smell (Fig. 5.9). It extends from the face to the end of the palate. In its simplest expla-nation the two nasal cavities are lined with a mucous membrane, kept moist by the secreted substance mucus. Chemicals in the air entering the nose must dissolve in this mucus before they can be detected. A small area – about the size of a small postage stamp – in the upper part of the nasal cavity contains *olfactory cells*, which are sensitive to the chemicals in the mucus solution. For a molecule to be detected it must bind specifically to the sensitive cells that act as *sensory receptors*. The sensory receptors situated in the olfactory epithe-lium (epithelium is the name given to the outer layer of covering cells) are believed to bind specifically with substances according to the shape of their molecules.

AROMAFACT

A very early theory based on 7 primary odours – musk, floral, camphor, peppermint, ether, pungent and putrid – is often quoted in aromatherapy books but has no scientific evidence and does not explain the range of odorants.

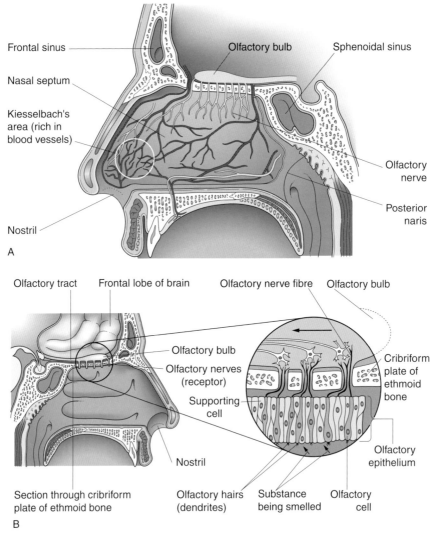

Figure 5.9 The human olfactory system. (A) Section through the nose. (B) Section through the cribriform plate. (C) The olfactory pathway to the cerebrum (forebrain). This shows the pathway of olfactory sensation. Nasal stimulation begins at the cilia of the olfactory receptor cells located at the ends of the olfactory nerves. The olfactory nerves then carry the impulse to the cerebrum, resulting in the sense of smell.

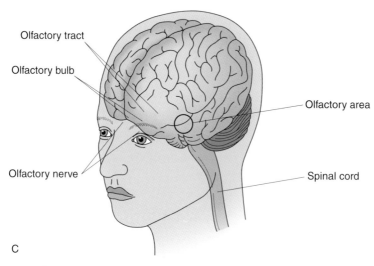

Figure 5.9   *Contd*

Molecular structure must be implicated as odorants bind specifically with the sensory receptors called odorant receptors (ORs). The olfactory mucus has proteins called odorant binding proteins (OBPs) that dissolve the odorant molecule in the aqueous/lipid interface of the mucus. The OBPs act as binder molecules to assist the transfer of odorant to the receptor and increase its relative concentration in the mucus relative to inhaled air. They also function to remove used odorants for breakdown and free up the receptor to detect other molecules.

When the odorant binds to the odorant receptor it changes the receptor structure and activates an olfactory protein called a G protein. This in turn converts ATP (adenosine triphosphate) to cAMP (cyclic adenosine monophosphate) that allows opening of ion channels, causing the receptor to become depolarized. Depolarization is an electrical change that triggers a nerve impulse. Impulses from the nasal receptors are sent along the olfactory nerve to the brain.

A number of receptors have been identified in the olfactory epithelium. These include TAARs (trace amine associated receptors) that detect important biological amines such as histamine, catecholamines (adrenaline, noradrenaline, dopamine) and VIRLIs, which are like the vomeronasal receptor of the nose. The vomeronasal organ (VNO) in humans is located as two tiny pits with ducts opening on both sides of the nasal septum just behind the opening of the nose. It is thought to be stimulated by airborne chemicals as opposed to those dissolved in the mucus. Its function is to detect pheromones. Among other theories is molecular vibration, which suggests that when odorants bind to receptor they cause a differential movement across the binding site. Each receptor is considered to be tuned to a specific vibrational frequency of the different odorants.

AROMAFACT

The importance of the scent molecule linking to a specific receptor in the nose is thought to be related to the shape of the molecule. The optical isomers *d*- and *l*-carvone are mirror images of each other, with different 3D molecular arrangements (Fig 5.10). This means that the *d*- and *l*-forms do not fit the same receptor sites and are responsible for different aromas. The *d*-carvone smells of caraway, while the *l*-form has a minty odour.

mirror

l-Carvone   *d*-Carvone

Figure 5.10   The relationship of *d*- and *l*-carvones as *non-superimposable* ('handed') mirror images of one another. C* is the asymmetric carbon atom, with four different groups attached, that gives rise to optical activity.

Brain and limbic system

AROMAFACT

If the areas of the brain that recognize and translate information about an odour are damaged or destroyed that person will experience impaired smell even when the nasal receptors are functioning normally.

When a molecule binds with its receptor site the olfactory cells become stimulated and send an impulse along the *olfactory nerve*. The olfactory nerve is the first cranial nerve. Cranial nerves that carry impulses into the brain are called sensory, while those that carry impulses away are called motor. Sensory information from the olfactory receptors of the nose is carried as a sensory impulse in the olfactory nerve to an area of the brain called the *olfactory bulb*. It is the olfactory regions of the brain that interpret this sensory information and distinguish different smells. Structures associated with the sense of smell are located in an area of the *fore-brain* (at the front) called the *rhinencephalon*. The rhinencephalon is not fully understood and its function is not restricted to olfaction or smelling. The *olfactory tract* then connects with another area called the *neocortex* that allows us to be aware of and to recognise odours or smells in the light of previous experience. In humans, with a relatively poor sense of smell, the olfactory bulb and tract are relatively small. (see Fig. 5.9C)

Other structures in this area make up the *limbic system* which is directly linked to the olfactory system. Areas called the *septal nuclei* and *amygdala* contain regions often called the 'pleasure centres', with the *hippocampus* concerned with motivational memory. Projections from the *cerebral cortex* connect with the *thalamus, hypothalamus* and *posterior pituitary gland*. The network of connections between all these different areas of the brain is highly complex. The role of the limbic system is significant in *autonomic* (involuntary or non-conscious) reactions that are implicated with emotional responses including fear, rage and motivation.

AROMAFACT

The limbic system is considered to be the most primitive part of the brain and thought to be the seat of our emotions and certain memories. These arrangements and links within the brain may explain the importance and complexity of the role of smell. Its contribution to our quality of life is often underestimated with many anosmics suffering depression, reduced libido and eating disorders. It has been estimated that up to 3% of the population has a reduced sense of smell yet it is given low priority in medicine.

The nose and its associated structures responsible for our sense of smell linking our nervous and endocrine (hormonal) systems serves to make our perception and reactions to an odour a unique experience. This reinforces its significance in the psychosomatic (mind–body) interchange. Scent can affect mood and emotion at a deep level. People often find that scents are powerfully effective in provoking long-forgotten memories.

AROMAFACT

An essential oil that a client likes probably has happy associations for them. Essential oils linked to summer flowers like rose, lavender and geranium are often used as antidepressants. It is also claimed that certain scents can assist learning and concentration. Basil and rosemary are attributed with stimulating mental clarity and have been shown to produce brain rhythms (measured with an instrument called an EEG – electroencephalograph) that are associated with alertness.

The sense of smell is not fully understood and no one theory adequately explains the range of smells we detect. Also, our interpretation of a scent is very subjective; it relies on past exposure and experiences which are linked up and associated within the brain. In many animals, a sense of smell is vital for survival, alerting them to food supplies or situations of danger. In humans smell is still used for such things, but anosmics do not usually have their lives directly threatened. We may be more distressed by our associated loss of taste, apparent when it is impaired by an infection such as a cold that inflames the mucous membrane of the respiratory tract. Absence of the ability to smell is not classified as a disability in the way that loss of sight or hearing are; however, it drastically limits our appreciation of the world and denies us a lot of information and pleasure.

The use of the sensory powers of the nose as an analytical tool is explored under odour purity in Chapter 7. It is a simple measure of quality but is subjective, as it requires insight and experience.

The technique and methods of analysis described in this chapter are used as a basis for the fuller explanation of essential oils used by aromatherapists in Chapter 7. Information from analytical data is also important in aspects of quality control and safety, which are considered in later chapters.

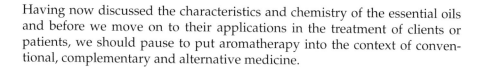

Chapter 6

Health, disease and therapy

Having now discussed the characteristics and chemistry of the essential oils and before we move on to their applications in the treatment of clients or patients, we should pause to put aromatherapy into the context of conventional, complementary and alternative medicine.

HEALTH

Health can be difficult to define and measure; the WHO (World Health Organization) describes it as 'a state of physical, mental and social well-being'. In the past it may have been viewed merely as freedom from disease or injury but this is too limited a definition for modern society. In fact lifestyle factors and our changing environment have given rise to new forms of ill-health.

Dietary choices, sedentary occupations and lack of exercise are responsible for obesity and associated conditions including cardiovascular diseases and diabetes. Smoking, excessive alcohol intake and improper drug use curtail both life and its quality. As life expectancy increases it is mirrored by the increase in degenerative diseases such as arthritis, osteoporosis, cardiovascular disease, cancer, hearing and eyesight decline, and brain cell deterioration (Alzheimer's).

If physical health is hard to define and subject to the pressures of modern society, mental health presents a more complex situation. Any variation from normal behaviour is tolerated less and there is an expectation that it should be controlled or cured but longer life expectancy and changes in social organization challenge the mental health and well-being of many individuals.

Stress and anxiety conditions affect both physical and mental health and are also associated with a modern lifestyle and its demands. Everyone experiences stress – some is normal and essential. But to be subject to stress over a long period can be very harmful. Stress is thought to exacerbate all other clinical conditions as it acts on the sympathetic branch of the autonomic nervous system. This system is responsible for the 'fight or flight' reactions in the body. It may cause changes to normal digestion, respiratory and cardiovascular system, poor immunity and exhaustion. Mentally it may be implicated with irritability, restlessness, mood swings, inefficiency, withdrawal and aggression. An estimated 60% of visits to GPs are thought to be due to stress related problems. It is responsible for a considerable loss of working days.

The solution to stress was very different for our ancestors and often involved simply attacking a threat or running away. Today the triggers can be more varied and the required reaction may not involve any actual physical activity. A modern definition, attributed to Richard Lazarus, is that of 'a condition or feeling experienced when a person perceives that demands exceed the personal and social resources the individual is able to mobilize'.

Dealing with the stress epidemic is an area where partnership between conventional medicine and complementary and alternative medicine (CAM) has been beneficial.

DISEASE

Disease can be defined as to be a lack of health with both physical and mental symptoms that cause a functioning outside the normal range of accepted values. It may be due to infections and infestations, injuries and genetic factors. In one sense disease is the measurable aspect of health; by measuring the symptoms of a disease and their severity we can see if an individual is becoming more or less healthy. By counting the number of cases of disease and the number of cures we can find out if health of the population is increasing or decreasing. Measurable results that give predictable reductions in disease are the basis for the development of what is called conventional medicine.

The study of the patterns of disease is called *epidemiology* and gives a wide range of information that can be used for medical, social and political ends. Biological, environmental and social are just some of the factors that need to be considered.

THERAPY

Therapy is the treatment of ill-health, be it due to disease, genetic factors, injury or lack of well-being. We will now look at how we can weigh up the merits of different kinds of therapy and what sort of evidence is useful in choosing conventional, complementary or alternative medicine, or a combination of them all, in an a particular case.

CAM is becomingly increasingly popular but there are a number of issues that need to be taken into consideration when evaluating the use and efficacy of any therapy. These include sources of information, research and clinical trials, safety, training and regulation. The situation relating to these is constantly evolving so there will be a need for it to be regularly reviewed and updated. For accurate, up-to-date information on these issues the speciality periodicals and appropriate organizations should be consulted.

SOURCES OF INFORMATION

We live in a world of information overload from which the field of essential oils and aromatherapy has not escaped. In addition to printed materials – such as textbooks, periodicals, research papers, magazines, general interest and hobby books – there is the internet and word of mouth. This information can range from the objective and reliable through to the subjective of dubious opinion. The internet is particularly prone to these contrasting styles with inputs from those who have vested interested and commercial motives. However, information from bona fide sources and organizations can be a useful tool. The plethora of information combined with our interest in our health has led to a recognizable group of people known as the 'worried well'.

It should also be remembered that there is pressure for research publication as a requirement for academic tenure. Some subjects are more amenable to producing results with a shorter time span. Scientific based research, and particularly clinical trials, necessitate a considerable investment in time and other resources so the quantity of information must be weighed against its quality.

RESEARCH AND CLINICAL TRIALS

In the past complementary therapies have been called 'alternative' or 'fringe' medicine but the position of conflict between complementary and conventional therapies is outdated. The term *allopathic* is used for the conventional, orthodox mainstream medicine and relies on gathering evidence through scientific research methodology. It examines outcomes, i.e. the results or consequences that follow from the action or intervention that we call the treatment. There is a clinical criterion called the *gold standard clinical variable*, which is often viewed as the measure of clinical improvement in a condition. This can be a simple quantitative measure for some conditions, e.g. blood sugar level for diabetes, peak air flow for asthmatics. Often there are multiple variables and simple quantitative criteria are inapplicable.

Research and its evaluation is a complex process relying on rigorous methods with statistical analysis. It is lengthy, expensive and relies on a team of professionals from different disciplines.

Six knowledge domains are identified in research methods and these can be applied to both mainstream and CAM. These are:

1. Laboratory methods – looking at scientific and molecular areas with testing 'in vitro' (lab methods like cell cultures) and 'in vivo' (on live test animals).

2. Qualitative – case studies investigating patient views of their illness.

3. Randomized controlled trials (RCTs) – seeking to isolate specific effects of different treatments on outcomes. Patients are randomly assigned to treatment groups to ensure comparability on all factors influencing outcomes with the exception of the treatment investigated. The treatment may or may not be delivered with patients unaware of which group they have been allocated to.

4. Observational methods – this describes the association between the treatment or intervention and the outcome. It uses monitoring techniques including epidemiological research, surveys and practice audits to assess the results.

5. Reviews – combination of systematic, expert and peer reviews evaluate accuracy and precision of research. Approaches are now protocol-driven and rely on statistical techniques.

6. Health Service research – explores the utilization and impact of interventions in the actual delivery setting. This involves consideration of feasibility, costs, practitioner competence and patient compliance. Again employing research, surveys and sample groups as appropriate at this stage.

The research methods and outcomes are examined, as they must also meet additional criteria for internal and external validity.

Internal validity is how likely the effects reported are due to the treatment or independent variable. This relies on:

- correct randomization
- baseline comparability of patient group (age, gender, other significant disease, lifestyle factors etc)
- change of intervention (poor compliance)
- blinding (did patients, practitioners and researchers know who got the treatment?)
- outcomes (was objectivity and reliability assessed?)
- analysis (was sample treated in valid numerical and statistical manner?).

External validification examines the likelihood of the observed effects occurring in different settings and outside the study. This looks at:

- generalizability (appropriate patient groups)
- reproducibility (clear and transferable treatments)
- clinical significance (sample size big enough, treatment appropriate for condition)
- therapeutic interference (flexibility in applying treatments and feedback from results)
- outcomes (clinically relevant from correctly reported and checked patient results).

The application of research-based medicine is a contentious issue in CAM. Though more interest and research is being directed into it this is not sufficient to compete with the funding allocated to mainstream medicine, particularly by pharmaceutical companies that invest millions in research, development and clinical trials.

In the case of aromatherapy, which uses genuine products of natural origin, there are additional features that make it difficult to apply rigorous research methodology. The composition of an essential oil from a specific species can vary for a number of reasons. This is the reason why chemical compositions are often quoted as a percentage range for a named essential oil. This means that its chemical profile will not be consistent. As the essential oils have distinctive odours which are significant when choosing blends for a client withdrawal of a particular oil will be obvious to them. This makes double blinds and random isolation impossible. Numbers needed for a statistically valid trial are also prohibitive. It should be realized that reporting back on a treatment used for a small number of clients is not clinical research. These case studies, though interesting and useful to other aromatherapists, should not be given unsubstantiated and widespread claims. Finally, the methodology and interaction between client and therapist is almost impossible to standardize. This is usually a significant factor in the experience and outcome of many treatments.

In evidence-based medicine there can be ambiguity in situations where patients give subjective answers to outcomes. For example the placebo effect is known to be significant in most areas of treatment. It is when a medicine or treatment is ineffective or inactive but helps to relieve a condition because the patient has faith in its powers. The 'specific and placebo' aspects of medicine are still subjects of research in both mainstream and CAM. It should always be remembered that many conditions are improved by a positive mental attitude. This can be triggered by appropriate support and encouragement from a variety of sources including the role of the therapist. Complementary practitioners often claim to offer a more holistic approach to patient care in which physical, mental and social factors in the patient's condition are taken into account rather than just the diagnosed disease. This is not excluded from mainstream medicine but time, financial and political constraints are often prohibitive. When both conventional and complementary approaches have been evaluated they often report similar percentage effectiveness.

SAFETY

Allopathic or mainstream medicine, practised by the medical profession relies heavily on pharmaceutical drugs. Drugs produce an effect on the body that directly opposes and alleviates symptoms of the disease. Prescription drug use has been estimated to have increased by 27% between the years 2002–2007 at a cost of billions to the NHS. Many patients look to a 'pill for every ill' and feel disappointed if a consultation with the doctor does not produce a prescription. Despite safeguards to monitor any problems with prescription drugs they have been linked with up to 15 000 deaths per year. These deaths are due to a number of factors including medication and dosage error, adverse reactions and improper use. It has been estimated that the health service foots a bill of over a billion pounds treating those who have experienced adverse drug incidents.

As well as increases in prescription drugs, nonprescription or over-the-counter (OTC) drug sales are also increasing. These also include herbal medicines, food supplements and essential oils. These products are periodically examined with directives to regulate their use, as they are not proved effective and safe in the same way as prescription drugs. Many OTC products make exaggerated claims and have inconsistent formulations of ingredients and unclear dosage. Some have been found to contain toxic contaminants and microbial pathogens. Improper use is also a cause for concern as some will interact with mainstream medicines and this should always be checked. Many people claim that complementary medicines are all natural and that this means they are a 100% safe alternative to prescription drugs. This is just not true and they should be used with care.

The safety of essential oils is always an important issue. They are potent chemicals and should be handled correctly. Their properties, toxicity and contraindications are addressed in a number of sources and textbooks that highlight safety issues in a systematic and responsible way. Safety is always under review and findings are published and disseminated. There have been scare stories in the media and there are individuals whose *raison d'etre* is to highlight the dangers of essential oils. They emphasize hazardous properties and concerns about certain components. There are essential oils that are best avoided but the vast majority of those used for aromatherapy have a good safety record.

The use and safety of essential oils needs to be put into perspective. Like many everyday household cleaning products bought in the supermarket they can contain some components that can be dangerous but the emphasis is on correct handling, dilution and application. If essential oils are bought by members of the public and are used without sufficient knowledge or understanding of their properties or quality then they can cause harm. A fully trained and qualified aromatherapist should have the knowledge and experience to handle oils in a safe and beneficial way. The internal use of essential oils in aromatic medicine and aromatology is another area of concern. Again, correct training with safe handling and dosage should address the problem.

TRAINING AND REGULATION

Training and qualifications in CAM therapies including aromatherapy is still developing. Anyone can buy essential oils and set themselves up as an aromatherapist with little knowledge of the human mind and body or of the use of essential oils. Many complementary therapists are working with little or no training. This is in contrast to mainstream medicine with high academic entry requirements, a structured career path and strictly monitored qualifications.

Courses for aromatherapy vary from short leisure course to degree level in institutions of higher education and entry qualifications are inconsistent. The background and experience of those delivering the courses is also variable. Currently there is only one chair of Complementary Medicine in the UK. This is at the Peninsula Medical School at the University of Exeter and Plymouth where they conduct scientific research and publish peer-reviewed articles. Many complementary therapists are self-employed and work in sole practice.

However, multidisciplinary clinics are increasing and complementary therapies are becoming integrated into the NHS.

The training and regulation situation is being addressed as the government and industry bodies are professionalizing CAM by setting National Occupational Standards (NOS) for training and qualifications. The voluntary self-regulatory body for aromatherapy is the Aromatherapy Council (AC). The council consists of aromatherapists from the register of members, elected by their peers, along with additional lay members. Its purpose is to protect the public from inadequately qualified aromatherapists who do not practice to the agreed levels of competence. The council's Code of Ethics and Professional Conduct coupled with Disciplinary and Complaints Procedures should give aromatherapists credibility by showing that they operate within a professionally regulated organization.

Chapter **7**

Composition of essential oils and other materials

This chapter will look at the composition of a number of popular aromatherapy materials. There is a lot of published data describing chemical compositions. This can be found in varying degrees of complexity in the aromatherapy books and, additionally, from a number of bodies such as ISO (International Organization for Standardization), RIFM (Research Institute for Fragrance Materials), IFRA (International Fragrance Association), AFNOR (Association Française de Normalisation) and the BP (British Pharmacopoeia).

QUALITY CONTROL

Quality control (QC) draws together the information concerning methods of analysis described earlier with that of the composition of the essential oils and shows how quality standards are used. This is important for the concept of quality control, which is an essential process in evaluating the composition and standards of many products including essential oils. Quality control in the production, blending, storage and packaging of essential oils ensures that the product is as described by the manufacturer at the time of supply. This control will include the taking of a number of samples of the product, which are then analyzed to confirm that the product is consistent and meets the composition requirements set for that oil. The requirements may be set by a professional body or standards organization or just by the manufacturer. The full set of requirements is called the *specification* of the oil and the testing shows whether the product conforms to the specification.

The complex nature of essential oils means that this specification is usually a list of acceptable *ranges* of composition for each of the main chemical components. The analysis used to assess compliance with specification is normally GC-MS, which can not only confirm the composition but also pick up impurities and adulteration in many cases.

AROMAFACT

The composition of commercially available essential oils cannot be artificially controlled as they are products of natural origin. However, when the essential oils are analyzed their composition should be within a range of acceptable values. If these values are not met, the oil should be rejected. This ensures a standard in the product supplied so that it should perform in a consistent manner when used therapeutically. QC is necessary to protect supplier, practitioner and client from any unforeseen effects of aromatherapy performed with oils that might present risks due to unknown properties.

BACKGROUND TO COMPOSITION

Analysis of an essential oil will tell us what compounds are present (qualitative analysis) and in what amounts (quantitative analysis). However, when considering the composition of any named oil it is difficult to lay down precise criteria. As with all products of natural origin, there will be variations according to growing conditions and how they are harvested, extracted and stored. Even if the species of plant is defined and the parts used for oil production are carefully controlled, variation in composition will occur. This has previously been explained in terms of *chemotypes* and will be examined in more detail for other essential oils later in this chapter. Even when examining a particular chemotype there will be differences in the amounts of constituents, although these are usually within a fairly narrow range.

It is important to remember that a typical essential oil may contain between 100 and 400 components. Most data and analytical information will relate to significant constituents and when constituents are listed it is not always the most abundant ones that contribute to their odour or properties.

AROMAFACT

Reputable suppliers should be able to supply information about their products along with analytical data. However, the analysis may only refer to a small number of the major components. At the time of writing, an analysis of the 10 most abundant components would cost approximately £40.00 per sample, rising to £85.00 for up to 20 of the most abundant components. Prices for up to the most abundant 50 components or an in-depth investigation are given on application. This is clearly out of the financial reach of the average aromatherapist, and represents a cost many times that of the purchase price of the oil.

It should be remembered that the analysis for any substance, including essential oils, can only be true for that substance at the time the tests were performed. The composition of oils can subsequently change with handling and storage, so by the time it reaches you, or by the time you use it, it may have a very different composition.

ORGANIC OILS

Organic agriculture is a huge environmental and political issue. Buying organic, in the context of things like food and oils refers to their method of production.

AROMAFACT

The scientific term organic means a compound containing the element carbon. Using this definition all essential and carrier oils are organic.

Organic agriculture is a move away from the large-scale aggressive methods in order to develop a safer and more sustainable method of farming. Its main features include the restricted use of artificial chemical fertilizers and pesticides; no genetically modified plants with farmers relying on developing healthy fertile soil growing a mixture of crops.

Strict regulations, known as standards, define their practice. The International Federation of Organic Agricultural Movements (IFOAM) lays down EU standards. In the UK the government sets the standards, which also meet the European and international standards set by their certifying bodies. Each one has its own symbol and EU code number. The main certifying body in the UK is the Soil Association, its UK code is 5 and its organic symbol appears on approximately 70% of organically produced food in the country. Others include The Organic Farmers and Growers Ltd (OF & G) UK code 2, The Scottish Organic Producers Association (SOPA) – UK3, The Irish Organic Farmers and Growers (IOFGA) – UK7 and the Quality Welsh Food Certification – UK13. Figure 7.1 shows two examples of organic organization logos.

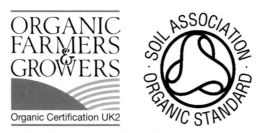

Figure 7.1   Two examples of organic association logos.

Symbols   Each EU country also has its own organic certification authority and code. For food and products imported from outside Europe the situation is more complex.

AROMAFACT

When you buy an organic oil there will not be an accompanying certificate. Currently essential oils and hydrosols do not come under the EU Directive for organic agriculture as it only covers food. It is the grower that has the certification and their literature should show the symbol of their certifying body. See the price list (Fig. 7.2) from a British company that grows and produces essential oils and products. The producer, in this case the farmer, has a UK Soil Association Licence number, which in this case is G4918 and they also have a licence H7677 which means they have been inspected and satisfy the Soil Association standards for organic health and safety products.

The analysis for chemical composition of an organically produced oil will be indistinguishable from that of a standard one. They contain the same range of compounds for any given oil. In a standard oil the possibility of trace compounds like pesticide residues is sometimes a cause of concern. The usual GC-MS type of analysis done on essential oils would not show such components. There are specialist companies that provide services to detect for such residues. This worry should be eliminated when buying genuinely produced organic oils.

AROMAFACT

If you are concerned about the quality and authenticity of your essential oils, your best guarantee is to buy from a reputable supplier whose integrity you can trust. The only way to differentiate between a conventional oil and an organic one is by the paper trail generated by inspection and validation from farmer to end product with certification by relevant bodies.

CERTIFIED ORGANIC ESSENTIAL OILS GROWN ON OUR HOME FARMS

Oil	Origin	2.5ml	qty	5ml	qty	10ml	qty	50ml	qty
Angelica Root *Angelica archangelica*	UK organic	£7.85		£12.83		£19.78		£76.74	
Angelica Seed *Angelica archangelica*	UK organic			£7.50		£12.16		£50.59	
Chamomile German *Matricaria recutita*	UK organic	£4.74		£7.36		£13.67		£46.20	

Figure 7.2   Price list showing Soil Association logo. (Courtesy of Jane Collins, Phytobotanica)

You will usually pay more for an authentic organic essential oil as the cost reflects its production. Typically, at the time of writing, an organic lavender (*Lavandula angustifolia*) would cost up to 81% more than the standard one. However price is not always a reliable guide and as the number of organic harvests expands prices are dropping. Also with organic wild harvested plants the prices are comparable. However, many aromatherapists are willing to pay a premium as they feel they are supporting a more sustainable and ecologically balanced environment for the future.

SPECIAL PROPERTIES OF ESSENTIAL OILS: SYNERGY AND QUENCHING

As has been emphasized, essential oils are made up of a mixture of a large number of chemicals. These chemicals are sometimes able to complement each other by having additive or synergetic effects influencing their properties. The combination of major components alone would not produce an oil resembling the natural product. The quality and characteristics rely on all components. This is one reason why the use of synthetic or adulterated oils is inappropriate for aromatherapy.

AROMAFACT

The holistic approach uses the idea that the whole is greater than the sum of its parts. In medicine it is the consideration of the complete person in the treatment of disease. The link between the body and the mind (the psychosomatic) and its significance to health are indisputable. A holistic healer considers all aspects of the patient's physical, mental, environmental and lifestyle factors as well as any pathological malfunction. When using an essential oil, the remedy relies on the complete oil rather than its individual components. This needs to be linked with the method of application and the skills of aromatherapists in interacting with their clients.

Thus interdependence means that although the chemical compounds and their individual amounts and properties are known in a particular oil, their interrelationships are often complex and may not reflect the properties of that whole oil in use. In most cases the whole oil is found to be more effective, with fewer side-effects than when using individual isolated components.

Although a knowledge of the individual components of the essential oils and their chemical and physiological properties is useful, it does not offer all the answers. Isolated compounds may have a specific action, which is described as the 'molecular approach'. However, properties shown by a natural and complete essential oil are not always predictable by considering the individual chemical properties of their components. This also explains why one essential oil may have a number of different actions.

This can be illustrated by the following considerations:

- Most ketones found in essential oils are toxic when isolated compounds are used. However, many oils high in ketones are considered safe to use; for example, camphor is found in *Rosmarinus officinalis* (rosemary) at 15–30% and in *Lavandula intermedia* (also known as *Lavandula hybrida*) (lavandin) at 5–15%, and carvone is the main component of *Mentha spicata* (spearmint) at up to 70%.

- In basil oil, methyl chavicol (also called estragole), a phenolic ether (p. 60), is considered to be a dermal irritant and to be carcinogenic. Linalool has an almost identical molecular formula but is a long chain rather than a benzene ring (p. 55) and is considered much safer.

- Thyme oil contains thymol and carvacrol (phenols; p. 59), which are also dermal irritants, but with linalool and other noncyclic alcohols the risks are significantly reduced.

- The oxide 1,8-cineole (also called eucalyptol) is often described as a skin irritant. It is a major component in *Eucalyptus globulus* (up to around 90%), which has GRAS (Generally Recognized As Safe) status. Within the oil it is attributed beneficial effects such as antiseptic and expectorant. The other components present are again the hydrocarbon terpenes α-pinene, limonene, cymene, phellandrene, terpinene and aromadendrene.

Synergy

Synergy or *synergism* describes the working together of two or more drugs to produce an effect greater than the sum of their individual effects. This occurs in the use of essential oils. Aromatherapists mainly use a number of different essential oils together in a blend. This means that the number of compounds applied increases significantly. An appropriate blend may work in such a way that the effect of the total number of essential oils is greater than that expected when considering the sum of their individual components. In a mixture of essential oils, the compounds when blended together have a mutually enhancing effect upon each other. However, it has been found that mixing or blending more than five essential oils is counterproductive.

Examples of synergism include the following.

- *Eucalyptus citriodora* has a strong antimicrobial activity, but tests on individual components showed relative inactivity. However, when combinations of the three major components in the same ratios occurring in the natural oil were mixed and used, antimicrobial activity was restored.

- In lavender essential oils, linalool and linalyl acetate are sedative and antispasmodic compounds; when lavender is used in blends with other essential oils, these effects can be enhanced.

Quenching

The term *quenching* is used when one component will suppress the harmful effects of another. A knowledge of this is used in safe applications of essential oils. The following are typical examples.

- The isolated aldehyde citral can be a skin irritant or sensitizer and has been implicated in reproductive disorders. In *Citrus limon* (lemon oil) it makes up to 5% of the composition. It has been shown that the hazardous effects are markedly reduced by the presence of the terpenes *d*-limonene and α-pinene also present in the oil.

- *Cymbopogan citratus* (lemongrass), with up to 70% citral, is irritant. Essential oils high in citral can be safely used when diluted by addition of an oil high in terpenes such as *d*-limonene, which will quench the citral. *Cymbopogan citratus* could be used with *Citrus paradisi* (grapefruit) as the latter contains up to 90% *d*-limonene.

- Cinammic aldehyde (cinnamaldehyde) is also a powerful skin sensitizer and the International Fragrance Association recommends its use with equal amounts of *d*-limonene as a quencher (see page **65**).

CHEMICAL PURITY AND STANDARD SAMPLES

A substance is said to be chemically pure when it is made up of identical atoms and molecules. This means that the concept of purity can only apply to a single element or compound. As essential oils are made up of mixtures of organic compounds, they cannot be strictly chemically pure. Chemical purity and composition have to be related to an 'odour profile' and be free from any contamination. Standard samples are used for reference when considering the purity of an essential oil, and the analytical techniques of GC-MS, refractive index and other methods previously described are applied. A standard sample or standard oil is a sample of a product that conforms to a specification for that product. It is kept for purposes of comparison with batch samples and used in quality evaluation.

Sensory analysis   The odour of an essential oil can be evaluated by conducting investigations on the evaporation of an essential oil under standardized conditions and comparing this to a standard sample of the oil. This is sometimes referred to as 'odour purity' but is a rather subjective method. It involves putting the essential oil and a standard sample onto separate smelling strips and allowing them to evaporate to a final dry-out under the same environmental conditions and time scale. This, along with a visual inspection of the oil, is the only immediate quality control measure available to the aromatherapist.

Definitions and regulations relevant to composition and purity   It is useful at this point to redefine and clarify the types of materials used in aromatherapy. The AOC – Aromatherapy Organizations Council, which represents 75%

of UK oil suppliers – has produced the following definitions to assist Trading Standards officers.

- An essential oil is an aromatic, volatile substance extracted by distillation or expression from a single botanical species. The resulting oil should have nothing added or removed.

- An absolute oil is an aromatic, volatile substance obtained by solvent extraction from a single botanical species, e.g. rose absolute, jasmine absolute. The resulting oil should have nothing added or removed during or after this process.

- An aromatherapy oil is not an essential oil. It is a product that meets the requirements of the profession of aromatherapy. It contains blends of undefined percentages consisting of vegetable oils and essential oils and sometimes absolutes.

The EC (European Community) requires cosmetic products to include a list of ingredients, in descending order of percentage composition, although percentages do not need to appear on the label.

AROMAFACT

In official EC labelling regulations, herbs and essential oils can only be described by their botanical names; for example, *Lavandula angustifolia* could refer to lavender herb extract, lavender water, lavender tincture or the essential oil. Every cosmetic ingredient has been given an INCI (International Nomenclature of Cosmetic Ingredients) name. Water is *aqua*, and fragrances including essential oils are *parfum*. This can make it difficult for consumers to distinguish between genuine aromatherapy products and those using synthetic materials unless each essential oil is named and listed.

REGULATORY AND ADVISORY BODIES

The organizations encountered when examining the composition of essential oils include the Research Institute for Fragrance Materials (RIFM), the International Fragrance Association (IFRA), the International Organization for Standardization (ISO), the Association Française de Normalisation (AFNOR) and the British Pharmacopoeia (BP). There is some overlap between recommendations for usage and safety by these bodies. The background and roles of RIFM and IFRA are described in the next chapter in relation to safety.

The International Organization for Standardization

This is a worldwide federation of national standards bodies drawn from 130 countries. It was established in 1974 and is based in Geneva, as a nongovernmental body with a mission to promote worldwide standardization. It aims to facilitate international exchange of goods and services and to develop intellectual, scientific, technological and economic activity. Its work has resulted in international agreements, which are published as International Standards that cover a wide range of technologies and services. Technical work is carried out in 218 technical committees (TCs) and the one covering essential oils is TC 54. Its activities cover a wide range of procedures such as packaging, conditioning and storage (ISO/TR210:1999), sampling (ISO212:1973), determination of optical rotation (ISO592:1998) and composition of oils. The composition of each essential oil will also have an individual reference and identification; e.g. oil of rosemary (*Rosmarinus officinalis* Linnaeus) is ISO1342:1988, and oil of basil, methyl chavicol type (*Ocimum basilicum* Linnaeus), is ISO11043:1998. These specifications were largely set up for the food and cosmetics industry to give specifications to ensure similarity of products.

AROMAFACT

It is accepted that genuine essential oils do not have a strictly consistent composition. Stipulation of an exact ISO specification may encourage adulteration, and this is contrary to the ethos of aromatherapy. However, ISO standards are often quoted and can be used as a general composition guideline.

The Association Française de Normalisation

Based in France and sometimes referred to as the 'Norme Française', AFNOR covers a wide range of services and goods with 17 major standardization programmes (GPNs). Each programme is piloted by a strategic orientation committee (COS) that is responsible for defining priorities, activities and cooperation within that area.

AFNOR publishes monographs on a number of essential oils relating to the chemical composition of a number of 'standard' oils. Compositions are presented as a percentage range for the main (approximately six) chemical components. In addition, the monographs are useful for safety recommendations and list physicochemical values for each oil.

AROMAFACT

This again illustrates the fact that defining percentage values for chemical components of an oil may act as a guideline for adulteration by unscrupulous suppliers.

British Pharmacopoeia

National pharmacopoeias were developed for the practice of pharmacy so that it should conform to standards laid down in the official pharmacopoeia of the relevant country. The British Pharmacopoeia (BP) is a government-approved list giving details of the manufacture, dosage, uses and characteristics of drugs. It is compiled by experts in pharmacy and pharmacology. The World Health Organization (WHO) has issued the Pharmacopoeia Internationalis in an attempt to standardize drug preparations throughout the world.

AROMAFACT

The BP lays down standards for drugs dispensed through a British pharmacy. These standards cover a number of essential oils that appear in the BP, e.g. clove, eucalyptus, peppermint, citronella. However, these are not always appropriate for aromatherapy use because specifications are too broadly based and do not reflect materials currently available and used. For example, the BP states that eucalyptus oil is required to have a 1,8-cineole content of 70%, whereas most natural eucalyptus oils contain less than this. To comply with the BP would encourage a redistillation to rectify the oil, which is entirely contrary to the ethos of aromatherapy.

British Herbal Pharmacopoeia

The British Herbal Pharmacopoeia (BHP) provides monographs of quality standards for 169 herbs commonly used in the United Kingdom for the preparation of botanical drugs. It is produced and regularly revised by a Scientific Committee of the British Herbal Medicine Association. The materials are the whole plant materials; for example, for marigold (*Calendula flos*) it refers to dried ligulate florets or dried composite flowers. It does not include essential oils. However, it may be of interest to aromatherapists as it covers an area of complementary medicine that is becoming increasingly popular and acceptable. It also illustrates an alliance between synergistic mixtures of natural materials with a scientific basis.

CHEMICAL COMPOSITION OF ESSENTIAL OILS

The chemical compositions of the essential oils are readily accessible from a wide range of aromatherapy books, periodicals and composition sheets, in the guidelines given by organizations and regulatory bodies, and from the data sheets and analyses obtainable from the oil suppliers.

This chapter looks at data drawn from a wide range of sources in order to illustrate the type of information available to the aromatherapist.

AROMAFACT

An aromatherapy-grade essential oil may contain up to 400 components. However, a typical GC analysis will detect over 200 but only chemically iden-tify up to 15 of the major components. These components may not include all those compounds that play a role in the action of the essential oil. The analysis is very useful, though, for identifying oils and detecting any adulteration.

Classification and species

When discussing essential oils and their composition, it is important to use the correct botanical Latin name. The general name is too vague and ambigu-ous in many cases. The botanical classification of plants is a taxonomic one: taxonomy is the classification of organisms into groups with similar struc-tures and origins. Plants are divided into 21 families; the family called the Labiatae or Lamiaceae is the one with the largest number of plants yielding essential oils. The families are then divided into taxonomic groups called *gen-era* (the plural of *genus*), which may contain one or many *species*. Species are a group of plants within a genus that are capable of interbreeding.

To describe an essential oil simply as lavender does not tell us enough about the particular species from which it comes and the consequent varia-tion in its composition. Its botanical name is needed. In the case of lavender, for example, the classification is

Family:	Labiatae or Lamiaceae
Genus:	*Lavandula*
Species:	*angustifolia* (true lavender)
	spica (spike lavender)
	hybrida (lavandin).

These would be written as *Lavandula angustifolia* or *L. angustifolia*; *Lavandula spica* or *L. spica*; and *Lavandula hybrida* or *L. hybrida*.

Developments in botanical classification

The botanical classification that we currently use is attributed to the Swedish botanist Carl Linnaeus. He developed the binomial (two-name) system as a simplification of previously used long Latin names, e.g. Wild Briar Rose was *Rosa sylvestris alba cum rubore, folio glabro* or *Rosa sylvestris indora seu canina* pre-Linnaeus – he changed it to *Rosa canina*, which we abbreviate further to *R. canina*. His groupings of plants were based on the arrangements and numbers of the stamens (male sex organs) and pistils (female sex organs). This could lead to a classification that did not always seem natural. The roses were associated with the genus *Saxifraga* (commonly known as the saxifrages) that are a wide range of perennials including alpines. However in spite of its limitations it was simple to use. With our understanding of DNA (deoxyribonucleic acid), which is the genetic material of most living organisms, and the progress in genome sequencing (the genes contained in the chromosomes of the organism) plant classification using this is being discussed. It shows an understanding of plants grouped according to their natural and evolutionary relationships. Under this new system roses are in the genus *Urtica* that contains nettles. However, classical taxonomy (which is the theory, practice and rules of classification) will continue to rely on morphology (structure) in plants as well as molecular data systems.

AROMAFACT

Familiar plant names based on the Linnaeus system will remain the basis for the foreseeable future.

Plants will have a specific DNA bar code, which will be a useful forensic tool. The DNA bar code is made up of a standard short region (or regions) of DNA selected from one or more of the genomes. It can be applied universally across land plants but is also variable enough to provide individual identification at species level. The bar code system can be applied to access a database for identification of known plants. It can be used to identify unknown samples from fragments of plant material by comparing them to the known standards and has applications for verification of material in natural products like herbal medicines and foodstuffs.

Chemotypes

A *chemotype* describes the subspecies of a plant that have the same morphological characteristics (relating to form and structure) but produce different quantities of chemical components in their essential oils. This again is widespread within the botanical family classification of the Labiatae or Lamiaceae. Examples of plants producing essential oils with different chemotypes include lavender, melissa, peppermint, basil, rosemary, sage and thyme.

AROMAFACT

When essential oils are described only by their common names, not only do these exclude the importance of the species but they also do not account for the chemotype; e.g. 'thyme' might be *Thymus vulgaris* CT thymol and 'rosemary' might be *Rosmarinus officinalis* CT camphor (CT after the name of the essential oil describes the chemotype, naming the significant compound within that oil).

Information found when looking at the different sources of data can be confusing, as the constituents are quoted in ranges (usually percentages, %), not in precise amounts.

AROMAFACT

The published data relating to the composition of a particular oil can vary owing to factors already outlined. It will also vary with the source of information and for each oil studied there may be different compounds and values quoted. Even the 'accepted' ranges quoted for the same compound will vary from source to source. This chapter will show this in the individual essential oils examined, and draws information and data from a variety of sources.

EXAMINATION OF ESSENTIAL OILS AND OTHER MATERIALS

The examination of a range of essences predominantly essential oils but also absolutes, resins and waxes, popular for use in aromatherapy. They are arranged in plant families, with common names and botanical names. For example, the essential oil commonly called clary sage belongs to the Lamiaceae (also called Labiatae) plant family and its botanical name is *Salvia sclarea*. Essences examined are:

Family	*Essence/Essential oil*
Lamiaceae (Labiatae)	1. The Lavenders
	2. Clary Sage (*Salvia sclarea*)
	3. Marjoram (*Origanum marjorana*)
	4. Rosemary (*Rosemarinus officianalis*)
	5. Thyme (*Thymus vulgaris*)
	6. Peppermint (*Mentha piperita*)
	7. Basil (*Ocimum basilicum*)
	8. Patchouli (*Pogostemon cablin*)
Rutaceae	9. Neroli (*Citrus aurantium*)
	10. Petitgrain (*Citrus aurantium*)
	11. Bitter orange (*Citrus aurantium*)
	12. Sweet orange (*Citrus sinensis*)
	13. Bergamot (*Citrus bergaia*)
	14. Lemon (*Citrus limon*)
	15. Mandarin (*Citrus nobilis*)
	16. Grapefruit (*Citrus paradisi*)

Graminae (Poaceae)	17. Lemongrass (*Cymbopogon citratus*)
	18. Vetivert (*Vetiveria zizanioides*)
Asteraceae (Compositae)	19. Chamomiles
Myrtaceae	20. The Eucalyptuses
	21. Tea Tree (*Melaleuca alternifolia*)
Geraniaceae	22. Geranium (*Pelargonium graveolens*)
Piperaceae	23. Black Pepper (*Piper nigrum*)
Apiaceae (Umbelliferae)	24. Fennel (*Foeniculum vulgare*)
Rosaceae	25. Roses
Oleaceae	26. Jasmine (*Jasminium grandiflorum*)
Annonaceae	27. Ylang-Ylang (*Cananga odorata*)
Santalaceae	28. Sandalwoods
Burseraceae	29. Frankincense (*Boswellia sacra*)
	30. Myrrh (*Commiphora myrrha*)
Styracaceae	31. Benzoin (*Styrax benzoin*)
Zingiberaceae	32. Ginger (*Zingiber officinale*)
Pinaceae	33. Cedarwoods
Cupressaceae	34. Cypress (*Cupressus sempervirens*)
	35. Juniper (*Juniperus communis*)

Uses and actions of essential oils The uses and actions of essential oils are briefly mentioned in the descriptions of the essential oils and are of paramount importance to the aromatherapist. There is a vast amount of published data, some the results of scientific work but much based in traditional folklore and anecdotal accounts. Information is often contradictory and many different oils appear to have the same properties. Information is beyond the scope of this book to go into clinical usage. A chemical or molecular approach is important for understanding properties and safe applications. However, aromatherapy is still an essentially holistic therapy and also needs experience, intuition and partnership between therapist and client.

POPULAR ESSENCES

Lamiaceae (Labiatae)

1. The lavenders (true, lavandin and spike) (Figs. 7.3, 7.4, 7.5)

AROMAFACT

Lavender is the mainstay of aromatherapy but represents a complex situation with different species, subspecies and chemotypes.

Lavender is a long-established essential oil, with a legendary folk tradition. The use of 'just lavender' is very misleading. The true lavender is from *Lavandula angustifolia* (also called *Lavandula officinalis*, *Lavandula vera*). This is divided into other subspecies *Lavandula delphinensis* and *Lavandula fragrans*. *Lavandula angustifolia* Miller is a lavender grown in France and is the only one recognized in the French Pharmacopoeia. Combined with the existence of many chemotypes, this gives an indication of the many possibilities for variation in the oil.

True lavender species grow at high altitudes (above 600 metres) on dry, limey soil from plants distinguished by small flower heads and no side shoots from the main stem.

Spike lavender comes from the *Lavandula latifolia* or *Lavandula spica* species. These grow at much lower altitudes, are easier and cheaper to cultivate and give high yields of oil. The main country of origin is Spain.

Lavandin is produced by a hybrid plant *Lavandula intermedia* or *Lavandula hybrida*, which was bred by crossing the true lavender (*Lavandula angustifolia*) with spike lavender (*Lavandula latifolia*). Lavandin is sometimes called 'bastard lavender'. Hybrids are widespread in horticulture, where they are bred to produce plants with the desired properties of the parents. The lavandin plants are easier to grow at lower altitudes (400–600 metres), yielding almost twice as much oil as the true lavender plant. Again, this is economically favourable and lavandin essential oil is particularly useful for the cosmetic and fragrance industries.

Chemically, all forms contain linalyl acetate, linalool and 1,8-cineole, along with many other compounds. Further analysis of each type reveals their differences in amounts of chemical components. The situation is illustrated by comparing published data for principal constituents and then seeing how these are reinforced by an actual GC chromatogram. This is shown in Table 7.1; the main figure is the published data while figures in brackets are those taken from the GC analysis of actual oil samples (*cis*- and *trans*-ocimene are minor hydrocarbon components, but are included as they are often used as markers for the authenticity of lavender oils). In all cases the amounts of compounds in the hybrid (*Lavandula intermedia*) are in between those of the true (*Lavandula angustifolia*) and the spike (*Lavandula latifolia*).

Table 7.1   Composition data (%) for lavender oil

Compound	*L. angustifolia*	*L. latifolia*	*L. intermedia*
Linalyl acetate	7–56 (33.29)	0.8–15 (5.37)	2–34 (23.1)
Linalool	6–50 (29.55)	11–54 (42.65)	24–41 (40.73)
Camphor	0–0.8 (0.21)	9–60 (12.39)	0.4–12 (3.51)
1,8-Cineole	0–5 (0.57)	25–37 (23.98)	6–26 (4.79)
cis-Ocimene	1.3–10.9 (6.2)	0.4–4 (0.55)	0.9–6 (1.63)
trans-Ocimene	0.8–5.8 (3.1)	0.1–2 (0.3)	1.0–4 (1.26)

The main figure represents published data (range), while the figures in parentheses are those taken from GC analyses illustrated in Figures 7.3, 7.4 and 7.5.

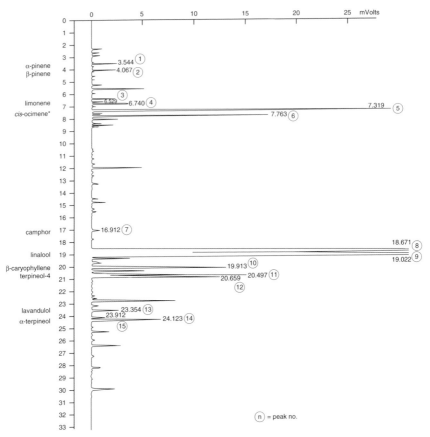

Run mode   : Analysis
Peak measurement : Peak area
Calculation type : Percent

Peak no.	Peak name	Result (%)	Retention time (min)	Time offset (min)	Area (counts)	Sep. code	Width 1/2 (s)	Status codes
1	α-Pinene	0.24	3.544	−0.000	4 084	PV	1.6	
2	β-Pinene	0.18	4.067	−0.000	3 106	BV	1.3	
3	Limonene	0.16	6.592	0.000	2 739	BV	2.4	
4	Cineole	0.57	6.740	−0.000	9 635	VV	2.5	
5	cis-Ocimene	6.62	7.319	−0.000	112 255	BB	3.9	
6	trans-Ocimene	3.16	7.763	−0.000	53 673	PV	3.0	
7	Camphor	0.21	16.912	0.000	3 645	VB	4.4	
8	Linalool	29.55	18.671	−0.001	501 125	BV	8.2	
9	Linalyl acetate	33.29	19.022	0.000	564 493	VV	10.2	
10	β-Caryophyllene	3.97	19.913	0.000	67 314	VV	5.2	
11	Terpineol-4	4.46	20.497	0.000	75 594	VV	4.9	
12	Lavandulyl acetate	3.55	20.659	0.000	60 266	VP	4.9	
13	Lavandulol	0.64	23.354	−0.000	10 856	VV	3.8	
14	α-Terpineol	0.32	23.912	−0.000	5 481	VV	4.1	
15	Borneol	1.91	24.123	0.000	32 470	VV	4.5	
	Totals:	88.83		−0.001	1 506 736			

Total unidentified counts: 189 093
Detected peaks: 160   Rejected peaks: 123   Identified peaks: 15

Figure 7.3   Lavender. A good-quality French lavender, true lavender *Lavandula angustifolia*. This shows a high linalyl acetate content (33.29%) and low camphor content (0.21%). This oil would meet the ISO standards. Courtesy of Jenny Warden, Traceability.

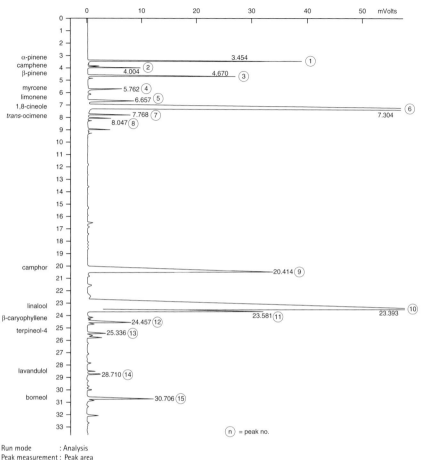

Run mode   : Analysis
Peak measurement : Peak area
Calculation type : Percent

Peak no.	Peak name	Result (%)	Retention time (min)	Time offset (min)	Area (counts)	Sep. code	Width 1/2 (s)	Status codes
1	α-Pinene	2.21	3.454	0.009	91 326	VV	2.0	
2	Camphene	0.56	4.004	0.004	23 304	VP	2.0	
3	β-Pinene	1.96	4.670	0.000	80 862	VB	2.7	
4	Myrcene	0.54	5.762	0.003	22 342	PV	3.0	
5	Limonene	1.44	6.657	−0.000	59 648	BV	6.4	
6	1,8-Cineole	23.98	7.304	0.000	991 194	VB	11.7	
7	cis-Ocimene	0.55	7.768	0.000	22 582	TS	0.0	
8	trans-Ocimene	0.30	8.047	−0.000	12 237	TS	0.0	
9	Camphor	12.39	20.414	0.000	512 202	VV	14.8	
10	Linalool	42.65	23.393	0.003	1 763 219	VV	24.5	
11	Linalyl acetate	5.37	23.581	0.001	222 129	VV	7.1	
12	β-Caryophyllene	1.21	24.457	−0.003	50 135	VV	6.1	
13	Terpineol-4	0.42	25.336	−0.000	17 435	VV	4.9	
14	Lavandulol	0.37	28.710	−0.000	15 215	VV	5.4	
15	Borneol	2.07	30.706	0.000	85 775	BV	6.5	
	Totals:	96.02		0.017	3 969 605			

Total unidentified counts: 164 424
Detected peaks: 164   Rejected peaks: 120   Identified peaks: 15

Figure 7.4   Lavender. This shows the GC analysis for spike lavender (*Lavandula latifolia*). The camphor level is high and that of linalyl acetate is low. Courtesy of Jenny Warden, Traceability.

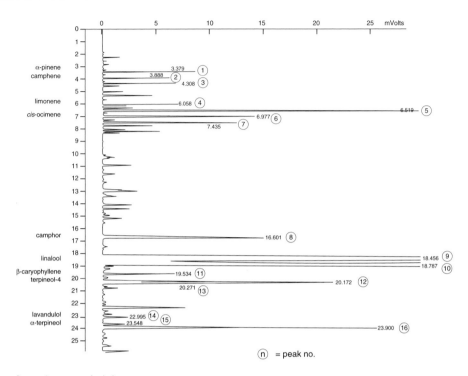

Run mode   : Analysis
Peak measurement : Peak area
Calculation type : Percent

Peak no.	Peak name	Result (%)	Retention time (min)	Time offset (min)	Area (counts)	Sep. code	Width 1/2 (s)	Status codes
1	α-Pinene	0.56	3.379	0.000	16 205	BB	1.5	
2	Camphene	0.30	3.888	−0.000	8 771	BB	1.3	
3	β-Pinene	0.33	4.308	−0.001	9 606	BB	1.3	
4	Limonene	0.70	6.058	0.000	20 051	BB	2.7	
5	Cineole	4.79	6.519	−0.000	137 953	VB	4.1	
6	cis-Ocimene	1.63	6.977	0.000	46 977	BP	3.2	
7	trans-Ocimene	1.26	7.435	0.000	36 250	VP	2.8	
8	Camphor	3.51	16.601	0.001	101 127	BB	6.5	
9	Linalool	40.73	18.456	0.000	1 172 300	BV	13.2	
10	Linalyl acetate	23.10	18.787	−0.002	664 836	VV	10.6	
11	β-Caryophyllene	0.98	19.534	0.000	28 239	VV	3.8	
12	Terpineol-4	4.63	20.172	−0.000	133 175	VV	5.9	
13	Lavandulyl acetate	1.17	20.271	−0.000	33 717	VV	4.2	
14	Lavandulol	0.42	22.995	0.000	11 992	VV	4.5	
15	α-Terpineol	0.33	23.548	−0.000	9 399	VV	4.2	
16	Borneol	6.80	23.900	−0.000	195 870	VP	7.8	
	Totals:	91.24		−0.002	2 626 468			

Total unidentified counts: 252 092
Detected peaks: 187   Rejected peaks: 134   Identified peaks: 16

Figure 7.5   Lavender. Analysis of *Lavandula hybrida*, showing a composition that is intermediate between the true lavender and spike lavender. Courtesy of Jenny Warden, Traceability.

The true lavender (*Lavandula officinalis*) shown in the chromatogram is high in linalyl acetate, conforming to the ISO standard composition range of 25–45% and linalool ISO standard of 25–38%. True lavenders also may have between 5% and 30% lavandulyl acetate; the GC for this sample shows quite a low value of 3.55%. Also characteristic of true lavender, the amounts of camphor and the oxide 1,8-cineole are low, but are increased in the other species. High ester and alcohol content makes this a desirable aromatherapy choice as it is gentle with no known contraindications.

For the spike (*Lavandula latifolia*) lavender the analysis shows a much lower acetate content and a high natural camphor and 1,8-cineole level. This makes it useful for respiratory infections, as an insecticide and for muscular pain. However, it must be used cautiously as it is a more vigorous oil.

The hybrid (*Lavandula intermedia*) lavender shows an intermediate composition between the true and spike for all major components. Ester content is lower and camphor content higher than in the true lavender. It is generally considered to be an inferior essential oil as it was initially bred for the perfumery industry. However, it has been attributed with many therapeutic applications with rare contraindications when used correctly.

Another type of lavender, *Lavandula stoechas*, is less commonly encountered. It has a very high camphor content (15–30%), which necessitates cautious handling. Its main component is fenchone (45–50%), a terpenoid ketone, which, although a ketone, is considered nontoxic, nonirritant and nonsensitizing.

2. Clary Sage *(Salvia sclarea)*

AROMAFACT

Clary sage has been shown to have powerful euphoric effects and should not be used if a client has consumed alcohol.

Several different chemotypes occur according to their geographical region of growth. They are mainly Mediterranean regions but also USA, Russia, Morocco and France. The essential oil has a heavy fragrance with herbal and nutty tones and pale green/yellow to clear colour. The odour can be attributed to the major component the ester linalyl acetate that can be present as up to 75% of the total composition. Also present alcohol linalool (up to 26%), terpenes β-caryophyllene (up to 3%), germacrene (up to 4%), neryl acetate (up to 1.7%). Box 7.1 shows a certificate of analysis which gives a more comprehensive insight to the chemical composition. Therapeutic applications are linked to antidepressive, spirit lifting and creative stimulating actions on the mind. Reputed to act as an antispasmodic and emmenagogue, and promoting the female hormone oestrogen it is used to ease PMS (pre-menstrual syndrome) and encourage and ease labour. Also used for respiratory conditions including asthma and for a range of skin conditions associated with

Box 7.1 Certificate of analysis for Clary Sage (*Salvia sclarea*)

CERTIFICATE OF ESSENTIAL OIL ANALYSIS 2007

ESSENTIAL OIL OF CLARY SAGE *(Salvia sclarea)*
COUNTRY OF ORIGIN – RUSSIA
METHOD OF EXTRACTION – Steam Distillation

Authenticated..

Peak No	Compound	% Composition
1	Myrcene	0.86
2	Limonene	0.51
3	E-Ocimene	0.35
4	α-copaene	0.75
5	linalol	9.90
6	linalyl-acetate	72.20
7	β-caryophyllene	2.11
8	germacrene D	2.57
9	α-terpineol	1.38
10	neryl acetate	1.17
11	alkene	0.34
12	geranyl acetate	2.06
13	nerol	0.52
14	geraniol	1.33
15	caryophyllene oxide	1.17
16	spathulenol	0.13
17	alcohol	0.68
18	alcohol	1.97

Courtesy of Jane Collins, Phytobotanica

greasy complexions such as acne, boils and dandruff. Although considered to be nontoxic, nonirritant and nonsensitizing it should be avoided during pregnancy.

3. Marjoram (Origanum marjorana)

AROMAFACT

Origanum marjorana is also called sweet marjoram. There are other species which may give rise to confusion. These include *Origanum vulgare* known as common or wild marjoram and *Thymus mastichina* which as its name suggests actually belongs to the Thyme species and is known as Spanish marjoram or oregano.

Sweet marjoram is a pale yellow oil with a warm, camphoraceous and spicy odour. Its main components are alcohols terpinen-1-ol-4 (14–20%), thujan-4-ol (4–13%), linalool (2–10%), α–terpineol (7–27%), hydrocarbon monoterpenes sabinene (2–10%) β-myrcene (1–9%), β-terpinolene (1–7%), α-pinene (1–5%), α–terpinene (6–8%), ester geranyl acetate (1–7%) and aldehyde citral (4–6%). Box 7.2 shows a GC analysis report. A versatile oil with many claimed therapeutic properties. Often called a comforting oil. Applied to the mind in situations of stress and grief where it calms and relaxes. For the body it is considered warming, analgesic, and antispasmodic suitable for muscle and joint pains. Also acting on the respiratory system for asthma and bronchitis, on the digestive system as a carmative relieving cholics and constipation and in skincare for bruising and chilblains. Considered a safe nontoxic, nonirritating and nonsensitizing essential oil but should be avoided during pregnancy.

Box 7.2   Certificate of analysis for Sweet Marjoram (*Origanum marjorana*)

GAS CHROMATOGRAPHY REPORT

Product Identification

Product Name :	Marjoram Sweet Oil
Botanical Name :	*Origanum marjorana*
Country of Origin :	Egypt
Agricultural Method :	Organic
Product Code :	E592
Batch Number :	764

Principal Constituents	Constituent %
α-Thuyene :	0.58
α-Pinene :	0.77
Sabinene :	7.55
Myrcene :	2.05
α-Phellandrene :	0.56
α-Terpinene :	8.00
Limonene :	1.04
1,8 Cineole :	1.95
β-Phellandrene :	trace
γ-Terpinene :	12.80
Terpinolene :	3.00
trans-Thuyanol-4 :	3.95
Linalool :	1.23
Linalyl acetate :	2.35
cis-Thuyanol-4 :	17.95
Terpinene-4-ol :	22.55
α-Terpineol :	3.17
β-Caryophyllene :	2.05
Neryl acetate :	1.27

Courtesy of Geoff Lyth, Quinessence Aromatherapy Ltd

4. Rosemary (Rosmarinus officinalis)

AROMAFACT

Rosemary oils are derived from one main species with well-documented cultivars that show variations in chemical composition due to the climate they are grown in.

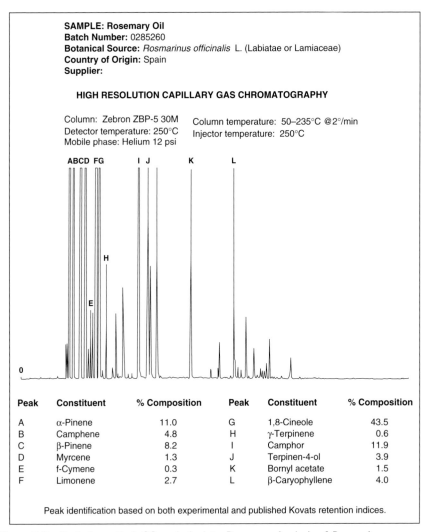

SAMPLE: Rosemary Oil
Batch Number: 0285260
Botanical Source: *Rosmarinus officinalis* L. (Labiatae or Lamiaceae)
Country of Origin: Spain
Supplier:

HIGH RESOLUTION CAPILLARY GAS CHROMATOGRAPHY

Column: Zebron ZBP-5 30M
Detector temperature: 250°C
Mobile phase: Helium 12 psi

Column temperature: 50–235°C @2°/min
Injector temperature: 250°C

Peak	Constituent	% Composition	Peak	Constituent	% Composition
A	α-Pinene	11.0	G	1,8-Cineole	43.5
B	Camphene	4.8	H	γ-Terpinene	0.6
C	β-Pinene	8.2	I	Camphor	11.9
D	Myrcene	1.3	J	Terpinen-4-ol	3.9
E	f-Cymene	0.3	K	Bornyl acetate	1.5
F	Limonene	2.7	L	β-Caryophyllene	4.0

Peak identification based on both experimental and published Kovats retention indices.

Figure 7.6   Typical supplier's GC analysis data. Rosemary. Analysis of *Rosmarinus officinalis.* Courtesy of Jasbir Chana, Phoenix Natural Products Ltd.

Rosemary has been used for a long time with extensive applications for culinary and medical purposes. *Rosmarinus officinalis* is the species used for the production of the essential oil.

Typically listed chemical components are:

Terpenes: camphene, pinene, limonene, myrcene
Sesquiterpenes: caryophyllene, humulene
Alcohols: borneol, linalool, terpineol
Ketones: camphor, thujone, verbenone
Aldehyde: cuminic aldehyde
Esters: bornyl acetate, fenchyl acetate
Oxide: 1,8-cineole

There are three principal chemotypes: verbenone, 1,8-cineole and camphor-borneol. These are examples of variation due to the climate they are grown in and are also called cultivars. The names of the cultivars are not Latinized and appear after the species name, often within quotation marks. For example, *Lavandula angustifolia* 'Maillette' is a type of lavender named after its originator. For rosemary the cultivars are named after their country of origin. As a consequence of this, the verbenone is also called French, the 1,8-cineole is called Tunisian and the camphor-borneol is called Spanish. A comparison of these in terms of their amounts of main components is shown in Table 7.2.

The essential oil has many beneficial effects and applications in aromatherapy for skin and hair care, as an antirheumatic, antispasmodic and calmative, for complaints of the respiratory, circulatory and digestive systems and for nervous disorders. The camphor type is best suited to the musculoskeletal system, and the 1,8-cineole for pulmonary congestion and efficient functioning of the liver and kidneys, with the verbenone being a safe nonirritant essential oil for skin and hair treatments.

Rosmarinus officinalis essential oil is usually regarded as nontoxic, nonsensitizing and nonirritant when used in sufficient dilution. It may cause dermatitis in hypersensitive individuals and there is some evidence to suggest it should not be used during pregnancy, by epileptics, or by those with high blood pressure. A material safety data sheet from an oil supplier (Box 7.3) shows the type of information available for a Spanish

Table 7.2   Main components (%) of three cultivars of *Rosmarinus officinalis*

	Cultivars		
Component	French	Tunisian	Spanish
Terpenes			
α-Pinene	10.5	10.3–11.6	19–27
β-Pinene	7.6	4.9–7.7	4.3–7.7
Camphene	4.2	4–4.3	7–9.9
Limonene	2.1	2–4.8	2.9–4.9
Alcohol (borneol)	3.1	2.8–4.3	2.4–3.4
Ketone (camphor)	Trace	9.9–12.6	12.4–20.8
Acetate (bornyl acetate)	13	1–1.4	0.4–1.6
Oxide (1,8-cineole)	49	40–44.5	17–25

Box 7.3   A typical supplier's data sheet: Rosemary

MATERIAL SAFETY DATA SHEET

ACCORDING TO EC LEGISLATION 91/155/E EC

Date created: June 1998   Date revised: June 1998

1. Identification
Commercial name: *Rosemary essential oil.*
Botanical nomenclature: *Rosmarinus officinalis.*
INCI name: *Rosmarinus officinalis.*
CAS number: *84604 – 14 – 8.*
EINECS/ELINCS number: *283 – 291 – 9.*

2. Composition
Main components: *1,8-cineole, camphor, α-pinene, β-pinene, β-caryophyllene, camphene, borneol, α-terpineol, bornyl acetate, myrcene, terpinen-4-ol.*
Additives (e.g. carriers, preservatives, antioxidants): *Nil.*

3. Potential health hazards
Inhalation: *None identified.*
Skin: *Concentrated liquid and vapours irritating to skin by prolonged exposure.*
Eyes: *Irritating to eyes with possible damage.*
Ingestion: *Harmful if swallowed.*

4. First aid
Inhalation: *If discomfort is felt, remove person to a well-ventilated area with plenty of fresh air.*
Skin: *Remove contaminated clothing. Wash affected area with plenty of soap and water.*
Eyes: *Flush immediately with plenty of cool water for 10 to 20 minutes. Seek medical advice from a medical doctor.*

Ingestion: *Seek immediate medical care.*

5. In case of fire
Extinguishing media: *Foam, carbon dioxide.*
Do not use: *Water.*
Special precautions: *Wear breathing apparatus as toxic vapours may be released during fire.*

6. Spill and leak procedure
Individual precautions: *Eliminate sources of ignition. Keep area well-ventilated and isolate the spill.*
Environmental protection: *Prevent the liquid from entering the drains and sewers.*
Cleaning methods: *Soak up the spill using inert absorbents. For large spills use pumps.*

7. Handling and storage
Store in a cool, dry and dark place in suitable containers (aluminium cans or lacquer-lined steel drums).
Handle in a well-ventilated area.
Keep away from sources of heat and ignition.

8. Personal protection/exposure control
Respiratory protection: *Wear breathing apparatus when working in an area of high vapour concentration.*
Skin protection: *Use protective gloves. Wear protective clothing when possibility exists of contact.*

continued

Box 7.3   A typical supplier's data sheet: Rosemary / Cont'd

Eye protection: *Goggles should be worn.*
General precautions: *Use good industrial hygiene practice.*

9. Physiochemical properties
Appearance: *Pale yellow liquid*
Odour: *Woody, herbaceous, camphor-like*
pH: *Neutral*
Boiling point: *Not available*
Flash point: *40 °C to 44 °C*
Autoignition temperature: *Not available*
Explosion limits: *Not available*
Vapour pressure (25 °C): *Not available*
Vapour density: *>1 (air = 1)*
Specific gravity (20 °C): *0.890–0.915*
Optical rotation (20 °C): *−5 ° to +10 °*
Refractive index (20 °C): *1.460–1.480*
Solubility in water (20 °C): *Negligible*
Partition coefficient log *Po/w*: *Not available*
Evaporation rate: *<1 (butyl acetate = 1)*

10. Stability and reactivity
Chemical stability: *Stable*
Conditions to avoid: *Normally stable. Not reactive with water.*
Hazardous decomposition products: *Not available.*

11. Toxicological information
According to RIFM-Monograph:
Acute toxicity: *Oral LD_{50}: 5 g/kg in rats.*
Dermal LD_{50}: 10 g/kg in rabbits.
Irritation: *Tested without irritation at 10%.*

Sensitization: *Tested without sensitization at 10%.*
Phototoxicity: *No phototoxic reaction reported.*

12. Ecotoxicological information
Fish toxicity: LCO/EC_{50}: *Not available.*
Bacteriotoxicity: ECO/EC_{50}: *Not available.*

13. Disposal method
Check Federal, State and Local Regulations.

14. Transport Information
UN Number 1993: Proper shipping name: Flammable Liquid N.O.S.
Hazard Class: 3.3 Packing group: III
Transport Safety: Air (ATA/ICAO) 2/PAX309/CA310/III
Sea (IMDG-Code): 3.3/III
Roll (R/D): 3.31c
Road (ADR): 3.31c
Symbol: Risk-Phrase
RIO, 22.38
Safety-Phrase: (24/25)

15. Legislation
Meets IFRA and RIFM guidelines.

Courtesy of Phoenix Natural Products Ltd

Rosmarinus officinalis. The sample conforms to the data in the table for the Spanish but also has compounds that would fit the ranges given for Tunisian.

Figure 5.6 also shows an IR spectral analysis of *Rosmarinus officinalis*.

5. Thyme (Thymus vulgaris)

AROMAFACT

Many species, subspecies and chemotypes of thyme exist. It represents a well-documented situation illustrating all these factors.

The main species are believed to originate from the wild type *Thymus serphyllum*, with the majority of oils coming from the *Thymus vulgaris* or common thyme species. However, there are over 150 species of the genus Thymus including *Thymus vulgaris* (common or red), *Thymus zygis* (Spanish), *Thymus serphyllum* (wild), *Thymus mastichina* (Spanish marjoram) and *Thymus capitatus* (Spanish oregano). Thyme belongs to the plant family Labiatae, whose members are easily hybridized: that is, there is interbreeding of different species, making it difficult to define species and subspecies. Exact botanical classification of the essential oil is also difficult and there are wide variations and conflicting data on the constituents for each species depending on the source of the information. Coupled with the fact that thyme is probably the aromatic plant with the most diverse range of chemotypes, these factors contribute to a very complex and often contradictory situation for these essential oils.

White thyme is not complete or natural, but is usually an adulterated and compounded oil made up of fractions of pine oils, rosemary, eucalyptus and red thyme, or it may be origanum with *p*-cymene, pinene, limonene and caryophyllene.

When considering the composition of the natural, whole essential oils, the environment the plants are grown in is an important factor in determining the chemical composition. Altitude is a significant factor in determination of chemotype. In general the gentler, alcohol chemotypes high in linalool, geraniol, thujanol-4 and α-terpineol are associated with growth at altitudes between 1000 and 1200 metres. They are called sweet thymes and owing to their high alcohol content are generally considered safe to use in a variety of conditions. This is in contrast to the phenolic chemotypes high in compounds such as carvacrol and thymol. These are called red thymes, and are extracted from plants growing at lower altitudes, usually close to the Mediterranean sea. The phenolics act as powerful antiseptics and need to be used with extreme care as they may cause skin irritation.

A 'typical' analysis of major components of these contrasting chemotypes for *T. vulgaris* shows this difference (Table 7.3). Typical analysis is

Table 7.3 A representative analysis (%) of phenolic and alcohol chemotypes (CT) of *Thymus vulgaris*

Compound	Red–phenolic CT	Sweet–alcohol CT
Thymol	30–48	2%
Carvacrol	0.5–5.5	
Linalool	0	30–80% linalool CT
Geraniol	0	30–80% or geraniol CT
Geranyl acetate	0	Up to 50%
p-Cymene	18.5–21.4	0
1,8-Cineole	3.6–15.3	0
β-Caryophyllene	1.3–7.8	4
α-Pinene	0.5–5.7	0
Terpinolene	1.8–5.6	0

again difficult to define, so 'representative' analysis might be a better description.

There are many published therapeutic uses of the thyme oils. Linalool CT, with very low phenol content, is attributed properties such as reviving, strengthening nerves and aiding concentration by stimulation of the cerebral regions of the brain. It is considered to be an immuno-stimulant and safe for use with children. The high ester content also contributes to its application as an antispasmodic for dry coughs.

In contrast the thymol CT varies widely with the alcoholic CTs in both olfactory and therapeutic properties. Thymol CT is also attributed immuno-stimulant action but it is strongly antiseptic and is used for infectious conditions like colds, coughs and bronchitis. It is also recommended for its warming analgesic properties for treatment of rheumatism, arthritis and sciatica. It stimulates the digestive and cardiovascular systems and may help raise the blood pressure.

The GC analysis (Fig. 7.7) shows a commercial white thyme with a high percentage of the phenols thymol (55.8%) and carvacrol (2.07%). This contrasts with that of sweet thyme (Fig. 7.8) with no phenolic compounds present and alcohols terpineol-4 (13%), α-terpineol (12.37%) and borneol (5.95%) making up a total of 31.34% for this particular sample.

6. Peppermint (Mentha piperita)

AROMAFACT

Mint covers numerous species with subspecies and chemotypes. Although an established and widely used oil, it should be handled with care.

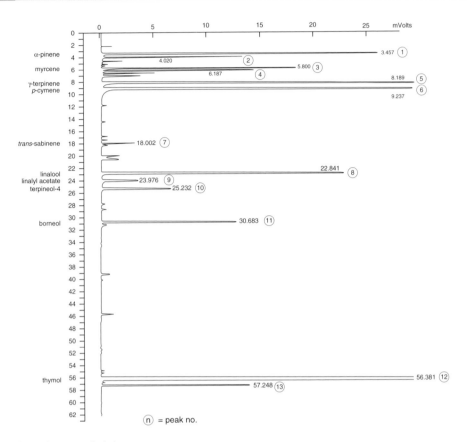

Run mode   : Analysis
Peak measurement : Peak area
Calculation type : Percent

Peak no.	Peak name	Result (%)	Retention time (min)	Time offset (min)	Area (counts)	Sep. code	Width 1/2 (s)	Status codes
1	α-Pinene	1.86	3.457	−0.000	83 940	VV	2.6	
2	Camphene	1.04	4.020	−0.000	46 737	VV	2.7	
3	Myrcene	1.77	5.800	0.000	79 750	BB	3.7	
4	α-Terpinene	1.29	6.187	−0.003	58 315	VV	3.5	
5	γ-Terpinene	6.38	8.189	0.009	287 469	PV	7.1	
6	r-Cymene	16.33	9.237	−0.003	735 642	VB	10.9	
7	trans-Sabinene	0.38	18.002	0.002	17 324	BV	4.9	
8	Linalool	4.95	22.841	0.001	222 803	BV	9.2	
9	Linalyl acetate	0.47	23.976	0.000	21 326	VV	8.6	
10	Terpineol-4	1.18	25.232	−0.000	53 335	VB	6.4	
11	Borneol	2.46	30.683	0.003	110 650	PB	7.6	
12	Thymol	55.58	56.381	0.000	2 503 672	BB	15.8	
13	Carvacrol	2.07	57.248	−0.002	93 021	TF	0.0	
	Totals:	95.76		−0.007	4 313 984			

Total unidentified counts: 190 517
Detected peaks: 123   Rejected peaks: 89   Identified peaks: 13

Figure 7.7   Thyme. A typical white Spanish thyme, showing the presence of thymol. Thymol has a retention time of 56.381 min and makes up 55.58% of the oil in this GC analysis of this particular sample. Courtesy of Jenny Warden, Traceability.

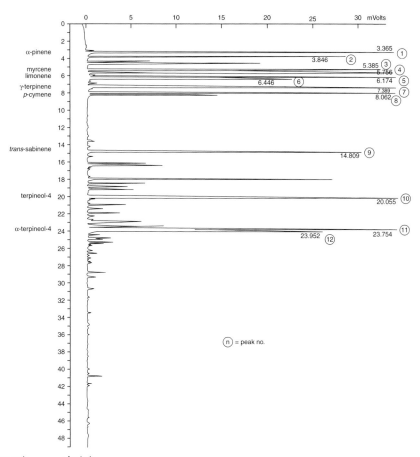

Run mode   : Analysis
Peak measurement : Peak area
Calculation type : Percent

Peak no.	Peak name	Result (%)	Retention time (min)	Time offset (min)	Area (counts)	Sep. code	Width 1/2 (s)	Status codes
1	α-Pinene	8.24	3.365	0.000	282 008	PB	2.8	
2	Camphene	2.03	3.846	−0.000	69 342	BB	2.1	
3	Myrcene	3.10	5.385	−0.000	105 971	BV	3.1	
4	α-Terpinene	3.76	5.756	0.000	128 648	BB	3.3	
5	Limonene	4.19	6.174	0.000	143 302	VV	3.7	
6	1,8-Cineole	2.15	6.446	0.000	73 728	VP	3.0	
7	γ-Terpinene	10.30	7.389	−0.000	352 521	PV	6.5	
8	p-Cymene	5.26	8.062	−0.000	180 050	VV	4.5	
9	trans-Sabinene	5.98	14.809	−0.000	204 528	VB	6.4	
10	Terpineol-4	13.00	20.055	0.000	444 691	VV	9.9	
11	γ-Terpineol-4	12.37	23.754	0.000	423 284	VV	5.9	
12	Borneol	5.95	23.952	0.000	203 602	VV	9.2	
	Totals:	76.33		0.000	2 611 675			

Total unidentified counts: 810 037
Detected peaks: 146   Rejected peaks: 68   Identified peaks: 12

Figure 7.8   Thyme. A typical sweet thyme, showing no thymol present. Courtesy of Jenny Warden, Traceability.

There are numerous species of mint including peppermint, *Mentha piperita*, spearmint, *Mentha spicata*, and cornmint, *Mentha arvensis*. *Mentha piperita* is actually a hybrid species bred from spearmint *Mentha spicata* and watermint *Mentha aquatica*. They all contain subspecies and chemotypes. Mints have a long tradition of culinary, fragrance, cosmetic and therapeutic applications.

Typical composition would be: menthol (27–51%), menthone (13–32%), isomenthone (2–10%), 1,8-cineole (5–14%), methyl acetate (2–4%), methofuran (2–12%), limonene (0.5–6%), pinenes (1.5–4%), germacrene (2.1–4.3%) and pulegone (0.1–1%). Box 7.4 shows a GC analysis for Mentha piperita.

Box 7.4   Analysis of Peppermint (*Mentha piperita*)

GAS CHROMATOGRAPHY REPORT

Product Identification

Product Name :	Peppermint (Mitcham) Oil
Botanical Name :	*Mentha piperita*
Country of Origin :	United Kingdom
Agricultural Method :	Organic
Product Code:	E622
Batch Number :	692

Principal Constituents	Constituent %
α-Pinene	0.66
β-Pinene	0.98
Sabinene	0.52
Limonene	1.44
1,8 Cineole	5.41
z-Ocimene	0.64
Menthone	14.13
cis-Sabinene-hydrate	1.70
Benzofuran, 4,5,6,7 etc	5.97
iso-Menthone	2.67
Menthyl acetate	6.30
Cyclohexanol	5.65
Menthol	50.98
Germacrene D	1.44
2-Cyclohexan-1-one, etc	0.70
Veridifloral	0.81

Courtesy of Geoff Lyth, Quinessence Aromatherapy Ltd

Therapeutic uses are widespread as peppermint has a skin toning effect and is most effective for digestive disorders such as indigestion and flatulence; it stimulates cardiovascular and lymphatic systems, works on ligaments for joint and muscle pain and has local antiseptic properties.

Most aromatherapy books state that peppermint is nontoxic, nonirritant when diluted and possibly sensitizing owing to its menthol content. It is often advised to use it in moderation. However, it should be used with caution and is contraindicated for use with babies and young children. The high menthol content has been shown to cause breathing problems in infants. It is irritant to mucous membranes and may exacerbate skin irritations and contact dermatitis. External use necessitates a concentration of not more than 3%. Internal use should be under the direction of a qualified medical practitioner, medical herbalist or pharmacist and is beyond the scope of aromatherapy.

7. Basil (Ocimum basilicum)

AROMAFACT

Basil essential oil contains the compound methyl chavicol (also called estragole) which has been a cause for concern. However, this should be viewed in the context of good safe aromatherapy practice.

Studies on laboratory rodents suggest methyl chavicol may be a carcinogenic compound. IFRA has a steering group for it and has set limits for amounts permitted in products. For fine fragrances it is 0.02%. It concluded that based on available data methyl chavicol was not likely to present a human cancer risk at current levels of exposure arising from its addition to fragrance products when added as the compound or from essential oils. Box 7.5 shows safety data for methyl chavicol. They are currently examining lower end doses so new permitted levels may be issued in the future. It should be remembered that the experimental dosage was up to 100,000 times higher than would be present in a correctly diluted aromatherapy blend and it does not follow that an observed effect in an experimental animal would also occur in humans. Essential oil is extracted from plants with many geographical origins and there are four principal chemotypes. Consequently amounts of chemical constituents can vary widely.

The French or sweet basil has a high linalool and lower methyl chavicol content with the exotic basil having the highest methyl chavicol content. It is for this reason that the sweet is often preferred for aromatherapy. Principal chemical components found in essential oils of basil include methyl chavicol (22–88%), methyl eugenol (0.3–6%), linalool (1.1–46%), limonene (2.0–4.9%), cis-ocimene (0.2–2.6%) and citronellol (0.6–3.9%). Analysis for a sample of

---

Box 7.5   Safety data for methyl chavicol (Estragole)

⚠ Estragole (= methyl chavicol)

Found in:	Amount:
Anise	1–4%
Basil (estragole CT)	40–87%
Basil (linalool CT)	1.3%–16.5%
Chervil (NCA)	70–80%
Fennel (bitter)	3–6.5%
Fennel (sweet)	1–5%
Ravensara anisata	88%
Star anise	0.3–5.5%
Tarragon (French)	70–87%
Tarragon (Russian)	0.1–17%

Terpenoid ether. Genotoxic in rat hepatocytes. Estragole is carcinogenic in mice because it is metabolised, in vivo, to the carcinogenic compound 1′-hydroxyestragole. The same metabolic process is believed to take place in humans. High doses are potentially carcinogenic, but very low doses are not, since they are readily detoxified. Estragole is not restricted by any regulatory agencies, even though its carcinogenic potential is similar to that of safrole, which is restricted. Acute oral LD_{50} in mice is 1.25 g/kg. Mildly irritating, non-sensitising.

Courtesy of Robert Tisserand-taken from Essential Oil Safety. A Guide for Health Care Professionals (Churchill Livingstone)

---

basil essential oil is shown in Box 7.6. The odour is spicy, sweet and herbaceous. It has a reputation as a powerful cephalic for clearing the head, stimulating and clarifying mental processes alleviating mental strain and disorder. It is claimed to benefit the respiratory system treating congested sinuses and infections, for muscle and joint problems like gout, as a calming cleanser for the digestive system and applied to menstrual problems. For the skin it is suited to acne-prone congested complexions and to cleanse insect bites. Generally considered relatively nontoxic on low dilutions, but may cause irritation and sensitization in some individuals. Should be avoided during pregnancy.

8. Patchouli (Pogostemon cablin)

AROMAFACT

An essential oil often associated with the flower power hippy generation of the 1960s. One of the few oils considered to improve with keeping.

Box 7.6   Analysis of essential oil of Basil (*Ocimum basilicum*)

CERTIFICATE OF ESSENTIAL OIL ANALYSIS 2007

ESSENTIAL OIL OF BASIL *(Ocimum basilicum)*
COUNTRY OF ORIGIN – Egypt
EXTRACTION–Steam Distillation

Authenticated...

Peak No	Compound	% Composition
1	α-pinene	0.51
2	0-pinene	0.69
3	1,8-cineole	6.20
4	linalol	16.04
5	l-bergamontene	4.41
6	methyl chavicol	59.45
7	α-terpineol	0.96
8	cl-copaene	1.28
9	cl-humulene	1.55
10	caryophyllene oxide	1.07
11	methyl eugenol	1.51
12	ester	1.50
13	T-cadinol	1.10
14	eugenol	2.21
15	cinnamaldehyde	0.61
16	sesquiterpine	0.91

Courtesy of Jane Collins, Phytobotanica

Closely related to Java patchouli (*P. heyneonus*) known as false patchouli and sometimes used to produce an essential oil. The true oil is a viscous amber colour with a sweet earthy odour. Its main component is patchouli alcohol (up to 40%) with bulnesene (14–17%), seychellene (8.5–9.5%), caryophyllene (3–4%), β-patchoulene (2.7–4%). There are a variety of attributed therapeutic properties. For the mind it is said to be a grounding oil helpful for those who feel depressed, detached and exhausted. Applied to the circulation it is considered stimulating, as a diuretic and for skin healing in conditions like acne and eczema. It is often used as a fixative in oriental perfumes, and a deodorizer as it masks unpleasant smells. Due to its very strong odour it is advisable to use in low proportions in a blend. Generally considered to be a safe oil as it is non-irritant and non-sensitizing.

Rutaceae

AROMAFACT

The species *Citrus aurantium* produces different essential oils depending upon which part of the plant is used. Expression of the outer peel of the almost ripe citrus fruit produces the Bitter orange essential oil, steam distillation of leaves and twigs produces Petitgrain, while steam distillation of the freshly picked flower produces Neroli or orange blossom essential oil.

9. Neroli (Citrus aurantium)

AROMAFACT

In addition to the essential oil produced by the steam distillation of the flowers, the neroli hydrolat (also called orange flower water) is a useful by-product. A concrete and absolute are also produced by solvent extraction of the freshly picked flowers.

The essential oil is a pale yellow with a light, bitter-sweet floral odour. The absolute is darker and more viscous with an odour closer to the original flower. The main chemical components of the essential oil are the alcohol linalool (30–37%), the ester linalyl acetate (6–17%) and monoterpenes limonene (12–18%) and β-pinene (12–15%). Also present geraniol (2–3%), nerol (1–3%), nerolidol (3–6%), citral and jasmone. Both the plant and the essential oil have many established uses. The essential oil is considered to be one of the most effective as a sedative, carmative and antidepressant and often used to treat insomnia. It is also claimed to be relaxant for smooth muscle (internal, involuntary muscles) especially those of the gut. Suitable for all skin types, both the essential oil and hydrolat are versatile materials for the aromatherapist. Considered safe as it is nonirritant and non-sensitizing and an example of a non-phototoxic citrus essential oil.

10. Petitgrain (Citrus aurantium)

AROMAFACT

The name petitgrain or little grains originates from the early use of unripe fruit rather than the current extraction from the leaves.

The essential oil is a pale yellow colour with a bright floral citrus with woody herbaceous undertones in its odour. Its chemical composition is high in ester often making up to 80% of the essential oil. A typical composition would be linalyl acetate (45%), geranyl acetate (3%), neryl acetate (0.5%), also present alcohols linalool (28%), geraniol (2.5%), α-terpineol (7.5%) and nerol (1%), terpenes myrcene (5%) and *trans*-ocimene (3.5%). Used extensively as a fragrance in cosmetics, soaps and detergents. In perfume manufacture it is a classic ingredient of eau de Cologne. It is applied to stress related conditions, insomnia and as a general restorative for convalescence. Antispasmodic and believed to ease digestive disorders such as indigestion and flatulence. Suited to most skin types, used as a tonic and helpful for pimples and acne. Considered to be a safe oil, non-irritant, non-sensitizing and non-phototoxic.

11. Bitter Orange (Citrus aurantium)

AROMAFACT

The bitter orange essential oil is very high, up to 90% in the monoterpene limonene due to its extraction by cold expression. Concern about the use of this oil in high concentrations is due to reported cases of contact dermatitis caused by the limonene levels. It is often used as a starting material for the isolation of natural limonene.

The essential oil is a yellowish brown liquid with a fresh floral odour with sweet undertones. Its main components are the monoterpenes limonene (up to 90%) β-myrcene (1–2%) and α-pinene (0.1–1.1%) with esters linalyl acetate (1%) and smaller amounts of geranyl acetate, neryl acetate and citronellal acetate. It also has small amounts of coumarins, aldehydes and alcohols. It finds application as a mild sedative calming oil for both mind and body in situations of anxiety. Believed to act on the circulatory system to combat palpitations and on the digestive system easing colic, indigestion and constipation. Considered to be a nontoxic, nonirritant and nonsensitizing when employed in low dilutions, however it is phototoxic. Box 7.7 shows the IFRA Guideline for Bitter Orange Peel Expressed.

12. Sweet Orange (Citrus sinensis)

AROMAFACT

An inexpensive oil which may have been produced by a variety of methods. An inferior quality essential oil is produced in large quantities from the by–products of fruit juicing processes.

Box 7.7   IFRA Guideline for Bitter Orange Peel Expressed

Cas N°:   68916–04–1   Empirical Formula: Not applicable
               72968–50–4
Synonyms: Orange Peel Oil, Bitter (Citrus aurantium L. subsp amara L.)
              Bitter orange oil (Citrus aurantium L. subsp. amara L.)
              Citrus aurantium peel oil
              Curacao peel oil (Citrus aurantium L.)
              Daidai peel oil (Citrus aurantium L.)

History: Initial Reviews: October 1975, June 1992
            Current Revision   July 2002
            Date:

            Implementation   July 3, 2002 for new submissions*
            Date: July 3, 2003 for existing fragrance compounds*
                               This date applies to the supply of fragrance
                               compounds (formulas) only, not to the finished
                               products in the marketplace
            Next Review   July 2007
            Date:

STANDARD: Restricted
Limits in the finished product:

Skin contact products:	Non skin contact products: No restriction
Leave-on products: 1.25%*	Purity: not Applicable
Rinse-off products: No Restriction (1)	Others: not applicable

Note box: (1): including household cleaning products
* Applications on skin areas exposed to sunshine. If combinations of phototoxic
fragrance ingredients are used, the use levels have to be reduced accordingly.
The sum of the concentrations of all phototoxic fragrance ingredients,
expressed in % of their recommended maximum level in the consumer product
shall not exceed 100. For Bitter orange peel oil expressed the general Standard
on "Citrus oils and other furocoumarin containing essential oils" also needs to
be taken into account.

Contribution from other sources:

Critical Effect: Photoirritation

RIFM Summaries:
Human Studies: The material was tested for phototoxic potential in human
volunteers (Kaidbey and Kligman, 1980). Five $\mu L/cm^2$ of 100% bitter orange oil
was applied to $2\,cm^2$ under occlusive tape. One cm circular sites were exposed to
visible light or $20\,J/cm^2$ UVA.
Reactions were read at 24 and 48 hours. All 8 subjects reacted.

continued

Box 7.7   IFRA Guideline for Bitter Orange Peel Expressed / Cont'd

Animal studies: The NOEL was based on studies conducted with pooled samples of bitter orange oil in one miniature swine and hairless mice, which showed NOEL of 6.25%.

Rexpan Rationale/Conclusion:
The RIFM Expert Panel reviewed the critical effect data for orange peel oil, bitter, and recommended that the skin contact level should change to 1.25%, incorporating a 5 fold uncertainty factor.

The term sweet orange essential oil can refer to a number of products, produced in a variety of methods, from the same plant species. These include cold expression of fresh ripe peel producing an orange coloured essential oil with a sweet, zesty fruit odour. Steam distillation of fresh peel gives a lighter very pale yellow coloured essential oil with a lighter sweet fruity odour. The main chemical components are monoterpenes with limonene (90–95%), β-myrcene (1.7–2.5%) α-pinene (0.5–0.9%), β-phellandrene (1–1.5%) and sabinene. Other measurable components include alcohols linalool (0.5–2%) and α-terpineol (0.1–0.8%), aldehyde citronellal (0.05–0.5%), ketone carvone (1.0–1.8%). The expressed oils will usually have the highest amounts of monoterpenes and also contain coumarins bergapten and auroptenol . The essential oil is bright, warm and cheerful and coupled with attributed sedative and carmitive properties give it applications for stress related problems by promoting relaxation and inducing sleep. Other claims are that it is hypotensive (lowers blood pressure), a digestive aid for dyspepsia and for bronchial conditions of the respiratory system. In skincare it is suited to oily acne-prone complexions. Although generally considered to be non-toxic, non-irritant and non-sensitizing the reports of dermatitis attributed to high limonene content should be remembered. The presence of coumarins and their implications in phototoxicity make avoiding use on skin prior to exposure to sunlight a sensible precaution.

13. Bergamot: Citrus bergamia (Citrus aurantium)

AROMAFACT

Bergamot is an essential oil with a potentially harmful constituent. Some aromatherapists choose to use ones with the bergaptene removed. However, many professional aromatherapists will use the expressed oil, observing the IFRA guidelines limiting a maximum concentration up to 0.04%.

Bergamot yields an essential oil made up of about 300 compounds. A typical analysis would show major components linalyl acetate (25–60%), linalool (4–29%), limonene (19–38%), α-terpinene (4–13%) and β-pinene (3–13%).

However, this is an example of an essential oil in which the minor components are of great significance; it contains a furocoumarin called bergaptene (0.2–0.5%), which is a phototoxic compound and needs to be used with caution. Many oils have it removed and are called FCF (furocoumarin-free) oils, even though this is technically a rectification of the whole oil. This is discussed under 'safety' in Chapter 8. The odour of this oil is also influenced by the presence of trace components guaienol, spathulenol, nerolidol, farnesol and β-sinensal. Box 7.8 shows safety data for bergamot oil and Box 7.9 shows a material data safety sheet.

Box 7.8   Safety data for Bergamot

Botanical name: *Citrus bergamia (= Citrus aurantium subsp. bergamia)*
Family: Rutaceae
Oil from: Fruit by expression

Notable constituents:

Linalyl acetate	36–45%
Limonene	28–32%
Linalool	11–22%
Bergapten	0.3–0.4%

Hazards:
Phototoxic (strong)
Photocarcinogenic

Contraindications (dermal): If applied to the skin at over maximum use level, skin must not be exposed to sunlight or sunbed rays for 12 hours.

Maximum use level: 0.4%

Toxicity data & recommendations: Phototoxicity is due to the presence of bergapten and some eight other furanocoumarins [216]. Several studies have shown that bergamot oil has carcinogenic properties when applied to mouse skin which is then irradiated with UV light. This photocarcinogenicity is due to bergapten. Bergamot oil, in the absence of UV light, is not carcinogenic; even low concentration sunscreens can completely inhibit bergapten-enhanced phototumorigenesis.

    IFRA recommends that, for application to areas of skin exposed to sunshine, bergamot oil be limited to a maximum of 0.4% in the final product, except for bath preparations, soaps and other products which are washed off the skin. See note on combinations of phototoxic oils.

Comments: A treated oil, sometimes rectified by distillation, is obtainable as bergapten-free oil. This oil is also known as furanocoumarin-free bergamot, or bergamot FCF. Its odour is inferior to that of the untreated, cold pressed oil, but it is not phototoxic or photocarcinogenic.

Compare: Angelica, cumin, lime, rue

Courtesy of Robert Tissetand-taken from Essential Oils Safety. A Guide for Health Care Professionals (Churchill Livingstone)

Box 7.9 Material data safety sheet for Bergamot

MATERIAL SAFETY DATA SHEET
ACCORDING TO EC LEGISLATION 91/155/E EC

Date created: August 2002   Date revised: June 2005

1. Identification:
Commercial name: *Bergamot FCF essential oil.*
Botanical Nomenclature: *Citrus bergamia.*
INCI name: *Citrus Aurantium var. bergamia.*
CAS number: 8007–75–8
EINECS CAS number: 89957–91–5.
EEC Number: 289–612–9.

2. Composition:
Main components: *Linalyl acetate, linalool, limonene, β-pinene, γ-terpinene.*
Additives (e.g. carriers, preservatives, antioxidants): *NIL*
Bergaptene less than 20 ppm.

3. Potential Health Hazards:
Inhalation: *None identified.*
Skin: *Concentrated liquid and vapours irritating to skin by prolonged exposure.*
Eyes: *Irritating to eyes with possible damage.*
Ingestion: *Harmful if swallowed.*

4. First aid:
Inhalation: *If discomfort is felt, remove person to a well ventilated area with plenty of fresh air.*
Skin: *Remove contaminated clothing. Wash affected area with plenty of soap and water.*
Eyes: *Flush immediately with plenty of cool water for 10 to 20 minutes. Seek medical advice from a Medical Doctor.*
Ingestion: *Seek immediate medical care.*

5. In case of fire:
Extinguishing Media: *Foam, Carbon dioxide.*
Do not use: *Water.*
Special precautions: *Wear breathing apparatus as toxic vapours may be released during fire.*

6. Spill and Leak Procedure:
Individual precautions: *Eliminate sources of ignition. Keep area well ventilated and isolate the spill.*
Environmental protection: *Prevent the liquid from entering the drains and sewers.*
Cleaning methods: *Soak up the spill using inert absorbents. For large spills use pumps.*

continued

Box 7.9   Material data safety sheet for Bergamot / Cont'd

7. Handling and storage:
Store in a cool, dry and dark place in suitable containers (aluminium cans or lacquer lined steel drums).
Handle in a well ventilated area.
Keep away from sources of heat and ignition.

8. Personal Protection/Exposure control:
Respiratory protection: *Wear breathing apparatus when working in an area of high vapour concentration.*
Skin protection: *Use protective gloves. Wear protective clothing when possibility exists of contact.*
Eye protection: *Goggles should be worn.*
General precautions: *Use good industrial hygiene practice.*

9. Physiochemical properties:

Appearance:	Clear, yellowish
Odour:	Fresh, fruity, lemony
pH:	Neutral
Boiling point:	Not available
Flash point:	+ 53°C–57°C
Autoignition Temperature:	Not available
Explosion Limits:	Not available
Vapour pressure (25 °C):	Not available
Vapour Density:	>1 (air = 1)
Specific Gravity (20 °C):	0.87–0.88
Optical Rotation (20 °C):	+8°–24°
Refractive Index (20 °C):	1.46–1.47
Solubility in water (20 °C):	Negligible
Partition Coefficient log P o/w:	Not available
Evaporation rate:	*<1 (Butyl Acetate = 1)*

10. Stability and Reactivity:
Chemical Stability: *Stable.*
Conditions to avoid: *Normally stable. Not reactive with water.*
Hazardous Decomposition Products: *Not available.*

11. Sensitisers:
Citral 0.7%, Limonene 45%, Linalool 15%, total 60.7%

12. Toxicological Information:
According to RIFM-Monograph:
Acute Toxicity: Oral LD_{50}:   *10 g/kg in rats.*
                             Dermal LD_{50}:   *20 g/kg in rabbits.*
Irritation: *Tested without irritation at 4%.*
Sensitisation: *Tested without sensitisation at 4%.*

continued

Box 7.9   Material data safety sheet for Bergamot / Cont'd

Phototoxicity: *Use should be limited to 20% as the expressed oil causes phototoxic reaction in sunlight.*

13. Ecotoxicological information:
Fish Toxicity: LCO/EC$_{50}$: *Not available.*
Bacteriotoxicity: ECO/EC$_{50}$: *Not available.*

14. Disposal Method:
Check Federal, State and Local Regulations.

15. Transport Information:
UN Number 1993: Proper shipping name: Flammable Liquid N.O.S.
Hazard Class: 3.3 Packing group: III
Transport Safety: Air (ATA/ICAO)
2/PAX309/CA310/III
                    Sea (IMDG-Code): 3.3/III
                    Rail (RID): 3.31c
                    Road (ADR): 3.31c

16. Regulatory Information:
The British Essential Oil Association Chip Regulations — 2002
Hazard Symbols: Xn
Risk Phrases: R10, 65
H/C %: 55
Safety Phrases: S62

DISCLAIMER: THE INFORMATION CONTAINED IN THIS MSDS IS OBTAINED FROM CURRENT AND RELIABLE SOURCES. HOWEVER, THE DATA IS PROVIDED WITHOUT WARRANTY, EXPRESSED OR IMPLIED, REGARDING ITS CORRECTNESS OR ACCURACY. IT IS THE USER'S RESPONSIBILITY TO DETERMINE SAFE CONDITIONS FOR USE AND TO ASSUME LIABILITY FOR LOSS, INJURY, DAMAGE OR EXPENSE RESULTING FROM IMPROPER USE OF THIS PRODUCT.

Courtesy of Jasbir Chana, Phoenix Natural Products

14. Lemon (Citrus limon)

AROMAFACT

Lemon essential oil has the potential to cause skin irritation and sensitization in some individuals. It is recommended that it should be used at a maximum of 1% in a massage blend. When extracted by expression the essential oil is phototoxic so its use should be avoided on the skin prior to exposure to the sun.

A pale yellow green liquid, its fresh, light and sharp citrus odour due to its main chemical component the monoterpene limonene (55–80%). Other monoterpenes present are β-pinene (10–17%), α-pinene (2.0–2.5%) and γ-terpinene (3–10%). Also found in much smaller amounts are alcohol linalool (0.1–0.9%), aldehydes geraniol (0.9–1.7%) and neral (0.5–1%). Coumarins and furanocoumarins, although usually accounting for less than 1%, are significant for the phototoxic properties of the bergapten. Box 7.10 shows a typical analysis for a lemon essential oil. The essential oil is reputed to be spirit uplifting and stimulating in times of mental fatigue. For the body it is helpful for dealing with digestive problems, for easing aches and pains in the joints and applied to conditions such as rheumatism and gout, for lowering blood pressure and helpful for easing headaches. It is believed to strengthen the immune system and be a good deodorizer for the body and breath. In skincare it is an efficient astringent suited to oily skins. However, caution must be exercised in use on the skin for the previously stated contraindications.

15. Mandarin (Citrus noblis)

AROMAFACT

Mandarin has the reputation as a gentle essential oil considered suitable for use with children and the elderly. In common with many other citrus oils it may be phototoxic so it is advisable to avoid use before exposure to sunlight.

A yellow/orange oil with a fresh, sweet citrus odour. Its main constituents are the monoterpenes limonene (65–77%), γ-terpinene (13–21%), α-pinene (1.5–3.0%), β-pinene (1.3–2.5%), β-myrcene (1.5–2.5%). Also present alcohols citronellol, geraniol and linalool (combined total 1–1.5%) and smaller amounts of aldehydes, esters and phenols. Refreshing, uplifting, claimed to be tonic to the digestive system stimulating appetite while calming when applied to hiccups, colic and flatulence. An essential oil associated with female problems and often used in blends for easing PMS (premenstrual syndrome) and on the skin for stretch marks. Suited to congested and oily skin acting as a toner. Considered to be a nontoxic, non-irritating and non-sensitizing with a possibility of phototoxicity.

16. Grapefruit (Citrus paradisi)

AROMAFACT

Citrus paradisi is a recent hybrid plant from Citrus maxima and Citrus sinensis (sweet orange). Native to Asia and the West Indies there are many different cultivars, which have been developed horticulturally to allow efficient growth in many other countries, like Australia, USA (California and Florida) and Israel. The cultivar is identified by the name added after the botanical name e.g. Citrus paradisi Macfad.

The essential oil is a pale yellowish green with a sweet, sharp refreshing citrus odour. Its chemical composition is very high in the monoterpene limonene (85–98%) with other monoterpenes β-myrcene (1.2–1.7%),

Box 7.10   Analysis of Lemon (*Citrus limonum*)

Product Identification

Product Name :	Lemon Oil
Botanical Name :	*Citrus limonum*
Country of Origin :	Italy
Agricultural Method :	Organic
Product Code :	E511
Batch Number :	996

Principal Constituents	Constituent %
α-Pinene + α - Thujene :	1.81
Camphene :	0.04
β-Pinene :	8.57
Sabinene :	1.62
Myrcene :	1.62
α-Phellandrene :	0.04
α-Terpinene :	0.17
Limonene :	70.58
β-Phellandrene :	0.32
cis-β - Ocimene :	0.07
γ-Terpinene :	8.52
p-Cymene :	0.35
Terpinolene :	0.38
Octanal :	0.05
Nonanal :	0.12
Citronellal :	0.07
Decanal :	0.04
Linalol :	0.12
Linalyl acetate :	0.05
α-Bergamotene :	0.34
Terpinene-4-ol & β-Caryophyllene :	0.24
Neral :	1.01
α-Terpineol :	0.37
Neryl acetate :	0.32
β-Bisbolene :	0.58
Geranial :	1.65
Geranyl acetate :	0.17
Nerol :	0.13
Geraniol :	0.06

Courtesy of Geoff Lyth, Quinessence Aromatherapy Ltd

phellandrene (1.0–1.5%), α-pinene (0.2–1.7%), smaller amounts of alcohols linalool (0.2–0.5%), geraniol (0.1–0.2%) and aldehyde citronellal (0.1–0.22%). Other analyzed components are usually present in much lower amounts. An analytical analysis and GC trace for a sample of grapefruit essential oil is shown in Box 7.11. Reputed to be excellent for lifting spirits in times of depression, stress, nervous and physical exhaustion. A big seller in airports for dealing with jet-lag symptoms of tiredness and headaches. Also found in preparations for minimizing cellulite due to claims that it detoxes, nourishes cells and acts as a diuretic. Also said to be balancing for the digestive system and for use on oily and congested skins. Non-toxic, non-irritant and non-sensitizing. Opinions differ about its phototoxicity so it is best to avoid use on skin prior to exposure to sunlight. It needs careful storage as it oxidizes rapidly.

Citrus oils should be used with care. The IFRA guidelines for their use and other furocoumarin containing essential oils are shown in Box 7.12.

Box 7.11   Analysis of Grapefruit (*Citrus paradisi*)

Product Identification

Product Name :	Grapefruit (white) Oil
Botanical Name :	*Citrus paradisi*
Country of Origin :	Florida USA
Agricultural Method :	Conventional
Product Code :	E420
Batch Number :	585

Principal Constituents	Constituent %
α-Thujene :	0.54
β-Pinene :	0.25
Myrcene :	1.90
Octanal :	0.45
Limonene :	95.00
β-Ocimene :	0.08
γ-Terpinene :	0.15
Octanol :	Trace
Linalol :	0.13
Nonanal :	0.06
Citronellal :	Trace
Decanal :	0.27
Neral :	Trace
Geranial :	0.09
Geranyl acetate :	0.09
β-Caryophyllene :	0.24
Valencene :	0.06
Nootkatone :	0.10

Courtesy of Geoff Lyth, Quinessence Aromatherapy Ltd

Box 7.12 IFRA guidelines for use of citrus oils and other furocoumarin containing essential oils

	Last Amendment	December 01, 1996
	First issued	December 01, 1996

CAS #	Recommendation	Skin Contact	Non-Skin Contact
	Restricted	15 ppm 5-MOP (excl. rinse-off pr)	No limitation

Where the bergapten (5-methoxypsoralen) content of all relevant oils present in a compound has been determined, it is recommended that for applications on areas of skin exposed to sunshine, excluding bath preparations, soaps and other products which are washed off the skin, the total level of bergapten in the consumer products should not exceed 0.0015% (15 ppm). This is equivalent to 0.0075% (75 ppm) in a fragrance compound used at 20% in the consumer product.

Where the level of bergapten has not been determined by appropriate methods, the limits specified in the guidelines on individual oils should apply.

In those cases, where such oils are used in combination with other phototoxic ingredients, the additive effect has to be taken into consideration and the use levels have to be reduced accordingly. The sum of the concentrations of all phototoxic fragrance ingredients, expressed in % of their recommended maximum level in the consumer product, shall not exceed 100.

Restrictions for furocoumarin containing essential oils have been recommended for Angelica root oil, Bergamot oil expressed, Bitter orange oil expressed, Cumin oil, Grapefruit oil expressed, Lemon oil cold pressed, Lime oil expressed, Rue oil.

The following essential oils contain small amounts of phototoxic furocoumarins. These levels are not high enough to require special restrictions if used alone, but if used in combination with one or the other phototoxic essential oil, attention should be paid that the total level of bergapten (5-MOP) in the consumer product does not exceed 15 ppm. This is equivalent to 75 ppm in a fragrance compound used at 20% in a consumer product. It is the responsibility of fragrance manufacturers to ensure that the level is observed. Typical levels of 5-MOP are the following: Petitgrain Mandarin oil – 50 ppm, Tangerine oil cold pressed – 50 ppm, Mandarin oil cold pressed – 250 ppm, Parsley leaf oil – 20 ppm.

These recommendations are based on the published phototoxic effects of bergapten and the established dose-effect relationships Young at al., J. Photochem. Photobiol. B, 7, 231 (1990); Dubertret et al. ibid 7, 251 (1990), idem, ibid, 7, 362 (1990).

These guidelines are regularly updated so it is advisable to check their website.

Courtesy of IFRA

Gramineae (Poaceae)

17. Lemongrass (Cymbopogon citratus)

AROMAFACT

Several species exist but two main ones are available to aromatherapists and these have differing properties. Each species again will have chemotypes.

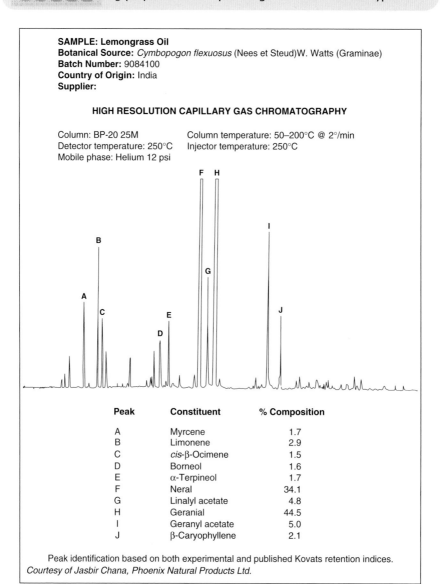

SAMPLE: Lemongrass Oil
Botanical Source: *Cymbopogon flexuosus* (Nees et Steud)W. Watts (Graminae)
Batch Number: 9084100
Country of Origin: India
Supplier:

HIGH RESOLUTION CAPILLARY GAS CHROMATOGRAPHY

Column: BP-20 25M
Detector temperature: 250°C
Mobile phase: Helium 12 psi

Column temperature: 50–200°C @ 2°/min
Injector temperature: 250°C

Peak	Constituent	% Composition
A	Myrcene	1.7
B	Limonene	2.9
C	*cis*-β-Ocimene	1.5
D	Borneol	1.6
E	α-Terpineol	1.7
F	Neral	34.1
G	Linalyl acetate	4.8
H	Geranial	44.5
I	Geranyl acetate	5.0
J	β-Caryophyllene	2.1

Peak identification based on both experimental and published Kovats retention indices.
Courtesy of Jasbir Chana, Phoenix Natural Products Ltd.

Figure 7.9 **Lemongrass.** Analysis of *Cymbopogon flexuosus*, showing a typical composition.

Although many species and varieties exist, the most commonly encountered ones are West Indian, *Cymbopogon citratus*, and East Indian,
Cymbopogon flexuosus. Within each variety there are a number of chemotypes. A generalized list of chemical components would include citral
(citral is a mixture of the isomers neral and geranial), myrcene, limonene,
linalool, geraniol, and geranyl acetate. *Cymbopogon flexuosus* is very high
in citral (up to 85%) and low in myrcene. *Cymbopogon citratus* is much
lower in citral, but higher in neral and myrcene. These variations are
reflected in the properties of the oils, with *Cymbopogon citratus* having
analgesic action due to the myrcene. Both have antimicrobial, antiseptic,
calmative, insecticidal and sedative actions with tonic effects on healing. Lemongrass is non-toxic but may cause dermal irritation or sensitization in some individuals. As one of the cheapest oils, it is not usually
adulterated.

A typical oil supplier's material data sheet is shown for *Cymbopogon flexuosus* in Box 7.13.

18. Vetivert (Vetivera zizaniodes)

AROMAFACT

An essential oil with a woody, earthy and smoky odour which can be very
overpowering. This odour is often strongly disliked despite being known in
India and Sri Lanka as the 'oil of tranquillity'. Better used in low concentrations
in blends as dilution makes it more subtle and acceptable.

Solvent extraction produces a resinoid employed in the perfume industry.
The essential oil is extracted from the root and rootlets by steam distillation.
Colour and scent can vary according to the source, the viscous liquid can
be pale yellow to olive, amber and even brown. Its chemical components
include alcohols vetiverol (0.2–21%), bicyclovetiverol (9–14%) and tricy-
clovetiverol (2.5–4.5%), the ester vetiverol acetate (1–2.3%), ketones α- and
β-vetivone (5–14%) and sesquiterpenes and organic aids. Commercially
used as a fixative and fragrance for oriental perfume, cosmetic, bathing
preparations and as a food preservative. In aromatherapy it is reputed to
have deep relaxing properties, an immuno-stimulant, for easing muscle
and joint pain and for dealing with menstrual and menopausal symptoms.
Suitable for oily skin prone to acne. Considered to be a non-toxic, non-
irritant and non-sensitizing.

Box 7.13   A typical supplier's data sheet: Lemongrass (*Cymbopogon flexuosus*)

MATERIAL SAFETY DATA SHEET
ACCORDING TO EC LEGISLATION 91/155/E EC

Date created: June 1998   Date revised: June 1998

1. Identification
Commercial name: *Lemongrass essential oil.*
Botanical nomenclature: *Cymbopogon flexuosus.*
INCI name: *Not available.*
CAS number: *Not available.*
EINECS/ELINCS number: *Not available.*

2. Composition
Main components: *Citral.*
Additives (e.g. carriers, preservatives, antioxidants): *Nil.*

3. Potential health hazards
Inhalation: *None identified.*
Skin: *Concentrated liquid and vapour irritating to skin by prolonged exposure.*
Eyes: *Irritating to eyes with possible damage.*
Ingestion: *Harmful if swallowed.*

4. First aid
Inhalation: *If discomfort is felt, remove person to a well-ventilated area with plenty of fresh air.*
Skin: *Remove contaminated clothing. Wash affected area with plenty of soap and water.*
Eyes: *Flush immediately with plenty of cool water for 10 to 20 minutes. Seek medical advice from a medical doctor.*
Ingestion: *Seek immediate medical care.*

5. In case of fire
Extinguishing media: *foam, carbon dioxide.*
Do not use: *Water.*

Special precautions: *Wear breathing apparatus as toxic vapours may be released during fire.*

6. Spill and leak procedure
Individual precautions: *Eliminate sources of ignition. Keep area well ventilated and isolate the spill.*
Environmental protection: *Prevent the liquid from entering the drains and sewers.*
Cleaning methods: *Soak up the spill using inert absorbents. For large spills use pumps.*

7. Handling and storage
Store in a cool, dry and dark place in suitable containers (aluminium cans or lacquer-lined steel drums).
Handle in a well-ventilated area.
Keep away from sources of heat and ignition.

8. Personal protection/exposure control
Respiratory protection: *Wear breathing apparatus when working in an area of high vapour concentration.*
Skin protection: *Use protective gloves. Wear protective clothing when possibility exists of contact.*
Eye protection: *Goggles should be worn.*
General precautions: *Use good industrial hygiene practice.*

9. Physiochemical properties
Appearance: *Reddish-brown liquid*
Odour: *Pungent, warm, heavy with lemon undertones*
pH: *Neutral*

continued

Box 7.13   A typical supplier's data sheet: Lemongrass (*Cymbopogon flexuosus*) / Cont'd

Boiling point: *Not available*
Flash point: *72°C*
Autoignition temperature: *Not available*
Explosion limits: *Not available*
Vapour pressure (25°C): *Not available*
Vapour density: *> 1 (air = 1)*
Specific gravity (25°C): *0.889–0.911 g/ml*
Optical rotation (25°C): *−3° to +1°*
Refractive index (25°C): *1.485–1.489*
Solubility in water (20°C): *Negligible*
Partition coefficient log $P_{o/w}$: *Not available*
Evaporation rate: *< 1 (butyl acetate =1)*

10. Stability and reactivity
Chemical stability: *Stable*
Conditions to avoid: *Normally stable. Not reactive with water.*
Hazardous decomposition products: *Not available.*

11. Toxicological information
According to RIFM-Monograph:
Acute toxicity: *Oral LD_{50}: 5 g/kg in rats. Dermal LD_{50}: 2 g/kg in rabbits.*
Irritation: *Tested without irritation at 4%.*

Sensitization: *Tested without sensitization at 4%.*
Phototoxicity: *No phototoxic reaction reported.*

12. Ecotoxicological information
Fish toxicity: LCO/EC_{50}: *Not available.*
Bacteriotoxicity: ECO/EC_{50}: *Not available.*

13. Disposal method
Check Federal, State and Local Regulations.

14. Transport information
Nonhazardous material transport in suitable containers.

15. Legislation
Meets IFRA and RIFM guidelines.

DISCLAIMER: THE INFORMATION CONTAINED IN THIS MSDS IS OBTAINED FROM CURRENT AND RELIABLE SOURCES. HOWEVER, THE DATA IS PROVIDED WITHOUT WARRANTY, EXPRESSED OR IMPLIED, REGARDING ITS CORRECTNESS OR ACCURACY. IT IS THE USER'S RESPONSIBILITY TO DETERMINE SAFE CONDITIONS FOR USE AND TO ASSUME LIABILITY FOR LOSS, INJURY, DAMAGE OR EXPENSE RESULTING FROM IMPROPER USE OF THIS PRODUCT.

Courtesy of Phoenix Natural Products Ltd

Asteraceae (Compositae)

19. The Chamomiles

AROMAFACT

The composition of essential oils depends upon species and chemotypes.

The general name chamomile is very misleading as there are three main species producing essential oils for aromatherapy. Each produces an essential oil with a different composition and properties. The species are Roman or English (*Anthemis nobilis*, also *Chamaemelum nobile*), German or blue (*Matricaria chamomila*, or *M. recutica*) and Moroccan (*Anthemis mixta*, or *Ormensis mixta*, or *Ormensis multicaulis*). The Moroccan is a more recently introduced oil with different properties from the other chamomiles and is sometimes called ormenis oil.

Typical compositions would be as follows:

- Roman: esters of angelic and tiglic acids (up to 85%), and pinene, farnesol, nerolidol, pinacarvone, cineole.
- German: chamazulene, farnesene, bisabobol, bisabobol oxide, *cis*-spiro ether. It also has four principal chemotypes.
- Moroccan: santolina alcohol, α-pinene, germacene, *trans*-spirocarveol.

The most expensive chamomile is the German and is distinguished by a dark blue colour. This is due to the presence of a sesquiterpene compound called chamazulene, which is formed by the decomposition of a colourless compound called matricene in the flowers during the distillation process. Chamazulene is not present in the plant. This can lead to adulteration of inferior quality Moroccan essential oil by the addition of synthetic chamazulene. Properties attributed to the Roman and German are anti-inflammatory (particularly the German), analgesic, calmative, antispasmodic and generally mentally soothing and relaxing. They are both regarded to be nontoxic and nonirritant but may cause dermatitis in susceptible individuals. There are fewer data available for the newer Moroccan chamomile but it is becoming more acceptable as an economical alternative as it emulates many of the properties of the others. It appears to be generally non-toxic and non-irritant due to its high level of alcohol.

The GC analysis data show samples of German chamomile, *Matricaria recutica*, with a presence of chamazulene at 3.27% (Fig 7.10). Typical values would be in the range of 2.5–7.5%. Analysis of the Roman/English, *Anthemis nobilis* (Fig. 7.11), does not show any chamazulene as it is below the level (0.01%) that would be detected by the GC analysis. However, the oil itself may show a pale blue tint due to traces of chamazulene.

Myrtaceae

20. The Eucalyptuses

AROMAFACT

Eucalyptus is a general name for up to 750 different species of the genus *Eucalyptus*, of which at least 500 produce essential oils. Even within the ones available to the aromatherapist there are many subspecies and chemotypes.

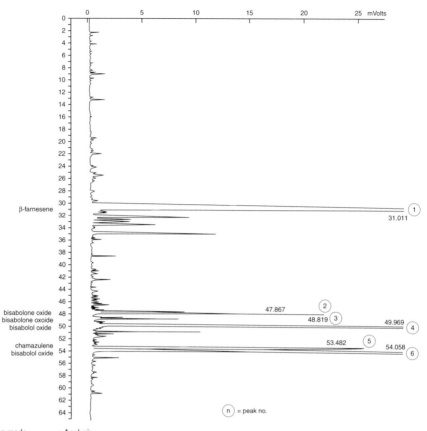

β-farnesene

bisabolone oxide
bisabolone oxoide
bisabolol oxide

chamazulene
bisabolol oxide

Run mode   : Analysis
Peak measurement : Peak area
Calculation type : Percent

Peak no.	Peak name	Result (%)	Retention time (min)	Time offset (min)	Area (counts)	Sep. code	Width 1/2 (s)	Status codes
1	b-Farnesene	30.46	31.011	0.000	1 448 129	VV	32.2	
2	Bisabolone oxide	3.30	47.867	0.007	156 988	VV	6.0	
3	Bisabolone oxide	2.87	48.819	0.009	136 542	VV	5.6	
4	Bisabolol oxide	24.17	49.969	−0.001	1 148 898	VV	12.1	
5	Chamazulene	3.27	53.482	0.002	155 378	VV	5.7	
6	Bisabolol oxide	15.06	54.058	0.008	716 130	VB	10.6	
	Totals:	79.13		0.025	3 762 065			

Total unidentified counts: 99 904
Detected peaks: 183   Rejected peaks: 65   Identified peaks: 6

Figure 7.10   Chamomile. Analysis of German *Matricaria recutica* or *M. chamomilla*, a blue chamomile, which has chamazulene present at between 2.5% and 7.5%. This sample has 3.27%. Courtesy of Jenny Warden, Traceability.

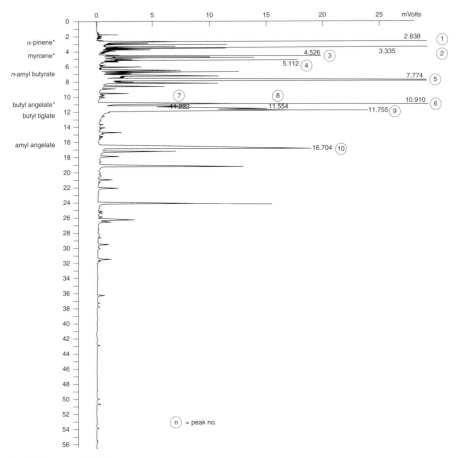

Run mode   : Analysis
Peak measurement : Peak area
Calculation type : Percent

Peak no.	Peak name	Result (%)	Retention time (min)	Time offset (min)	Area (counts)	Sep. code	Width 1/2)	Status codes
1	α-Pinene	10.24	2.638	−0.000	309 996	VV	2.4	
2	β-Pinene	2.82	3.335	0.000	85 191	VV	2.1	
3	Myrcene	1.98	4.526	−0.000	60 000	VV	2.8	
4	Limonene	2.36	5.112	0.000	71 385	VV	3.5	
5	n-Amyl butyrate	13.68	7.774	0.000	413 906	VV	9.3	
6	Butyl angelate	9.50	10.910	0.000	287 633	BV	9.1	
7	Butyl angelate	2.35	11.222	−0.000	71 094	VV	9.4	
8	Butyl tiglate	6.42	11.554	−0.000	194 350	VV	23.2	
9	Butyl tiglate	6.49	11.755	0.000	196 491	VV	10.0	
10	Amyl angelate	9.76	16.704	0.002	295 209	BV	14.9	
	Totals:	65.60		0.002	1 985 255			

Total unidentified counts: 1 040 952
Detected peaks: 206   Rejected peaks: 132   Identified peaks: 10

Figure 7.11   Chamomile. Analysis of *Anthemis nobilis*, Roman (or English) chamomile. The chamazulene level is often below the level detected by the GC analysis of about 0.01%. Courtesy of Jenny Warden, Traceability.

The main essential oil-producing species of *Eucalyptus* include *Eucalyptus globulus*, also called blue gum eucalyptus; *Eucalyptus dives*, known as broad-leaved peppermint eucalyptus; *Eucalyptus citriodora*, known as lemon-scented eucalyptus; *Eucalyptus radiata*, known as narrow-leaved peppermint gum; *Eucalyptus smithii*, known as gully gum; and *Eucalyptus polybractea*, known as blue mallee. Within each species there are many subspecies and chemo-types. This illustrates a very complex situation, producing essential oils with varying compositions and properties.

Major components listed under a general heading for eucalyptus would be citronellal, cineole, camphene, fenchene, limonene, phellandrene and pinene. The individual species show the different proportions (amounts shown are approximate percentages):

- *Eucalyptus globulus*: α-pinene (11%), β-pinene (0.15%), α-phellandrene (0.09%), 1,8-cineole (69%), limonene (3.3%), aromadendrene (1.6%), globu-lol (5.33%).
- *Eucalyptus dives*: piperitone (40–50%), phellandrene (20–30%), globulol (6%), 1,8-cineole (0.45%), limonene (0.3%), terpineol-4 (4%), *p*-cymene (3.4%).
- *Eucalyptus citriodora*: citronellal (56%), citronellol (8%), 1,8-cineole (2%), γ-terpinyl acetate (2%), citronellic acid (5.5%), citronellyl acetate (11.5%).
- *Eucalyptus radiata*: α-pinene (15–21%), 1,8-cineole (57–71%), limonene (5%), *p*-cymene (0.3–1%).
- *Eucalyptus smithii*: α-pinene (4.1%), β-pinene (0.1%), 1,8-cineole (81%), terpineol-4 (0.1%), globulol (2.4%).
- *Eucalyptus polybractea*: α-pinene (0.9%), β-pinene (0.25%), 1,8-cineole (92%), limonene (1.1%), terpineol-4 (0.5%), globulol (0.05%).

The eucalyptus essential oils find widespread applications in pharmaceuti-cal formulations like mouthwashes, inhalers, hygiene and cleansing prod-ucts such as soaps and detergents, for room sprays and insect repellents, as a flavouring in foods, in perfumery and as a starting material for indus-trial compounds that are extracted, mainly by distillation. For aromather-apy, the oils can be used for skin care, the respiratory system, the immune system, the nervous system, the urino-genital system and the musculo-skel-etal system.

The essential oils have also been shown to have bacteriostatic activity. They are generally considered to be safe when used correctly externally but there is a possibility of sensitization by *Eucalyptus globulus* in some individuals. Taken internally, eucalyptus oils are toxic. When choosing a eucalyptus essential oil the varying compositions and properties must be carefully considered in the context of the client's condition.

The GC analysis shows samples of *Eucalyptus citriodora* (Fig 7.12) and *Eucalyptus radiata* (Fig 7.13). Both of these traces show that published data are not always found in actual samples of essential oil. The *Eucalyptus citri-odora* shows a high level of citronellal (73.94%), while the *Eucalyptus radiata* has a high level of 1,8-cineole (76.37%); both of these are higher than in the published data. However, for *Eucalyptus radiata* values of 1,8-cineole

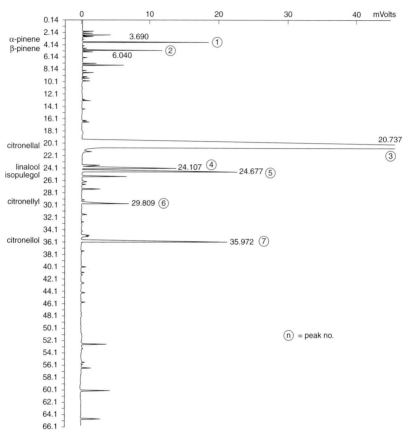

Run mode   : Analysis
Peak measurement : Peak area
Calculation type : Percent

Peak no.	Peak name	Result (%)	Retention time (min)	Time offset (min)	Area (counts)	Sep. code	Width 1/2 (s)	Status codes
1	α-Pinene	0.78	3.690	0.000	34 344	PV	1.7	
2	β-Pinene	0.64	5.040	−0.000	27 892	VV	2.2	
3	Citronellal	73.94	20.737	−0.003	3 235 287	BB	27.6	
4	Linalool	2.53	24.107	−0.003	110 529	VV	7.5	
5	Isopulegol	5.33	24.677	−0.003	233 442	VV	10.1	
6	Citronellyl	1.40	29.809	−0.001	61 144	VB	7.2	
7	Citronellol	5.95	35.972	0.002	260 394	VP	11.8	
	Totals	90.57		−0.008	3 963 032			

Total unidentified counts: 412 638
Detected peaks: 327   Rejected peaks: 276   Identified peaks: 7

Figure 7.12   Eucalyptus. Analysis of *Eucalyptus citriodora*, showing a typical composition with a high level of citronellal (73.94%). Courtesy of Jenny Warden, Traceability.

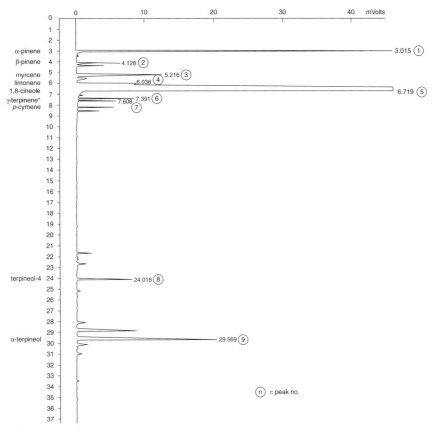

Run mode   : Analysis
Peak measurement : Peak area
Calculation type : Percent

Peak no.	Peak name	Result (%)	Retention time (min)	Time offset (min)	Area (counts)	Sep. code	Width 1/2 (s)	Status codes
1	α-Pinene	3.88	3.015	0.000	127 394	BB	2.0	
2	β-Pinene	0.67	4.128	−0.000	22 123	BV	2.8	
3	Myrcene	2.60	5.216	−0.000	85 517	BV	6.7	
4	Limonene	2.08	6.036	0.000	68 290	BV	8.3	
5	1,8-Cineole	76.37	6.719	0.001	2 509 625	VB	13.3	
6	γ-Terpinene	0.69	7.391	0.001	22 511	BV	2.5	
7	p-Cymene	0.44	7.608	0.000	14 553	VB	2.4	
8	Terpineol-4	1.49	24.018	−0.002	49 024	PB	5.4	
9	γ-Terpineol	6.04	29.569	0.001	198 329	VB	9.3	
	Totals	94.26		0.001	3 097 366			

Total unidentified counts: 188 593
Detected peaks: 222   Rejected peaks: 199   Identified peaks: 9

Figure 7.13 Eucalyptus. Analysis of an Australian sample of *Eucalyptus radiata*. The level of 1,8-cineole is quite high, 76.37%. The quoted range is 64–75%. Levels above 75% indicate *Eucalyptus globulus* or another variety. Courtesy of Jenny Warden, Traceability.

in the range 64–75% are often quoted, with values above this indicating *Eucalyptus globulus* or another species. The charts show a marked difference in the 1,8-cineole levels: the level is very high in *Eucalyptus radiata* but the compound is not shown in the major components of *Eucalyptus citriodora*.

21. Tea tree (Melaleuca alternifolia)

AROMAFACT

Tea tree is a misleading name. Tea tree is the general name given to all melaleuca trees (of the family Myrtaceae), usually associated with Australia. The species *Melaleuca alternifolia* is the one producing the essential oil. Many chemotypes exist and standards set for composition may encourage adulteration.

The tea tree, or sometimes ti-tree, is actually a general name for members of the *Melaleuca* plant genus. The term tea tree comes from local usage as a type of herbal tea prepared from the leaves. *Melaleuca alternifolia* is a worldwide top-selling essential oil. Other oils from this family include cajeput (*Melaleuca cajeputi*) and niaouli (*Melaleuca viridiflora*), which are distinctive essential oils with their own characteristics.

A typical listing for major components would be α-pinene (2.0–2.3%), β-pinene (0.2–0.5%), myrcene (0.3–0.5%), α-phellandrene (0.6–0.9%), α-terpinene (7.0–7.6%), limonene (1.0–1.6%), 1,8-cineole (2.0–14.5%), γ-terpinene (14.0–17.5%), *p*-cymene (2.5–6.5%), terpinolene (2.8–3.9%), terpineol-4 (35.0–47.0%), α-terpineol (2.9–5.6%) (Fig. 7.14 show actual analytical data).

The Australian standard for *Melaleuca alternifolia* tea tree oil sets levels for 1,8-cineole that should not exceed 15% and for terpineol-4 that should not be less than 30%. The components of this type of tea tree oil vary considerably owing to the existence of different varieties of the same plant species; there are also many chemotypes and it has been shown that even trees growing next to each other can produce oils with differing composition. Imposing chemical standards can encourage adulteration; commonly oils of various cultivars and species are blended and terpineol-4 is often added.

Melaleuca alternifolia has a long history of use by Australian aborigines and was put into military first aid kits during World War II. It has impressive antimicrobial properties, acting on viruses, bacteria and fungi. Clinical studies have shown it to be effective as an antiseptic in dentistry, various skin conditions including acne, boils, dandruff, vaginal thrush (a fungus), foot infections and coughs and colds. The antimicrobial activity is attributed to the terpineol-4 and *p*-cymene. It is additionally attributed with immuno-stimulant activity aiding the body to respond to and resist infections.

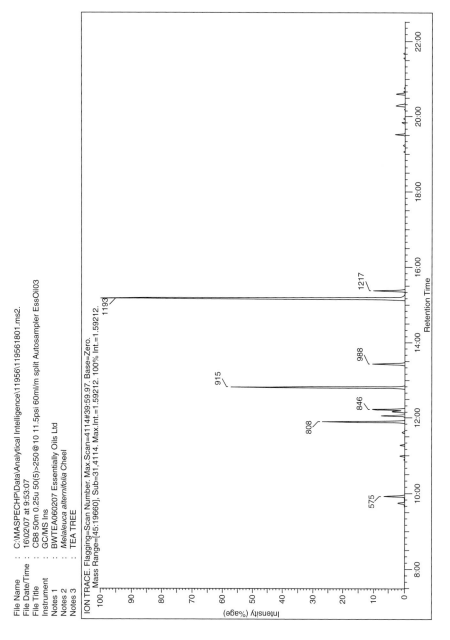

File Name   : C:\MASPECHP\Data\Analytical Intelligence\119561\119561801.ms2.
File Date/Time : 16\02\07 at 9:53:07
File Title   : CB8 50m 0.25u 50(5)>250@10 11.5psi 60ml/m split Autosampler EssOil03
Instrument   : GC/MS Ins
Notes 1   : BWTEA060207 Essentially Oils Ltd
Notes 2   : *Melaleuca alternifolia* Cheel
Notes 3   : TEA TREE

ION TRACE. Flagging=Scan Number. Max.Scan=4114#39:59.97. Base=Zero.
Mass Range=[45:19660]. Sub=31,4114. Max.Int.=1.59212. 100% Int.=1.59212.

Figure 7.14   See legend next page

Peak Area	Peak Time	Peak Scan	Marker Text
0.83	9:44.57	554	α-Thujene
2.28	9:55.28	575	α-Pinene
0.11	10:53.92	690	Sabinene
0.59	10:59.53	701	β-Pinene
0.55	11:16.87	735	β-Myrcene
0.36	11:37.27	775	Probably α-Phellandrene
9.80	11:54.10	808	α-Terpinene
2.72	12:03.79	827	p-Cymene
0.43	12:09.91	839	Limonene
1.27	12:10.42	840	β-Phellandrene
3.96	12:13.47	846	Eucalyptol
20.46	12:48.66	915	γ-Terpinene
3.52	13:25.89	988	α-Terpinolene
41.99	15:10.43	1193	Terpinen-4-ol
3.56	15:22.66	1217	α-Terpineol
0.09	18:31.85	1588	Copaene
0.19	19:04.49	1652	Possibly a Gurjunene isomer
0.25	19:14.18	1671	trans-β-Caryophyllene
1.27	19:31.52	1705	Probably Aromadendrene
0.42	19:50.90	1743	Probably Alloaromadendrene
0.23	19:57.01	1755	Unidentified C15H24
1.08	20:17.92	1796	Probably Ledene
0.74	20:18.43	1797	Germacrene B
1.20	20:36.28	1832	d-Cadinene
0.18	20:40.36	1840	Unidentified
0.11	20:45.97	1851	Unidentified
0.20	21:33.39	1944	Caryophyllene Oxide
0.20	21:40.02	1957	Unidentified

Courtesy of Charles Wells and Bill Morden, Analytical Intelligence

Figure 7.14   Tea tree. Analysis of *Melaleuca alternifolia*, showing a typical composition.

Melaleuca alternifolia is generally considered to be nontoxic and nonirritant. However, it may cause sensitization in some individuals and several components have been found to be responsible. One of these, 1,8-cineole, is restricted by regulation to a maximum of 15% as it is a sensitizing substance.

A more detailed examination of *Melaleuca alternifolia* is shown in Box 7.14. This information, in this format, is aimed at healthcare professionals.

Geraniaceae

22. Geranium (Pelargonium graveolens)

AROMAFACT

There are over 700 varieties of geranium, with two main ones used for essential oil production.

Generally *Pelargonium graveolens* gives a rose aroma while *Pelargonium odorantissimum* has an apple-like fragrance. Although there are over 700 varieties of cultivated pelargoniums, the main commercial oil-producing one is *Pelargonium graveolens*.

Box 7.14   A typical data sheet aimed at healthcare professionals: Tea tree

Melaleuca alternifolia fol. [Tea tree]
Myrtaceae

Representative constituents

Hydrocarbons
Monoterpenes (25–40%) α-pinene 0.8–3.6%, β-pinene 0.1–1.6%, α-terpinene
4.6–12.8%, γ-terpinene 9.5–28.3%, p-cymene 0.4–12.4%, limonene
0.4–2.77%, terpinolene 1.6–5.4%, α-thujene 0.1–2.1%, sabinene 0–3.2%,
myrcene 0.1–1.8%, α-phellandrene 0.1–1.9%, β-phellandrene 0.4–1.6%,
terpinolene 3%
Sesquiterpenes β-caryophyllene 1%, aromadendrene 0.1–6.6%, viridiflorene
0.3–6.1%, d-cadinene 0.1–7.5%, allo-aromadendrene 0.3%, α-muurolene 0.1%,
bicyclogermacrene 0.1%, α-gurjunene 0.2%, calamenene 0.1%

Alcohols
Monoterpenols terpineol-4 28.6–57.9%, α-terpineol 1.5–7.6%
Sesquiterpenols globulol 0.1–3.0%, viridiflorol 0.1–1.4%, cubenol 0.1%

Oxides
1,8-cineole 0.5–17.7%, 1,4-cineole trace

Properties and indications
analgesic	
antibacterial	
antifungal	Candida
anti-infectious	abscesses, skin infections, intestinal infections, bronchitis, genital infections
anti-inflammatory	abscesses (including dental), pyorrhoea, vaginitis, sinusitis, otitis
antiparasitic	lamblias, ascaris, ankylostoma
antiviral	viral enteritis
immunostimulant	low IgA and IgM
neurotonic	debility, depression, PMS, anxiety
phlebotonic	haemorrhoids, varicose veins, aneurism
radioprotective	radiotherapy burns (preventative)

Observations
- no known contraindications
- no irritation or sensitization at 1% dilution when tested on humans
- no phototoxic effects reported

continued

> **Box 7.14** A typical data sheet aimed at healthcare professionals: Tea tree / Cont'd
>
> - said to prevent post-operative shock due to anaesthetic
> - tea tree oil has a low cineole content and is nonirritant to the skin or the mucous surfaces
> - in a single blind randomized study on 124 patients with mild to moderate acne, tea tree oil was compared with benzoyl peroxide: both treatments produced a significant improvement, while fewer patients using the tea tree oil reported unwanted effects.
>
> *Courtesy of Len and Shirley Price, taken from Aromatherapy for Health Professionals (Churchill Livingstone)*

Typical chemical composition would show: citronellol (21–28%), geraniol (14–18%), linalool (10–14%), geranyl acetate (0.3–4.5%), menthone (0.7–2.2%), limonene (0.1–0.6%), geranyl butyrate (0.5–1.3%), myrcene (0.2–0.4%), α-pinene (0.18–0.4%).

A GC analysis is shown in Chapter 5 (Fig. 5.2). The oil is non-toxic, non-irritant and generally non-sensitizing, but there is a chance of contact dermatitis with sensitive individuals. It has many uses in cosmetics, fragrances and flavourings. In aromatherapy it has been attributed beneficial effects in a variety of conditions including menstrual disorders, and as an anti-inflammatory, diuretic, antiseptic, antidepressant, calmative and balancing for the endocrine system.

Piperaceae

23. Black Pepper (Piper nigrum)

AROMAFACT

The essential oil is extracted from steam distillation of the fully grown unripe fruit which are then dried to form the familiar black peppercorns. Black peppercorns contain higher amounts of oil and are more aromatic than the white pepper.

A pale olive green essential oil with a sharp, warm, woody spicy odour. Principal constituents are monoterpenes limonone (15–17%), sabinene (9–19%), β-pinene (5–14%), α-pinene (2–11%), β-myrcene (1.5–2.5%), carene (0.2–14.0%), α-phellandrene (0.5–5.0%), sesquiterpenes β-caryphyllene (9–31%), β-bisabolene (0.1–5.1%) and β-farnescene (1–3%). Box 7.15 shows a chemical analysis and Box 7.16 is a material safety data sheet from a supplier. Traditionally used as a warming and stimulating essential oil for mind and body coupled with analgesic and vasodilating properties make it a good choice for muscular aches and pains and in pre-sport preparations. In herbal medicine black pepper has been used for digestive problems such as nausea, colic, heartburn, diarrhoea and flatulence. Although it is believed to be nontoxic and nonsensitizing it can be irritant with a rubefacient ('making red' by increasing localized blood circulation) effect. It is also said to be incompatible with homeopathic treatments.

Box 7.15   Certificate of analysis for Black Pepper (*Piper nigrum*)

CERTIFICATE OF ESSENTIAL OIL ANALYSIS 2007
ESSENTIAL OIL OF BLACK PEPPER (*Piper nigrum*)
COUNTRY OF ORIGIN – INDIA
EXTRACTION – STEAM DISTILLATION FROM CRUSHED BLACK PEPPERCORNS

Authenticated..

Peak No	Component Name	Amount (%)
1	α pinene	10.16
2	α-phellandrene	1.35
3	β pinene	10.43
4	sabinene	13.75
5	δ-3-carene	9.20
6	α-phellandrene	0.80
7	myrcene	1.67
8	limonene	16.42
9	β-phellandrene	2.27
10	ρ-cymene	2.15
11	δ elemene	1.98
12	α-copaene	2.74
13	linalol	0.57
14	β-caryophyllene	18.00
15	terpinen-4-ol	0.85
16	α-humulene	1.21
17	(z)-β-farnesene	0.42
18	β-selinene	0.47
19	α-muurolene	0.46
20	β-bisabolene	1.20
21	δ-cadinene	0.68
22	caryophyllene oxide	3.22

Courtesy of Jane Collins, Phytobotanica

Box 7.16 Material safety data sheet for Black Pepper (*Piper nigrum*)

1. Identification of substance/preparation & company
PRODUCT NAME;   PEPPER OIL BLACK
COMPANY NAME: Phytobotanica UK Ltd, Mill House Organic Medicinal and
Aromatic Plant Farm, Greens Barn, Greens Lane, Lydiate, Merseyside L31 4HZ
Emergency Tel No: 01695 420 853   Emergency Contact: Dr. Jane Collins

2. Composition/Information on Ingredients
Chemical Identification Pepper Oil Black *Piper Nigrum*
CAS Number   8006–82–4
EINECS Number

3. Hazards Identification
GENERAL   When undiluted and not properly handled, can be irritating to the
skin and eyes and upon inhalation. Combustible material that can
sustain a fire.
ENVIRONMENT   When spilled, can contaminate the soil, ground and surface water.

4. First-Aid Measures

Inhalation:	Remove from exposure site to fresh air. Keep at rest. Obtain medical attention.
Eye exposure:	Rinse immediately with plenty of water for at least 15 mins. Contact a doctor if symptoms persist.
Skin exposure:	Remove contaminated clothes. Wash thoroughly with soap & water, flush with plenty of water. If irritation persists, seek medical advice.
Ingestion:	Rinse mouth out with water. Seek medical advice immediately.
Other:	Take Risk and safety phrases (section 15) into consideration

5. Fire Fighting Measures

Extinguishing media:	Carbon dioxide, dry chemical, foam. Do not use a direct water-jet on burning material.

6. Accidental Release Measures

Personal precautions:	Avoid inhalation and contact with skin and eyes. A self-contained breathing apparatus is recommended in case of a major spill.

continued

Box 7.16   Material safety data sheet for Black Pepper (*Piper nigrum*) / Cont'd

Spillage:	Remove ignition sources. Provide adequate ventilation. Avoid excessive inhalation of vapors. Gross spillage should be contained immediately by use of sand or inert powder and disposed of according to local regulations.
Environment precautions:	Keep away from drains, soils, surface & ground waters.

7. Handling & Storage

Handling:	Apply good manufacturing practice & industrial hygiene practices, ensuring proper ventilation. Observe good personal hygiene, and do not eat, drink or smoke whilst handling.
Storage conditions:	Store in tightly closed original container, in a cool, dry & ventilated area away from heat sources & protected from light. Keep air contact to a minimum. Avoid plastic and uncoated metal containers.
Fire protection:	Keep away from ignition sources & naked flames. Take precautions to avoid static discharges in working area.

8. Exposure Controls/Personal Protection

Respiratory protection:	Avoid excessive inhalation of concentrated vapours.
Eye protection:	Wear safety glasses.
Skin protection:	Avoid skin contact. Use chemically resistant gloves as needed.

9. Physical & Chemical Properties

Appearance:	Almost colourless liquid
Odour:	Characteristic herbal
Flash-point °C:	47 °C (CC)
Oxidising property	none expected
Relative density	0.88745 to 0.8750 @ 20 °C
Refractive index	1.4805 to 1.4810 @ 20 °C

continued

> **Box 7.16**   Material safety data sheet for Black Pepper (*Piper nigrum*) / Cont'd

10. Stability & Reactivity

Reactivity:	It presents no significant reactivity hazards, by itself or in contact with water. Avoid contact with strong acids, alkali or oxidising agents.
Decomposition:	Carbon monoxide and unidentified organic compounds may be formed during combustion.

11. Toxicological Information
This material is according to EEC Directive 67/548/EEC classified as:
Safe when used as directed

12. Ecological Information
General: This material is unlikely to accumulate in the environment and environmental problems under normal use conditions are unexpected.

13. Disposal Considerations
Dispose of according to local regulations.
Avoid disposing to drainage systems and into the environment.

14. Transport Regulations

	Class	Pack group	Sub risk	UN no	IMDG page
Road (CDGRR):	3		111	1993	
Air (IATA):	3		111	1993	
Sea (IMDG):	3		111	1993	

15. Regulatory Information
Classification Packaging/Labelling (Directive 88/379/EEC)
Risk phrases   R10 Flammable

16. Other Information
Conc % Limits (*)

In-line with general product specification. Always satisfy suitability for specific application. The data provided in this material safety data sheet is meant to represent typical data/analysis for this product and is correct to the best of our knowledge. The data was obtained from current and reliable sources, but is supplied without warranty, expressed or implied, regarding its' correctness or accuracy. It is the user's responsibility to determine safe conditions for the use of this product, and to assume liability for loss, injury, damage or expense arising from improper use of this product. The information provided does not constitute a contract to supply to any specification, or for any given application, and buyers should seek to verify their requirements and product use.

Courtesy of Jane Collins, Phytobotanica

Apiaceae (Umbelliferae)

24. Fennel (Foeniculum vulgare)

AROMAFACT

There are two types of fennel, bitter and sweet. It is only the sweet that is used in aromatherapy. They differ chemically in that the bitter fennel contains between 15–23% of the ketone fenchone, which is practically absent in the sweet fennel.

Extracted by steam distillation of the crushed seeds gives a very pale yellow essential oil with a floral, herby, anise-like odour. It is from the same family as aniseed and coriander. Main chemical components include methyl ethers *trans*-anethole (50–90%) and methyl chavicol (2–12%), mono-terpenes limonene (1.3–17.0%), α-pinene (1.5–3.5%), phellandrene (0.4–4.9%) and sabinene (0.2–2.0%), aromatic hydrocarbon p-cymene (0.3–4.8%), ketone fenchone (trace to 23%), alcohol fenchol (2–4%) and oxide 1,8-cineole (0.8–6.0%). Box 7.17 shows the analytical data from an oil supplier. Many of the therapeutic properties attributed to it are due to the oestrogen mimicking action of the *trans*-anethole. It can be helpful for both menstrual and menopausal women. For the digestive system it is used as a carmative for hiccups, colic, vomiting and flatulence. Also reputed to have a diuretic and cleansing properties applied to cellulite and poor circulation. In skin it is suited to greasy, dull and mature complexions. Although extracts of fennel plant have been used extensively in drinks like gripe water for babies and young children, there are a number of safety issues, especially with the essential oil. Sweet fennel essential oil is powerful and it is advisable to use it with care and in moderation. Considered nonirritating, nonsensitizing and nonphototoxic. It is also generally considered to be relatively nontoxic but due to high levels of *trans*-anethole it should be avoided during pregnancy, breast feeding, endometriosis and oestrogen-dependent cancers. It should also not be used by epileptics, people with respiratory difficulties and those with liver problems and paracetamol takers.

Rosaceae

25. Rose otto (Rosa damascena)

AROMAFACT

Rose extracts are expensive but generally safe. There are variations due to the method of extraction: steam distillation produces the essential oil, while solvent extraction give a concrete or absolute.

Box 7.17   Analysis data for Sweet, Fennel (*Foeniculum vulgare*)

Product Identification

Product Name :	Fennel Sweet Oil
Botanical Name :	*Foeniculum Vulgare*
Country of Origin :	France
Agricultural Method :	Organic
Product Code :	E360
Batch Number :	859

Principal Constituents	Constituent %
α-Pinene :	1.69
Camphene :	0.13
β-Pinene :	0.79
Myrcene :	0.27
p-Cymene :	0.70
Sabinene :	0.05
α-Phellandrene :	4.51
Limonene :	8.10
1,8 Cineol :	0.85
γ-Terpinol :	0.70
cis-b-Ocimene :	0.92
α-Cymene :	0.30
Terpinolene :	0.18
α-Fenchone :	2.27
Camphor :	0.06
Methyl chavicol :	2.30
p-Anisaldehyde :	0.20
tr-Anethol :	73.45
Anisaldehyde :	0.12
cis-Anethole :	0.16

Courtesy of Geoff Lyth, Quinessence Aromatherapy Ltd

Two major species are used for oil production: *Rosa damascena*, which yields rose otto, Bulgarian rose oil and Turkish rose oil; and *Rosa centifolia*, which yields French rose oil or Moroccan rose oil. There are also many different subspecies.

The method of extraction has an important influence on the composition of the final product. The fresh flower petals produce the essential oil after steam distillation and produce rose water as an important by-product. Solvent extraction produces a concrete or absolute. The chemical composition of rose oils is considered to be one of the most complex, with much still to be identified. A general list of principal constituents of distilled products would list mainly citronellol (35–55%), geraniol and nerol (30–40%), stearopten (16–22%), phenylethyl alcohol (1.5–3%) and farnesol (0.2–2.0%), with trace constituents including rose oxide, damascone, damascenone and ionone. A comparison of the essential oil from distillation and the absolute from solvent extraction shows a marked difference in amounts of principal constituents. These are most notably the phenylethyl alcohol which is 60–65% in the absolute but is lost in distillation and as low as 1–3% in the essential oil; the stearopten is not usually detected in the essential oil but can be 8–22% in the absolute. The alcohols citronellol and geraniol are higher in the oil, 18–55% and 12–40% respectively, compared to 18–22% and 10–15% in the absolute.

The significance of a minor component having an important contribution to the odour qualities is illustrated by β-damascenone. Although only present at about 0.14%, it gives 70% of the total odour.

As the rose essential and absolute oils are some of the most expensive oils in the market, they are likely to be adulterated. True essential oils may be diluted by the addition of chemicals such as phenylethyl alcohol, diethyl phthalate (DEP), citronellol and geraniol and with fractions from other essential oils such as geranium. The absolute may be adulterated with synthetic fractions of oils such as Peru balsam and clove bud absolute.

The essential oil, absolute and floral water have extensive culinary, perfumery and cosmetic applications. In aromatherapy they are excellent for skin care, gynaecological conditions and digestive disorders and are particularly noted for their uplifting psychological effects, acting as calming agents and antidepressants (see page **225**).

Rosa damascena is considered to be one of the safest choices of aromatherapy oil as it is non-toxic, non-irritant and non-sensitizing.

Oleaceae

26. Jasmine (Jasminium grandiflorum)

AROMAFACT

Jasmine flowers for the production of essences are picked at night as the plants biochemical reactions cause odorous compounds to be at their most intense after dark. It is an expensive essential oil to produce and this is reflected in the price of a good quality product.

Different products are available from jasmine according to the method of extraction. Solvent extraction gives the concrete; use of alcohol, followed by filtration of insoluble waxes, on the concrete separates the absolute and an essential oil is produced by steam distillation of the absolute. The absolute is most commonly used in aromatherapy. It is a viscous orange brown liquid with a powerful, warm, heady, floral and exotic odour. Chemical analysis reveals a complex composition with a large number of compounds. The ester benzyl acetate makes up to 67%, with alcohols linalool (12–16%) benzyl alcohol (3–6%) and geraniol (8–11%) the heterocyclic indole (1.9–2.7%) and ketone *cis*-jasmone (2.6–3.4%). The many other compounds, although present in low amounts, are important to the overall floral odour of the essential oil. Jasmine type essences are often produced synthetically but do not compare to the genuine product of natural origin. Also due to the high price of genuine jasmine it is often adulterated. Considered to be a particularly feminine oil it is often used for menstrual problems, easing labour and childbirth and post natal recovery. Reputed to be antidepressant, good for muscular aches and pains and suitable for all skin types. Considered to be non-toxic, non-irritant and generally non-sensitizing.

Ammonaceae

27. Ylang ylang (Cananga odorata)

AROMAFACT

There are a number of products sold as ylang ylang. Although botanically less ambiguous than most of the other examples, they show considerable variation in composition. This is due to the extraction process.

The situation is botanically less ambiguous than for thyme, say, with ylang ylang produced from *Cananga odorata* variety *genuina* giving the high-quality essential oil used for aromatherapy and perfumery. It is closely related to *Cananga odoratum* variety *macrophylla*, which gives cananga oil. The ylang ylang essential oil is produced by steam distillation of the freshly picked flowers. It is the variation in the times and temperatures employed during this processing that gives rise to a range of essential oils sold as ylang ylang. The 'complete' oil is unfractionated (Fig. 7.15) and is further processed to give separate products. The top grade is called Ylang Ylang Extra Superior, with successive grades Extra (Fig. 7.16), Grade 1, Grade 2 and Grade 3 (Fig. 7.17). Sometimes a complete essential oil is made up of a blend of ylang ylang 1 and 2.

An analysis of major components present in a ylang ylang essential oil would include sweet smelling esters methyl benzoate, benzyl benzoate, benzyl acetate and geranyl acetate; alcohols linalool, geraniol, farnesol and eugenol; sesquiterpenes germacrene, β-caryophyllene and cadinene; monoterpene pinene; and ethers *p*-cresyl methyl ether and safrole. This, however, is a gross generalization and the amounts present in each grade vary considerably.

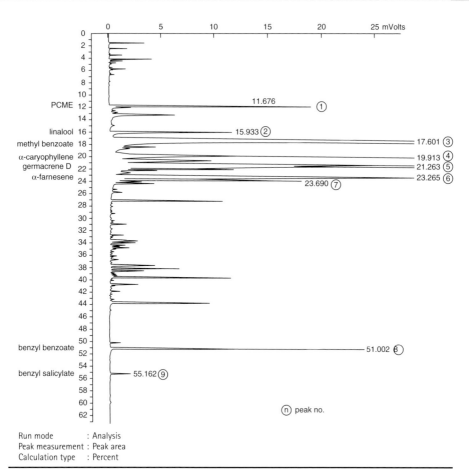

Run mode   : Analysis
Peak measurement : Peak area
Calculation type : Percent

Peak no.	Peak name	Result (%)	Retention time (min)	Time offset (min)	Area (counts)	Sep. code	Width 1/2 (s)	Status codes
1	PCME	1.90	11.676	0.046	102 648	VV	4.8	
2	Linalool	2.17	15.933	−0.004	117 121	VV	7.0	
3	Methyl benzoate	37.32	17.601	−0.023	2 018 861	VV	26.0	
4	α-Caryophyllene	8.95	19.913	−0.018	483 985	VV	13.7	
5	Germacrene D	6.43	21.263	−0.012	347 678	VV	13.9	
6	α-Farnesene	10.37	23.265	−0.013	561 032	VV	12.5	
7	Geranyl acetate	2.33	23.690	−0.013	126 142	VV	6.2	
8	Benzyl benzoate	3.04	51.002	−0.012	164 181	PB	6.8	
9	Benzyl salicylate	0.28	55.162	0.000	15 233	BB	6.9	
	Totals:	72.79		−0.049	3 936 881			

Total unidentified counts: 1 472 222
Detected peaks: 168   Rejected peaks: 118   Identified peaks: 9

Figure 7.15   Ylang ylang, *Cananga odorata.* Analysis of whole oil before distillation. Courtesy of Jenny Warden, Traceability.

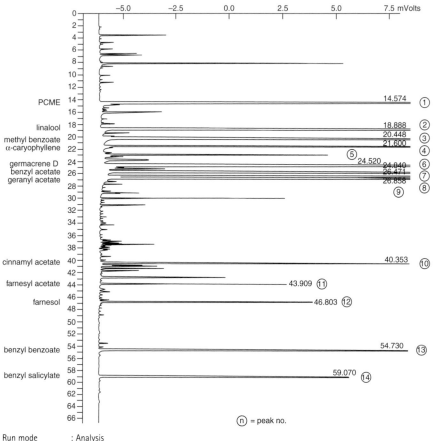

Run mode   : Analysis
Peak measurement : Peak area
Calculation type : Percent

Peak no.	Peak name	Result (%)	Retention time (min)	Time offset (min)	Area (counts)	Sep. code	Width 1/2 (s)	Status codes
1	PCME	7.71	14.574	0.004	277 158	PB	6.1	
2	Linalool	13.14	18.888	0.008	472 427	BB	9.1	
3	Methyl benzoate	7.71	20.448	0.008	277 052	VB	10.1	
4	α-Caryophyllene	5.91	21.600	0.000	212 653	PB	6.4	
5	Germacrene D	2.36	24.520	−0.000	84 841	VV	7.7	
6	Germacrene D	12.19	24.840	0.000	438 343	VV	14.6	
7	Benzyl acetate	11.26	25.845	0.005	404 794	VV	8.5	
8	α-Farnesene	5.85	26.471	0.001	210 477	VV	10.2	
9	Geranyl acetate	7.26	26.858	−0.002	260 956	VB	8.8	
10	Cinnamyl acetate	3.45	40.535	0.005	124 133	VV	5.9	
11	Farnesyl acetate	1.48	43.909	−0.001	53 271	BB	5.6	
12	Farnesol	1.71	46.803	0.003	61 307	VB	5.2	
13	Benzyl benzoate	5.69	54.730	−0.000	204 696	PB	7.6	
14	Benzyl salicylate	2.51	59.070	−0.000	90 291	BB	7.6	
	Totals	88.23		0.031	3 172 399			

Total unidentified counts: 422 779
Detected peaks: 223 Rejected peaks: 183 Identified peaks: 14

Figure 7.16   Ylang ylang, *Cananga odorata.* Ylang Ylang Extra: typical profile high in esters and linalool but lower in sesquiterpenes. Courtesy of Jenny Warden, Traceability.

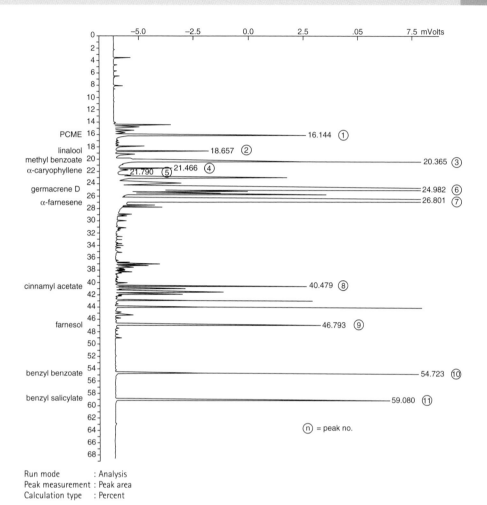

Run mode   : Analysis
Peak measurement : Peak area
Calculation type : Percent

Peak no.	Peak name	Result (%)	Retention time (min)	Time offset (min)	Area (counts)	Sep. code	Width 1/2 (s)	Status codes
1	PCME	1.59	16.144	0.000	56 062	PB	5.4	
2	Linalool	0.53	18.657	0.001	18 805	BP	3.8	
3	Methyl benzoate	7.69	20.365	0.000	271 494	VB	10.3	
4	α-Caryophyllene	0.39	21.466	0.000	13 756	BV	4.7	
5	Benzyl acetate	0.17	21.790	−0.305	6 129	VB	11.5	
6	Germacrene D	28.50	24.982	0.002	1 005 741	VV	20.5	
7	α-Farnesene	31.70	26.801	0.001	1 118 819	VB	22.2	
8	Cinnamyl acetate	1.34	40.479	−0.001	47 252	VV	4.9	
9	Farnesol	1.45	46.793	0.003	51 264	VB	5.2	
10	Benzyl benzoate	5.29	54.723	0.001	186 665	PB	7.5	
11	Benzyl salicylate	2.84	59.080	0.002	100 198	BB	7.5	
	Totals	81.49		−0.296	2 876 185			

Total unidentified counts: 653 238
Detected peaks: 175   Rejected peaks: 134   Identified peaks: 11

Figure 7.17   Ylang ylang, *Cananga odorata.* Ylang ylang Grade 3, showing typical profile – esters low, sesquiterpenes high. Courtesy of Jenny Warden, Traceability.

Box 7.18 Certificate of analysis for Sandalwood (*Santalum album*)

ESSENTIAL OIL OF SANDALWOOD *(Santalum album)*
COUNTRY OF ORIGIN - AUSTRALIA

EXTRACTION - STEAM DISTILLATION OF THE DRIED ROOTS AND HEARTWOOD
Authenticated...

Peak No	Compound	% Amount
1	α-santalene	1.58
2	β-santalene	27.44
3	alkene	1.50
4	alkene	1.05
5	ketone	4.44
6	alcohol	0.77
7	α-santalol	46.21
8	alkene	4.74
9	β-santalol	5.12
10	alkene	1.03
11	cedrene	0.83
12	sesquiterpene	0.70
13	alcohol	4.59

Courtesy of Jane Collins, Phytobotanica

Box 7.19 Material safety data sheet for Sandalwood (*Santalum album*)

1. Identification of substance/preparation & company
PRODUCT NAME; SANDALWOOD OIL
COMPANY NAME: Phytobotanica UK Ltd, Mill House Organic Medicinal and
Aromatic Plant Farm, Greens Barn, Greens Lane, Lydiate, Merseyside L31 4HZ
Emergency Tel No: 01695 420 853 Emergency Contact: Dr. Jane Collins

2. Composition/Information on Ingredients
CHEMICAL IDENTIFICATION SANDALWOOD OIL
CAS Number 8006–87–9

3. Hazards Identification
GENERAL   When undiluted and not properly handled, can be irritating to
                the skin and eyes and upon inhalation. Combustible material
                that can sustain a fire.
HAZARD SYMBOL   Xn Harmful
RISK PHRASES   R22, Harmful if swallowed
                R43 May cause sensitization by skin contact
                R36/38 Irritating to eyes and skin

continued

ENVIRONMENT   When spilled, can contaminate the soil, ground and surface water.

4. First-aid measures

Inhalation:	Remove from exposure site to fresh air. Keep at rest. Obtain medical attention.
Eye exposure:	Rinse immediately with plenty of water for at least 15 mins. Contact a doctor if symptoms persist.
Skin exposure:	Remove contaminated clothes. Wash thoroughly with soap & water, flush with plenty of water. If irritation persists, seek medical advice.
Ingestion:	Rinse mouth out with water. Seek medical advice immediately.
Other:	Take Risk and Safety phrases (section 15) into consideration

5. Fire fighting measures

Extinguishing media:	Carbon dioxide, dry chemical, foam. Do not use a direct water-jet on burning material.

6. Accidental release measures

Personal precautions:	Avoid inhalation and contact with skin and eyes. A self-contained breathing apparatus is recommended in case of a major spill.
Spillage:	Remove ignition sources. Provide adequate ventilation. Avoid excessive inhalation of vapours. Gross spillage should be contained immediately by use of sand or inert powder and disposed of according to local regulations.
Environment precautions:	Keep away from drains, soils, surface & ground waters.

7. Handling & storage

Handling:	Apply good manufacturing practice & industrial hygiene practices, ensuring proper ventilation. Observe good personal hygiene, and do not eat, drink or smoke whilst handling.
Storage conditions:	Store in tightly closed original container, in a cool, dry & ventilated area away from heat sources & protected from light. Keep air contact to a minimum. Avoid plastic and uncoated metal containers

continued

Box 7.19   Material safety data sheet for Sandalwood (*Santalum album*) / Cont'd

8. Exposure controls/personal protection

Respiratory protection:	Avoid excessive inhalation of concentrated vapours.
Eye protection:	Wear safety glasses
Skin protection:	Avoid skin contact. Use chemically resistant gloves as needed.

9. Physical & chemical properties

Appearance:	Pale yellow liquid
Odour:	Sweet Woody
Flash-point °C:	110 °C (CC)
Oxidising property	none expected
Relative density	0.9714 @ 20 °C
Refractive Index	1.5403 @ 20 °C

10. Stability & Reactivity

Reactivity:	It presents no significant reactivity hazards, by itself or in contact with water. Avoid contact with strong acids, alkali or oxidising agents.
Decomposition:	Carbon monoxide and unidentified organic compounds may be formed during combustion.

11. Toxicological information
This material is according to EEC Directive 67/548/EEC classified as:
Harmful if swallowed
Irritating to eyes and skin
May cause sensitization by skin contact

12. Ecological information

General:	This material is unlikely to accumulate in the environment and environmental problems under normal use conditions are unexpected.

13. Disposal considerations
Dispose of according to local regulations.
Avoid disposing to drainage systems and into the environment.

14. Transport regulations

	Class	Pack group sub risk	UN no	IMDG page
Road (CDGRR):	not restricted			
Air (IATA):	not restricted			
Sea (IMDG):	not restricted			

continued

> **Box 7.19**   Material safety data sheet for Sandalwood (*Santalum album*) / Cont'd
>
> ### 15. Regulatory Information
> Classification Packaging/Labelling (Directive 88/379/EEC)
>
> | | |
> |---|---|
> | Hazard symbol | Xn Harmful |
> | Risk Phrases | R22, Harmful if swallowed |
> | | R43, May cause sensititsaton by skin contact |
> | | R36/38 Irritating to eyes and skin |
> | Safety phrases | S13, Keep away from food, drink and animal feeding stuffs |
> | | S20/21 When using do not eat, drink or smoke |
>
> ### 16. Other information
> Conc % Limits (*)
> In-line with general product specification. Always satisfy suitability for specific application. The data provided in this material safety data sheet is meant to represent typical data/analysis for this product and is correct to the best of our knowledge. The data was obtained from current and reliable sources, but is supplied without warranty, expressed or implied, regarding its' correctness or accuracy. It is the user's responsibility to determine safe conditions for the use of this product, and to assume liability for loss, injury, damage or expense arising from improper use of this product. The information provided does not constitute a contract to supply to any specification, or for any given application, and buyers should seek to verify their requirements and product use.
>
> *Courtesy of Jane Collins, Phytobotanica*

respiratory system for coughs, laryngitis and catarrh, and for urinary complaints such as cystitis. Versatile in skin care, effective for oily skin and acne as well as dry damaged mature complexions. Considered to be non-toxic, non-irritant and non-sensitizing.

Burseraceae

29. Frankincense (Boswellia sacra)

AROMAFACT

Frankincense is also known as Olibanum and is sold for respiratory problems such as colds, coughs laryngitis and bronchitis

Incisions made into the bark of the shrub produce a natural oleo-gum resin. Depending on the quality of this resin, different grades of essential oil are produced when it is steam distilled. There is also an absolute that is widely employed as a fixative. The essential oil is very pale yellow or green with a balsamic, sweet woody odour with fresh top notes due to its monoterpene content. A typical composition would be α-pinene (15–23%), α-thujene (19–28%), limonene (6–9%), sabinene (4–8%), octanol (10–14%), linalool (1–4%), octyl acetate (50–60%), incensyl acetate (2–4%) and incensole (1.5–2.5%). Frankincense and its extracted products have a long history in religious ceremonies and have been used over the centuries in perfume, cosmetics, soaps and pharmaceuticals. In aromatherapy, in common with other oils extracted from resins, it is applied to the respiratory system. Reputed to slow down the breathing rate it has a calming and soothing effect on both mind and body. Also used for urinary infections and menstrual problems including heavy periods. Suited to oily skin and said to benefit mature complexions by its soothing and antiwrinkle action. The distilled essential oil is considered to be gentle, non-toxic, non-irritant and non-sensitizing.

30. Myrrh (Commiphora myrrha)

AROMAFACT

Myrrh has well known biblical connections and widespread use in the ancient world. Its drying and mummification properties made it a commonly used embalming oil.

A gum resin (oleoresin) exudes from the cut bark of the shrub and is used to produce either a resinoid and resin absolute by solvent extraction or the essential oil by steam distillation. The essential oil is an amber liquid with a spicy, warm, balsamic and slightly medicinal odour. It contains a large number of compounds, which have not been fully identified yet. A typical chemical composition would be sesquiterpenes δ-elemene (25–30%), α-copaene (9–12%), β-elemene (5–7%), bourbonene (4–6%), α-bergamotene (4.0–5.5%), lindestrene (3–4%) ketones curerenone (10–13%) and methyl isobutyl ketone (5.5–6.5%), nitrogen heterocyclic methylfurans (5–8%). In common with other essential oils extracted from resins it is said to have beneficial effects on the respiratory system with a cleansing action for colds, sore throats, catarrh, laryngitis and bronchitis. Considered effective in treating mouth ulcers, weak teeth and gums, it is often formulated into toothpastes where its bitter taste is masked by peppermint. A tonic for the digestive system easing diarrhoea and flatulence and a uterine stimulant relieving painful periods. For this reason it should be avoided during pregnancy. Applied to the skin its healing properties are suited to eczema, ulcers, boils, bedsores and often used in topical creams. Although non-irritant and non-sensitizing it may be toxic in high concentrations.

Styracaceae

31. Benzoin (Styrax benzoin)

AROMAFACT

The Styracaceae family does not produce an essential oil but a solid gum resin (oleo-resin) called benzoin. The resinous solid needs to be melted before use. Commercially benzoin is sold as the solid dissolved in a suitable solvent. A 'true' absolute is also produced in much smaller quantities. It is well known as an ingredient of Friars Balsam.

Crude benzoin comes directly from the trees as a sap which is exuded from the bark. There are different types of crude, Sumatra and Siam, with differing chemical compositions. Sumatra is made up of mainly coniferyl cinnamate sumareinolic acid with benzoic acid, cinnamic acid and traces of styrene, vanillin and benzaldehyde. The Siam is high in coniferyl benzoate (up to 75%) with benzoic acid, cinnamyl benzoate, vanillin and siaresinolic acid. The benzoin resinoid can be produced from either or from a mixture of the two types. The crude gum is processed to make a tincture by macerating with alcohol, a resin absolute by extraction with hot or cold alcohol or the resinoid by extraction with a hydrocarbon solvent. It is the resin absolute that is considered most superior and preferred for use in aromatherapy. Box 7.20 shows a typical analysis. The odours are rich, sweet and balsamic. Used for de-stressing, comforting yet rejuvenating for both mind and body, calming the digestive system and easing muscular aches and pains. It has a good reputation for respiratory disorders like asthma bronchitis, coughs and situations where fluid needs expelling from the body. Used on dry, cracked skin applied to conditions like wounds, sores, irritated, itching and chapping. Non-toxic, non-irritant but with possible sensitization. The tincture has some reports of contact dermatitis and has been implicated as moderately toxic.

Zingiberacae

32. Ginger (Zingiber officinale)

AROMAFACT

There are several essential oil producing species available according to their country of origin. Consequently their chemical analysis will show a resultant variation in composition.

Box 7.20   Certificate of analysis for Benzoin (*Styrax benzoin*)

CERTIFICATE OF ESSENTIAL OIL ANALYSIS 2007

ESSENTIAL OIL OF BENZOIN (Styrax benzoin)
COUNTRY OF ORIGIN – SUMATRA
EXTRACTION – FROM THE GUM EXUDED FROM THE TREES

Authenticated..

Peak No	Compound	% Composition
1	α-copaene	0.18
2	alkene	0.05
3	benzaldehyde	0.11
4	β-caryophyllene	0.19
5	β-cedrene	0.09
6	formic acid, phenylmethyl ester	0.05
7	delta-cadinene	0.19
8	benzyl alcohol	59.03
9	ethyl cinnamate	1.00
10	eugenol	0.09
11	diethly phthalate	31.51
12	vanillin	0.73
13	benzyl benzoate	0.10
14	benzoic acid	1.06
15	trans cinnamic acid	2.60
16	alcohol	0.37
17	benzyl cinnamate	0.20
18	1,4-dihydroxy-5, 8-bis (ethylamino) etc	2.45

Courtesy of Jane Collins, Phytobotanica

Extracted from the pungent dried and unpeeled roots or rhizome by steam distillation. A pale amber or greenish liquid with a spicy, woody, fresh and warm odour. Its chemical components include the sesquiterpenes zingiberene (1.9–50.9%) and β-sesquiphellandrene (1.4–9.1%), monoterpenes α-pinene (0.3–4.4%), camphene (1.1–8.2%), limonene (1.2–3.1%) and β-phellandrene (1.2–4.3%), alcohols citronellol (4.1–6.4%), linalool (1–5.8%) and geraniol (3.0–23.1%), aldehyde geranial (12–37%) and acetate geranyl acetate (0.1–28.0%). Ginger and its products are used extensively in perfumes, cosmetics, digestive preparations and many food product categories. The essential oil, which is stimulating and warming, has a long history as a remedy for digestive system disorders and is useful for situations like travel sickness that cause nausea. Its stimulating properties are also applied to the circulation and for aching joints and muscles. Non-toxic and non-irritant in low concentrations but possibly slightly sensitizing and phototoxic so it may be advisable to dilute well before using on the skin.

Pinaceae

33. Cedarwood, Atlas (Cedrus atlantica)

AROMAFACT

Many essential oils come under the name cedarwood. These commonly include Atlas cedarwood (*Cedrus atlantica*) and Virginian cedarwood (*Juniperus virginiana*). They share some similar properties although some authorities feel the Atlas to be superior and safer.

Atlas cedarwood essential oil is extracted from the wood by steam distillation to produce an orange coloured liquid with a camphoraceous, warm and woody odour. Its main components are sesquiterpene cedrene (up to 50%), alcohols atlantol and cedrol, ketone atlantone (10–14%) and numerous other compounds. Box 7.21 shows analysis of a Virginian cedarwood which also has cedrene as its main component. Properties attributed to Atlas cedarwood include mind balancing for anger, stress and exhaustion, as an expectorant for the respiratory system and an antiseptic in treatment of kidney and bladder disorders. For the skin its astringent actions are beneficial for oily skin, conditions such as psoriasis, scalp irritations and dandruff. Considered to be a nontoxic, nonirritating, nonsensitizing but not recommended for use during pregnancy. Data published for Atlas cedarwood aimed at health professionals is shown in Box 7.22.

Cupressaceae

34. Cypress (Cupressus sempervirens)

AROMAFACT

Sempervirens means 'ever living'. Many species of cypress are used for essential oil production with *C. sempervirens* considered to be the superior one.

Steam distillation of needles and twigs produce a yellow to pale green oil with a spicy, woody, slightly sweet and sharp odour. Its chemical composition

---

Box 7.21   Certificate of Analysis for Virginian Cedarwood *(Junipus virginiana)*

CERTIFICATE OF ESSENTIAL OIL ANALYSIS 2007

ESSENTIAL OIL OF CEDARWOOD (VIRGINIAN)
(Junipus virginiana)
COUNTRY OF ORIGIN – USA
EXTRACTION – STEAM DISTILLATION OF THE TIMBER

Authenticated..

Peak No	Compound	% Composition
1	α-pinene	0.84
2	α-cedrene	39.98
3	β-cedrene	9.08
4	thujopsene	19.23
5	alkene	0.59
6	β-chamigrene	1.99
7	alkene	2.06
8	alkene	0.45
9	cedrene isomer	1.99
10	cuparene	1.35
11	alkene	0.34
12	cedrol	16.55
13	widdrol	3.62
14	alkene	0.54
15	alkene	0.59
16	ketone	0.40
17	alcohol	0.40

Courtesy of Jane Collins, Phytobotanica

---

is high in mono-terpenes including α-pinene (34–58%), β-pinene (2.7–3.1%), careen (14–24%), limonene (2.3–5.5%), α-terpinolene (2.2–6.1%), sesquiterpene cadinene (1.2–3.1%), aromatic hydrocarbon *p*-cymene (0.1–1.8%), alcohols cedrol (5.3–22.0%) and borneol (1.0–8.9%), and ester terpenyl acetate (3.8–5.2%). Used in aromatherapy for nervous tension and stress relief. Reputed to be vaso-constricting and astringent finding therapeutic applications for conditions such as oedema, cellulitis, varicose veins, cramp, haemorrhoids and poor circulation. Thought to be beneficial to the respiratory system and to have a regulatory effect on the menstrual cycle and for menopausal symptoms. Suitable for oily skin and often used as a deodorizer checking profuse perspiration. Considered to be non-toxic, non-irritant and non-sensitizing.

Box 7.22 Typical Data Sheet aimed at healthcare professionals: Atlas Cedarwood (*Cedrus atlantica*)

CEDRUS ATLANTICA LIG. *[ATLAS CEDARWOOD, SATINWOOD]* A BIETACEAE

Representative constituents

Hydrocarbons
sesquiterpenes (50%) cedrene

Alcohols
sesquiterpenols (30%) atlantol, α-caryophyllene alcohol, epi-β-cubenol

Ketones
sesquiterpenones (20%) α-atlantone, γ-atlantone *other* α-ionone

Other
epoxy-β-himachalene and its epimer deodarone

Properties	Indications
antiseptic	skin problems, scalp (with cade oil), urinary tract, eczema, pruritus (with bergamot oil)
arterial regenerator*	arteriosclerosis*
cicatrizant	skin problems, wounds
lipolytic*	cellulite*
lymph tonic*	cellulite*, lymph circulation problems, water retention
mucolytic	bronchitis*
stimulant	scalp problems

Observations
- it is important to specify this oil accurately: the term cedarwood oil has little meaning, because many oils are sold under this name, many of them from the Cupressaceae family
- considered in France to be neurotoxic and abortive, and not normally used there for pregnant women and infants
- leave internal use of this oil to a doctor
- the Moroccan oil *C. atlantica* showed no irritation or sensitization at 8% dilution when tested on humans (Opdyke *1976g*)
- has no phototoxic effects reported, although the use of toilet preparations containing unspecified cedarwood oils followed by exposure to various wavelengths sometimes causes dermatitis (Winter 1984)

Courtesy of Len & Shirley Price, taken from Price & Price Aromatherapy for Health Professional (Churchill Livingstone)

35. Juniper (Juniper communis)

AROMAFACT

The essential oil extracted from the berries by steam distillation is considered to be superior to that from the twigs and leaves. The wood oil is often adulterated with turpentine oil and it is advisable to avoid it for aromatherapy.

The water white essential oil has a slightly woody-balsamic and refreshing odour. Its main chemical components are the monoterpenes α-pinene (26–71%), β-pinene (1.5–13.9%), limonene (2.3–41%), sabinene (0.2–8.9%), β-myrcene (2.5–9.8%) and others in lower amounts, the aromatic hydrocarbon p-cymene (1.1–5.2%), alcohol terpinene-4-ol (2.1–9.7%) and oxide 1,8-cineole (0.5–4.0%). A certificate of analysis is shown in Box 7.24 with the accompanying spectra in Box 7.25. Historically juniper was used to treat contagious diseases and the British Herbal Pharmacopoeia cites its use for cystitis and rheumatism. Its partnership with gin is well known. It is regarded as an efficient detoxifier and diuretic with extracts used commercially in diuretic and laxative preparations. It is frequently applied to problems of the urino-genital system. However, it has been suggested that the essential oil may be a kidney irritant when levels of pinenes are high, as found in essential oil extracted from needles and branches. The essential oil from the berry is also employed for stress and anxiety relief and believed to ease menstrual pains. In skincare it is suited to oily and congested complexions and conditions such as eczema, psoriasis and dermatitis. It is considered to be nontoxic and nonsensitizing but there have been reports of irritant reactions. It should not be used on anyone with kidney disease or during pregnancy as it may stimulate the uterine muscles. Safety data is illustrated in Box 7.23.

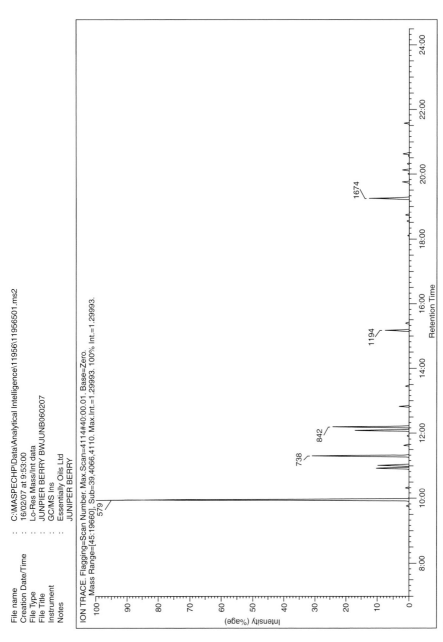

File name : C:\MASPECHP\Data\Analytical Intelligence\11956\11956501.ms2
Creation Date/Time : 16/02/07 at 9:53:00
File Type : Lo-Res Mass/Int data
File Title : JUNPIER BERRY BWJUNB060207
Instrument : GC/MS Ins
Notes : Essentially Oils Ltd
JUNIPER BERRY

ION TRACE. Flagging=Scan Number. Max.Scan=4114#40:00.01 . Base=Zero.
Mass Range=[45:19660], Sub=39,4066,4110. Max.Int.=1.29993. 100% Int.=1.29993.

Figure 7.18 See legend next page

Peak Area	Peak Time	Peak Scan	Marker Text
0.40	9:46.13	557	α-Thujene
41.96	9:57.35	579	α-Pinene
0.54	10:19.28	622	Camphene
4.03	10:55.48	693	Sabinene
3.95	11:01.09	704	β-Pinene
12.06	11:18.43	738	β-Myrcene
0.76	11:37.81	776	Probably a-Phellandrene
0.26	11:55.15	810	α-Terpinene
7.01	12:05.35	830	p-Cymene
9.83	12:11.47	842	Limonene
1.31	12:50.22	918	g-Terpinene
0.49	13:27.45	991	α-Terpinolene
3.07	15:10.97	1194	Terpinen-4-ol
0.55	15:24.23	1220	α-Terpineol
0.10	17:02.13	1412	Possibly Bornyl Acetate
0.24	18:05.88	1537	α-Cubebene
0.32	18:33.42	1591	Copaene
0.49	18:44.63	1613	Probably β-Elemene
5.28	19:15.74	1674	trans-β-Caryophyllene
1.01	19:45.83	1733	α-Caryophyllene
1.04	20:07.75	1776	Germacrene D
0.43	20:19.48	1799	Probably α-Muurolene, or isomer
0.19	20:33.76	1827	Probably γ-Cadinene
1.01	20:37.84	1835	d-Cadinene
0.77	21:34.96	1947	Probably Caryophyllene oxide

Courtesy of Charles Wells and Bill Morden, Analytical Intelligence Ltd.

Figure 7.18 Juniper berry. Analysis of *Juniperus communis*, showing a typical composition.

Box 7.23 Safety data for *Juniperus communis*

Juniper

Botanical name: *Juniperus communis*

Family: Cupressaceae (= Coniferae)

Oil from: Berries

Notable constituents:

α-pinene	40%
Myrcene	12%
β-pinene	7%
Terpinen-4-ol	6%
Sabinene	5%
Limonene	3%

Acute oral LD$_{50}$: > 5 g/kg [422]

Hazards: None

Contraindications: None

Toxicity data & recommendations: Juniper is the only profile included which the authors do not regard as hazardous. It is included because other sources have frequently flagged juniper as being contraindicated in both pregnancy and kidney disease. A vigorous attempt was made to trace the source of these contraindications. There is evidence that juniper berries are abortifacient, but there is no evidence that juniper oil is responsible for this effect. No evidence could be found to support the contraindication of juniper oil in kidney disease.

Most of the above referenced sources refer to 'juniper' generically, without specifying a particular preparation. None of them refer to what seems to be the

continued

Box 7.23   Safety data for *Juniperus communis* / Cont'd

only scientific basis for the abortifacient activity of juniper. Ethanolic and acetone extracts of juniper berries have a significant antifertility effect in rats. An ethanolic extract of juniper berries was found to demonstrate both an early and a late abortifacient activity in rats.

An ethanolic extract would contain some essential oil, but there is no evidence that the essential oil is responsible for these effects. Since the oil constitutes only some 1.5% of the raw material, and since all the major components of the essential oil are apparently non-toxic (see Chemical Index), it seems inconceivable that juniper oil could be responsible for the reproductive toxicity noted above.

Nutmeg oil, which is apparently non-abortifacient, contains 10–25% α-pinene, 2–3% myrcene, 12% β-pinene, 5–6% terpinen-4-ol, 15–35% sabinene and 3–4% limonene. These same components constitute some 75% of juniper oil. The administration of up to 0.56 g/kg of nutmeg oil to pregnant rodents for 10 consecutive days had no effect on nidation or on maternal or fetal survival; no teratogenic effect was observed. Myrcene showed no reproductive toxicity when tested on pregnant rats at 250 mg/kg, which is equivalent to a human dose of 135 g of juniper oil.

Comments: There are two likely reasons why juniper oil acquired a 'tainted' reputation, which has since been quoted and re-quoted. Firstly, there has undoubtedly been some confusion between juniper (*Juniperus communis*) and savin (*Juniperus sabina*).

One research paper, published in 1928, has the sub-heading: 'Emmenagogue Oils (Pennyroyal, Tansy and Juniper)'. In the body of the text it later states: 'The popular idea has always been that pennyroyal, tansy, savin and other oils produce abortion'. It is very obvious that savin and juniper oils have been confused. Any such confusion would readily explain why juniper oil might have been thought of as being dangerous in pregnancy, since savin certainly is so.

Secondly, if juniper berries are abortifacient, and if the component responsible for this is unknown, then suspicion could naturally fall on the essential oil. Gin has a reputation as an abortifacient, but again juniper oil is very unlikely to be responsible for any such effects, since the average maximum concentration of juniper oil in alcoholic beverages is only 0.006%.

The authors believe, therefore, that there is no reason to regard juniper oil as being hazardous in any way.

Courtesy of Robert Tisserand - taken from Essential Oil Safety. A Guide for Health Care Professional (Churchill Livingstone).

CARRIERS

The substances that are used to transport the essential oils into the body are called *carriers*. Carriers include a range of substances such as the air when inhaling, water in a bath and all the lotions, creams, shampoos and other products that are used to apply preparations containing essential oils to the skin.

When using essential oils on the skin in a massage, the essential oils are diluted in a carrier oil. There are very few exceptions to this. Carrier oils are vegetable oils, also called fixed vegetable oils, in which the essential oils dissolve easily and efficiently. The carrier oils enhance the absorption of the essential oils through the skin and provide lubrication to allow the therapist's hand to move smoothly over the client's skin. In addition, some carrier oils have beneficial and therapeutic properties of their own.

General structure and properties of carrier oil molecules

Edible oils and fats come under the biochemical classification of lipids owing to their insolubility in water. They are composed of two chemically bonded components, a fatty acid and glycerol; there are many different fatty acids. When fats and oils are digested in the body, the fatty acids are liberated. Fatty acids are vital in the diet to act as starting materials for cell structures, for other important bodily chemicals including hormones and as an energy source.

The fatty acid molecule is made up of a hydrocarbon chain whose length varies according to the particular fatty acid, which is water-insoluble, or *hydrophobic*, with a terminal carboxylic acid group, which is water-soluble, or *hydrophilic*.

```
┌ ─ ─ ─ ─ ─ ─ ─ ─ ─ ─ ─ ─ ─ ─ ─ ─ ─ ┐
│ HYDROCARBON CHAIN                  │     ╱  CARBOXYLIC ACID  ╲
│                                    │    (      GROUP          )
└ ─ ─ ─ ─ ─ ─ ─ ─ ─ ─ ─ ─ ─ ─ ─ ─ ─ ┘     ╲                   ╱
```

The hydrocarbon chain structure differs between different fatty acids not only in the length of the chain, which is determined by the number of carbon atoms, but also in the type of carbon-to-carbon bonding. Saturated chains contain all single bonds, while the unsaturated ones have one (monounsaturated) or more (polyunsaturated) double bonds. The number of hydrogen atoms in the formula of an unsaturated structure will be less than that for the corresponding saturated one with the same number of carbon atoms. This can be seen when looking at four different fatty acids, all with 17 carbon atoms in the hydrocarbon chain.

Stearic acid
$C_{17}H_{35}COOH$

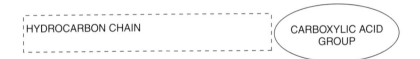

Saturated (all single, no double bonds)

Oleic acid
$C_{17}H_{33}COOH$

$$H-C-C-C-C-C-C-C-C-C=C-C-C-C-C-C-C-C-COOH$$

Monounsaturated (one double bond)

Linoleic acid
$C_{17}H_{31}COOH$

$$H-C-C-C-C-C-C=C-C-C=C-C-C-C-C-C-C-C-COOH$$

Polyunsaturated (two double bonds)

Linolenic acid
$C_{17}H_{29}COOH$

$$H-C-C-C=C-C-C=C-C-C=C-C-C-C-C-C-C-C-COOH$$

Polyunsaturated (three double bonds)

Note that for each extra double bond in the chain there are two fewer hydrogen atoms in the molecular formula.

Table 7.7 shows the names, hydrocarbon chain lengths and number of double bonds present in fatty acids commonly occurring in dietary fats and oils.

The presence of the double bonds in the hydrocarbon chains of the unsaturated fatty acids means that they can exist as either *cis* or *trans* isomers (see Ch. 2). The molecules can be represented as

trans   *cis*

This relationship can apply at *each* double bond of a polyunsaturated chain; hence such designations as 'all-*trans* fatty acid'.

The *trans* form of the molecule is more stable than the *cis* but will still fit onto many of the sites on the enzymes and membrane structures of the cells. When it does this, it blocks the sites and prevents the normal reactions of the *cis* molecules, which would usually be accepted at these sites. *Trans* fatty acids have been implicated in adverse health warnings. They are believed to be

Table 7.7 Chain lengths and degrees of unsaturation in fats and oils commonly occurring in the diet

| Hydrocarbon chain length | Fatty acid | | | |
| | | Unsaturation | | |
	Saturated	Mono	Poly (2)	Poly (3)
9	Capric			
10	Lauric			
11	Myristic			
15	Palmitic	Palmitoleic		
16	Heptadecenoic	9-Heptadecenoic		
17	Stearic	Oleic	Linoleic	Linolenic
19	Arachidic	Eicosenoic		
21	Behenic	Erucic		
23		Lignoceric	Tetracosaenoic	

detrimental because of their interference with the normal biochemical pathways of the *cis* molecules within the cells.

Saturated fatty acids are characteristic of fats of animal origin, which are usually solids at room temperature, while vegetable oils contain unsaturated fatty acids and are usually liquids at room temperature. Certain fatty acids must be supplied in the diet, as the body is unable to manufacture them. They are called the essential fatty acids. Linoleic and linolenic acids are probably the best documented of these owing to their role in the human diet and their relevance to health. Appreciable amounts are absorbed into the bloodstream only after the complete oil has been ingested and chemically digested. However, the properties of the fatty acids present in the carrier oils used are significant for their suitability in aromatherapy. There is an ever-increasing choice of available vegetable oils and only a few representative ones are described here.

AROMAFACT

Pure carrier oils or fixed vegetable oils should always be used for aromatherapy massage. Baby oils, which are mineral oils, are not suitable; they act as skin protectors and moisturizers, holding water in the skin. This makes it more difficult for the essential oil to enter the body by this route.

THE FIXED CARRIER OILS

These are arranged in their botanical family classification. Amounts quoted are either % typical ranges or typical analysis amounts.

Rosaceae

1. Sweet Almond (Prunus amygdalus var dulcis)

Sweet almond does not produce essential oil but the 'fixed' carrier oil is extracted during processing the kernels.

This is a relatively inexpensive oil used extensively in skin care products; it is nourishing to the skin and suitable for use with conditions such as eczema. It contains a high proportion of mono- and polyunsaturated fatty acids, including oleic (65%), linoleic (26%), palmitoleic (0.5%) and linolenic (0.2%) acids. Saturated fatty acids found include palmitic (6.5%) and stearic (1.3%). Vitamins present are A, B1, B2 and B5, with vitamin E contributing to storage through its antioxidant properties. Antioxidants are often added to foods, including fats and oils, where they prevent slow oxidation by atmospheric oxygen. An oxidized fat or oil becomes rancid owing to formation of unpleasant-smelling acids.

AROMAFACT

Do not confuse sweet almond with bitter almond (*Prunus amygdalus* var *amara*). The essential oil is extracted by steam distillation after maceration of pressed nuts. A major component is benzaldehyde (95%), which is moderately toxic. Hydrocyanic acid is also formed, which is poisonous. It is not suitable for aromatherapy but is used in the food industry.

2. Apricot Kernel (Prunus armeiaca)

A light textured oil, which is virtually clear with a tinge of yellow and a strong marzipan odour. Used for sensitive skins making it suitable for facial blends. Rapidly absorbed and a good choice for dry mature and inflamed skin.

It is high in polyunsaturated fatty acids; its main components are oleic acid (up to 62%) and linoleic acid (up to 31%) with palmitic (up to 5%) and others, in order of descending amount stearic, palmitoleic and linolenic acids. There are no known reports of toxic effects from the oil, however, the apricot kernels are poisonous if ingested and have been reported to cause contact dermatitis.

3. Peach Kernel (Prunus vulgaris)

A practically odourless, pale green oil extracted from the nut kernel. Acting as an efficient emollient which aids elasticity and suppleness of skin, making it an ideal choice for dry and mature skin. Physically and chemically it is similar to sweet almond and apricot oils. Fatty acids present: oleic acid (62%) linoleic acid (29%) and palmitic acid (5%). It also has vitamins A and E. Considered a safe non-sensitizing and non-irritating oil.

Fabaceae/Leguminosae

4. Soya (Glyine max)

Extracted from the bean and often called Soyabean oil. A versatile carrier suitable for all skin types. It is comparatively high, up to 17%, in unsaturated fatty acids with the unsaturated linoleic (54%), oleic (24%), palmitic (10%), linolenic (7%) and stearic (4%). It also contains the highest amount of lecithin of any vegetable oil and the cold pressed oil is particularly high in vitamin E. It needs careful storage as it oxidizes easily. Soya oil may cause allergic reactions and has been reported to damage hair.

5. Peanut (Arachis hypogaea)

Peanut is also known as groundnut or arachis oil. Sometimes used as a cheap alternative to almond oil. Criticised as being quite oily and slow to absorb into the skin. Used externally it has been attributed therapeutic properties to help deal with arthritis and rheumatism. Fatty acids present are oleic acid (35–72%), linoleic acid (13–43%), stearic acid (1.3–6.5%), behenic acid (1–5%), lignoceric acid (0.5–3.0%) and ecosenoic acid (0.5–2.1%). The unrefined oil has vitamin E and various minerals but these are very low in the commercial product. The peanut is the most common and highly documented nut causing allergic reactions which can give rise to fatal anaphylaxis. Caution should be exercised when using the oil especially with babies, young children and nursing mothers.

Asteraceae/Compositae

6. Sunflower (Helianthus annus)

A practically odourless clear oil with a faint yellow tinge. Inexpensive, thin and non-oily it is especially suitable for blending with other carriers. Extracted from the seeds, which have a long tradition in culinary applications. The oil is available in a range of qualities and is also a favourite for cooking but this is the highly refined oil, which is not usually recommended for aromatherapy. External use is believed to be beneficial for skin problems such as ulcers, bruises, acne and seborrhoea. Fatty acid composition linoleic acid (up to 74%), oleic acid (up to 15%), palmitic acid (up to 6.4%), stearic acid (4.2%), linolenic acid (0.2%) and palmitoleic acid (0.1%). It is also high in vitamins A, B-complex, D and E, with minerals calcium, potassium, iron, zinc and phosphorus. Considered to be a safe oil with no reported contraindications.

Vitaceae

7. Grapeseed (Vitis vinifera)

An almost colourless and odourless oil which is inexpensive and becoming an increasingly popular choice for both culinary and massage applications. It is non-greasy, hypoallergenic and a common ingredient for skin creams. It blends well with other more viscous carriers. High in polyunsaturated fatty acids especially linoleic (58–81%), with oleic (12–20%), palmitic (5–11%) and stearic (3–6%). It is a safe and versatile oil, nontoxic with no reported contraindications.

Oleaceae

8. Olive Oil (Olea europaea)

This is a heavier oil used in soaps and cosmetics but less favoured for massage unless blended with less viscous oils. It is traditionally used as a culinary oil, with many researched beneficial health effects due to the high level of monounsaturated fatty acids. Fatty acid composition is oleic (75.5%), palmitic (11%), linoleic (8%), stearic (2.7%), palmitoleic (1.2%) and linolenic (0.7%).

Lauraceae

9. Avocado (Persea americana)

Avocado produces a rather viscous oil that penetrates the upper skin layers well and is beneficial for dry skin and is often found in sun preparations. It is versatile, with applications ranging from soothing nappy rash to an ideal choice for damaged, dry and mature skin. It is a mixture of monounsaturated and saturated fatty acids, with oleic (60–70%), linoleic (8–15%), palmitoleic (4–7%), linolenic (2%), palmitic (12–16%) and stearic (2%). Vitamins A, B and D are found along with lecithin. Lecithin is one of the major phospholipids (a lipid combined with a phosphate group) of the body. Phospholipids are vital chemicals needed in the body for structural and metabolic functions.

Pedaliaceae

10. Sesame Oil (Sesamum indicum)

Oils can be extracted from raw or roasted seeds. The best grade oil coming from cold pressing and filtering. Most sesame oils are practically odourless with a pale yellow colour. Usually blended with other carriers, as it is a thicker oil. Cosmetically it is used in hair products, shampoos and brilliantine, soaps and sunscreens and lubricating creams. It has good keeping properties and is not readily prone to oxidation from the air. Typical fatty acid composition would be oleic (33–46%), linoleic (41–52%), palmitic (5.5–9.5%), stearic (4–6%)

with a trace of linolenic. It contains the phospholipid lecithin and is high in vitamins E and B-complex, with minerals calcium, magnesium and phosphorus. Some caution may be advisable, as some hypersensitivity has been reported.

Linaceae

11. Linseed Oil (Linum usitatissimum)

The Latin name for the flax plant, from which the oil is extracted, means most useful. The versatility of the plant, its seeds and oil are well documented in history. There are two common names used for the products of the same plant – linseed oil and flaxseed oil. Linseed oil is extracted from the seeds by a hot, steam and high-pressure method to produce the commercial product. This is the oil that is used in making paints, wood preservatives, varnishes, stains, linoleum and putty. Flaxseed oil is extracted by the cold pressing of the seeds. The resultant oil is not filtered, deodorized or refined. Internally linseeds and oils were used for digestive disorders such as stomach problems and as a laxative. Linseed oil is used in cosmetic preparations such as emollients, soaps and shaving creams and is thought to be a useful ingredient for skin poultices treating burns and scalds. Chemically it is high in omega-3-fatty acids in common with fish oils. Typical fatty acid composition would be linolenic (57%), oleic (19%), linoleic (15%), palmitic (6%) and stearic (3.5%). The flaxseed oil contains vitamin A and beta-carotene (a precursor to vitamin A).

The oils both oxidize rapidly so care must be taken with storage in a refrigerated airtight bottle.

Corylaceae

12. Hazelnut (Corylus avellana)

An amber-yellow coloured oil with a pleasant characteristic odour. Particularly suited to greasy complexions as it rapidly penetrates the skin, having an astringent and circulatory stimulating effect in addition to its nutritive properties. When diluted with other carriers like sunflower or grapeseed the blend may benefit conditions like acne. Cosmetically hazelnut oil is used in sun filter lotions and creams, soaps, shampoos and other hair products. Its main fatty acids are oleic (70–84%), linoleic (9–19%) and stearic (1–4%). It has been reported to cause immunological urticaria (a skin condition also known as hives) and in common with other nut oils there is a possibility of anaphylactic shock.

Juglandaceae

13. Walnut (Juglans regin)

The oil has a characteristic walnut smell with the cold pressed oil a deep golden brown. The refined oil is lighter in colour and has a longer shelf life.

Cosmetically it is utilized in hair and skin preparations. In aromatherapy it may be externally beneficial to treat itchy and peeling scalp conditions. As a minor emollient with other oils it can be used as a relieving treatment for a range of skin disorders including superficial burns and sunburn. High in polyunsaturated fatty acids a typical composition would be linoleic acid (40–70%), linolenic acid (11–14%), oleic acid (16–36%), palmitic acid (7–8%) and stearic acid (2–3%), with minerals calcium, sodium, potassium, magnesium, iron, copper, manganese, zinc, sulphur, chlorine and phosphorus. The advantage of walnut, unlike some other nut oils, is it has no reported contraindications.

Proteaceae

14. Macadamia (Macadamia ternifolia)

A peach coloured oil with a delicate nutty aroma. Emollient and highly nourishing it is particularly suited to dry and mature skins. It is unusual in that it is comparatively high in the unsaturated fatty acids oleic acid (55–67%), palmitoleic acid (18–25%), palmitic acid (7.0–9.5%), stearic acid (2.0–5.5%) and myristic acid (0.6–1.6%). It has good keeping properties, as it is quite resistant to oxidation. There are no reported irritation or allergy reactions in skin testing.

Arecaceae

15. Coconut (Cocus nucifera)

The initially produced 'coconut oil' is actually a white solid highly saturated fat with a characteristic odour. It is extracted by either cold pressing or solvent extraction of the coconut flesh. This fat has a melting point of 25 °C and is reasonably stable to oxidation when exposed to the air. Chemically it is very high in saturated fats, typically up to 85%.

When the solid is further treated by fractionating it gives a clear oil. This commercial product is referred to as Fractionated Coconut oil. It contains more fatty acids of a shorter chain length, like octanoic (8 carbon atoms) and decanoic (10 carbon atoms), than the solid.

Due to its emollient properties it is found in products like soaps, hair conditioners, skin moisturizers and lipsticks. It is also employed as a hair pomade, particularly popular in tropical regions where it is reputed to prevent hair from going grey; unfortunately there is no scientific evidence to support this. In aromatherapy the emollient properties of the oils are put to use for massage blends and skin creams. Coconut oil, particularly the solvent extracted, has been implicated in allergic reactions so a cautionary approach is advisable.

Onagraceae

16. Evening Primrose Oil (Oenthera biennis)

This is a much favoured and highly publicized oil attributed with many beneficial properties when taken internally. The range of conditions that it benefits includes inflammatory ones like rheumatoid arthritis, Crohn's disease and multiple sclerosis, which are affected by levels of hormone-like substances called prostaglandins. The oil is particularly high in gamma linolenic acid (GLA 8.5–11.5%), which affects enzyme activity and ultimately the prostaglandins. Other fatty acids present include linoleic acid (65–74%), oleic acid (7%) and palmitoleic acid. It is also claimed to be beneficial for alleviating PMS (premenstrual syndrome). For its use as a massage oil there is some anecdotal evidence that it reaches the blood, making it effective for rheumatoid arthritis and PMS sufferers. It has also been shown to be beneficial to clients with eczema and psoriasis.

Graminae

17. Wheatgerm (Triticum vulgare)

This is a fairly heavy oil, high in the antioxidant vitamin E, making it suitable for use with other carrier oils, where it extends their keeping properties. It is useful for dry and mature skins and suitable for some types of dermatitis, and helpful for repairing sun-damaged skin. It contains a mixture of unsaturated and saturated fatty acids: linoleic (54%), oleic (19%), palmitic (16%), linolenic (7%), ecisadenoic (1.5%) and stearic (1%).

AROMAFACT

Wheatgerm oil is extracted by warm pressing or solvent extraction from the germ of the wheat. The wheatgerm is approximately 25% protein, so the oil will also contain some protein. Owing to this it may be contraindicated in a number of allergy sufferers and a test should always be carried out before use.

Euphorbiaceae

18. Castor (Ricinus communis)

A viscous oil not currently widespread in use for aromatherapy. Its traditional uses are well documented ranging from laxative when taken internally to external cosmetic applications in hair products and nail and lipsticks. Industrially it is used for treating leather and production of dyestuff oils.

LIQUID WAX

Simmondsiaceae

Jojoba (Simmondsia chinensis)   This is not actually an oil but a liquid wax. It is good for cosmetic use with moisturizing properties and ideal for dry skin and conditions like eczema and psoriasis. It is similar chemically to sebum and able to dissolve it. The oil keeps well owing to a stable molecular structure and analysis shows both saturated and unsaturated fatty acids, with eicosenoic (71%), oleic (14%), stearic (10%) and palmitic (1.5%). The presence of a compound called myristic acid is thought to confer anti-inflammatory properties.

BUTTERS

Shea butter

A creamy substance sometimes used as a low cost substitute for cocoa butter. Shea butter is a solid fatty oil from the nuts of Karite nut trees found in central and West Africa. Their botanical name is *Butyrospermum parkii* or *Vitellaria paradoxa* Gaertner. Extracted by cold pressing the product can be used raw or further refined. Nontoxic with a host of African folklore properties. It is an excellent moisturizer ideal for ageing skin due to its range of vegetable oils and claimed to benefit cell regeneration and circulation. Also used for skin conditions such as burns, ulcers and stretch marks. Due to its deep penetrating nature it is thought to soothe painful joints and aching muscles. Employed widely for culinary purposes and in cosmetic manufacture of soaps, sun protectors and lip balms. It contains five principal fatty acids, predominantly stearic and oleic together making up to 85–90% of the total, the others being palmitic, linoleic and arachidic. It also contains tocopherols (vitamin E) steroids, triterpenes, cinnamic acid, keratin and a number of phenolic compounds that give it antioxidant properties. It is generally considered a safe material but there have been warnings that latex allergy suffers would be wise to check with a patch test before use.

Cocoa butter (*Theobroma cacao*)

Made from the cocoa bean it is a low melting solid with a slight yellowish colour but only a very faint chocolate smell. It has a very wide range of culinary, pharmaceutical and cosmetic applications. Its melting point of 38 °C, close to that of core body temperature, means it is utilised in suppositories. It is a quickly absorbed, rich skin emollient. It gives softness, nourishment and protection and is found in ointments, creams, lip balms, body butter, massage bars and bath melts. Frequently recommended for prevention of stretch marks and chapped skin. Although found in many sun products it is not a protection factor. It contains a high proportion of saturated fatty acids (62%)

with monounsaturated (34%) and polyunsaturated (3%). Major fatty acids present are oleic (29–35%), palmitic (20–30%) and linoleic acid (1–3%). It is a stable fat with no cholesterol and high in antioxidants including vitamin E and alpha tocopherol.

INORGANIC CARRIER MATERIALS

Clays

Clays are a mixture of minerals. They come in a number of colours according to their individual mineral content. A typical composition would be silica (up to 52%), iron (4–6%), calcium (7–9%), potassium (3–5%), magnesium (2–3%), manganese (0.3%), sodium (0.1–0.3%), phosphorus (0.2%) plus various other trace elements.

They can be used both internally (correctly diluted with water) and externally.

- **Green Clay** – the most widely used as it has especially absorbent properties believed to be beneficial for drawing out skin toxins and promoting tissue repair. Fuller's earth, a grey-green powder, is hydrated aluminium silicate and aluminium magnesium sulphate. Employed for its absorbing properties in cleansing products. Sulphur may be added to treat oily skins. A typical chemical analysis of a commercially available Ionised Green Clay would be silica (44.5%), water (25%), aluminium (13.5%), calcium (5.5%), iron (4%), carbon (3.5%), magnesium oxide (2%), potassium (1%), phosphorus (0.37%), sulphur (0.15%), sodium (0.04%), manganese (0.03%), zinc (0.03%), chlorine (0.01%) and others (0.37%).

- **Red Clay** – colour due to iron (Fe) content; taken internally for anaemia and fatigue.

- **White Clay** – used in beauty preparations suitable for sensitive skin.

- **Kaolin** or **China Clay** – a white powder; hydrated aluminium silicate with good absorbent properties suitable for greasy complexions prone to acne.

- **Pink Clay** – a mixture of red and white clays. Used in facemasks for dry and sensitive skin.

- **Calamine** – a pale pink powder; zinc carbonate and zinc oxide. With a long tradition of use for inflamed and sensitive skins due to its soothing action. An established stalwart of home first aid boxes.

- **Yellow Clay** – used for joint and skin problems.

Clays disperse easily in water, but not with hydrophobic oils. They are particularly suited for use with the hydrolats.

COSMETIC AGENTS AND TOILETRIES

A variety of other materials are suitable as carriers of essential oils. These include gels, lotions, creams, soaps and shampoos. Collectively they can be referred to as cosmetic bases and toiletries. Their formulations are quite complex and varied, and this – along with marketing claims – is big business.

Many creams and lotions act as a moisturiser, which is an example of an emollient. Emollient means softening and soothing to the skin. An emollient provides protection to the skin against moisture loss. They do not actually put water into the skin but protect it from warm and dry conditions and in cold windy weather. Typical natural substances that act as emollients are almond oil and lanolin (from sheep wool). The term humectant is also used to describe the action of some ingredients found in cosmetic bases. This is defined as something that produces moisture or as a substance added to another to keep it moist. Examples are glycerine and sorbitol. Nourishing creams act predominantly as moisturizers but also deliver substances to feed and benefit the skin. These substances include vitamins, anti-oxidants, sun protection factors, proteins and a host of other ingredients that claim a variety of benefits. Many of these claims are unsubstantiated and in chemical terms substances usually need to be hydrophobic (lipid-soluble) to penetrate the epidermis of the skin.

Cleansing or washing the body is important not only for hygienic purposes but also as a pleasurable and relaxing experience. Cleansing products include soaps, detergents, shampoos, bath preparations, skin cleansers, face packs and masks. Soap and water can be an excellent cleansing agent. Soap is produced by the chemical reaction called saponification between an animal fat (tallow which is beef or sheep fat) or a vegetable oil (such as coconut or palm) with an alkaline. Salt is added during manufacture to form the solid. A typical soap might contain sodium stearate. Soaps dissolve in water to form an emulsion which can penetrate and dissolve the grease on the skin surface. Synthetic detergents are not derived from plant or animal materials but usually from petroleum products. They differ chemically in a number of ways with the advantage of not forming a solid 'scum' when used in hard water. Their action is similar to that of soap as they act as a surface-active agent for removing grease. Many contain TLS (triethanolamine lauryl sulphate), which is a clear liquid and found in many shampoos and bathing preparations acting as the actual detergent or surface-active molecule. Many beauty therapists and aromatherapists do not favour this and alternative formulations are available.

Table 7.8 shows a range of cosmetic bases, along with their chemical composition, that are available from an aromatherapy supplier.

The addition of appropriate essential oils can tailor these cosmetic bases, which are acting as carrier substances, and extend their use into a variety of useful applications.

Table 7.8   Cosmetic bases

PRODUCT
ALOE VERA GEL BASE - Water (Aqua), Aloe barbadensis Gel, Glycerin, Polysorbate 20, Triethanolamine, Phenoxyethanol, Carbomer, Caprylyl Glycol, Chlorphenesin, Potassium Sorbate
ALOE VERA MOISTURISING LOTION - Water (Aqua), Caprylic/Capric Triglyceride, Glycerin, Vitis vinifera, Aloe barbadensis Gel, Glyceryl Stearate SE, Stearic Acid, Phenoxyethanol, Triethanolamine, Catearyl Alcohol, Caprylyl Glycol, Carbomer, Tocopheryl Acetate, Chlorphenesin, Potassium Sorbate
AQUEOUS GEL BASE - Aqua, Propylene Glycol, Triethanolamine, Phenoxyethanol, Carbomer, Caprylyl Glycol, Chlorphenesin
BATH MILK BASE - Aqua, Helianthus annuus Caprylic/Capric Triglyceride, Ceteareth-20, Glyceryl Stearate SE, Phenoxyetanol, Caprylyl Glycol, Xanthum Gum, Chlorphenesin
BATH OIL BASE - Helianthus annuus, Polysorbate 20
BUBBLE BATH BASE - Water (Aqua), Cocoamidopropylbetaine (coconut foaming agent) Hydroxyethylcellulose (vegetable wax) and Methyldibromoglutaronitrile & Plenoxyethanol (preservative)
CLEANSING LOTION BASE - Water (Aqua), Caprylic/Capric Triglyceride, Glycerin, Stearic Acid, Cetearyl Alcohol, Persea americana, Prunus dulcis, Glyceryl Stearate, PEG-100 Stearate, Phenoxyethanol, Triethanolamine, Caprylyl Glycol and Chlorphenesin
CONDITIONER BASE (HAIR) - Water (Aqua), Cetrimonium chloride (palm oil based conditioning agent) Cetearyl alcohol (coconut based wax), Brassica napus 'Canola'
CREAM BASE - Water (Aqua), Caprylic/Capric Triglyceride, Cetyl alcohol, Glyceryl Stearate, PEG-100 Stearate, Glycerin, Prunus dulcis, Vitis vinifera, Benzyl alcohol, Phenoxyethanol, Potassium sorbate, Tocopheryl acetate, Sodium benzoate, Citric acid, Tocopherol
DEAD SEA SALTS (Fine)
EXFOLIATING SCRUB - Water (Aqua), Prunus dulcis(grains), Cetyl alcohol, Glycerin, Glyceryl Stearate, PEG-100 Stearate, Prunus dulcis, Vitis vinifera, Benzyl alcohol, Phenoxyethanol, Potassium sorbate, Sodium benzoate, Citric acid, Tocopherol
LIGHT FACE CREAM - Water (Aqua), Cetyl alcohol, Glycerin, Glyceryl stearate, PEG-100 stearate, Cocos nucifera, Persea americana, Prunus dulcis, Benzyl alcohol, Phenoxyethanol, Potassium sorbate, Sodium Benzoate, Citric acid, Tocopherol
LIQUID SOAP BASE - Water (Aqua), Cocamide DEA, Sodium Lauryl Glucose Carboxylate, Lauryl Glucoside, PEG-120 Methyl Glucose Dioleate, PEG-75, Limnanthes alba, Cocoamidopropyl
LOTION BASE - Water (Aqua), Cetyl alcohol, Glycerin, Glyceryl Stearate, PEG-100 Stearate, Prunus dulcis, Vitis vinifera, Benzyl alcohol, Phenoxyethanol, Potassium sorbate, Sodium benzoate, Citric acid, Tocopherol
MASSAGE OIL BASE - Coocos nucifera, Borago officinalis

continued

PRODUCT

MOISTURISING CREAM BASE - Water (Aqua), Cetyl alcohol, Caprylic/Capric Triglyceride, Glyceryl stearate, PEG-100 Stearate, Glycerin, Cocos nucifera, Persea americana, Vitis vinifera, Benzyl alcohol, Phenoxyethanol, Potassium sorbate, Sodium benzoate, Citric acid, Tocopherol

MOISTURISING LOTION BASE - Water (Aqua), Cetyl alcohol, Glycerin, Glyceryl stearate, PEG-100 stearate, Cocos nucifera, Persea americana, Prunus dulcis, Benzyl alcohol, Phenoxyethanol, Potassium sorbate, Sodium Benzoate, Citric acid, Tocopherol

'ORMAGEL' SEAWEED GEL BASE - Water (Aqua), Glycerin, Fucus vesiculosus (Bladderwrack) Extract, Propylene Glycol, Polysorbate 20, Phenoxyethanol, Triethanolamine, Carboner, Caprylyl Glycol, Chlorphenesin

SHAMPOO BASE CLEAR - Water (Aqua), Cocoamidopropylbetaine (coconut foaming agent) Hydroxyethylcellulose (vegetable wax) and Methyldibromoglutaronitrile & Plenoxyethanol (preservative)

SHOWER GEL BASE - Water (Aqua), Cocoamidopropylbetaine (coconut foaming agent) Hydroxyethylcellulose (vegetable wax) and Methyldibromoglutaronitrile & Plenoxyethanol (preservative)

SURFACTANT - (dispersant/emulsifier) - Polysorbate 20 (derived from Lauric Acid).

Our range of unfragranced cosmetic base products use wholly naturally derived ingredients, except where non-natural preservatives/stabilisers are crucial for the integrity and effectiveness of the product over time, and are guaranteed Sodium Laureth Sulfate and Paraben free.

All of our bases are formulated so that essential oils can be added to them directly and easily mixed into finished products. Itemised ingredients listings are given above. The majority of these products are water and vegetable oil based and can be extended with distilled water to obtain the required consistency.

The ingredients used are considered environmentally friendly, mild and not tested on animals. No animal-derived ingredients are used.

Courtesy of Justin Wells, Essentially Oils Ltd.

AQUEOUS PRODUCTS OF PLANTS

The use of aqueous (water-based) plant products, especially the Hydrolats, is becoming more popular with widespread applications. Although many of these have been used for hundreds of years their composition and range of properties is still the subject of research.

AROMAFACT

Their properties are said to mirror the properties of their essential oil. They are often considered to be milder and safer due to their dilute nature, however, they still need to be handled with care and insight. Purity is an important factor and a reliable source of material essential.

The definition and term essential oil is widely understood and accepted. However the associated aqueous products currently present a more confusing situation. The most commonly encountered names are Hydrosols, Hydrolats and Floral Waters.

AROMAFACT

The terminology is often used in a totally illogical and interchangeable way. This can be confusing for the aromatherapist as many suppliers use different names for the same products.

There are many different associated aqueous products with varying methods of production and composition. Simple working definitions of the three most commonly encountered are:

Hydrolat A term favoured in France and Germany. This is the aqueous product of distillation, it is the condensed steam that has passed through the plant material when extracting the essential oil. They are the true partial extracts of the plant material from the distillation process and may be considered to be a by-product of the volatile essential oil.

Hydrosol The term commonly used in the UK and USA and often interchangeable with Hydrolat. However, hydrosol can be an imprecise name and does not always restrict itself to aqueous distillation by-product. Some hydrosols are made by infusing the complete essential oil in water.

Fragrant waters   This is a very vague term as it covers a range of products, including those synthetically prepared, which are not appropriate to aromatherapy. Also the term Floral Water can be confusing as it implies a product made exclusively from flowers. This leaves a situation with a varying quality and composition of available waters ranging from the genuine product of distillation to an artificially chemically synthesized one. Some floral waters have compounds such as alcohol (ethanol) and glycerine added.

Chemically, apart from their high water content, the hydrolats can differ significantly from their associated essential oils. It is estimated that the volatile organic compounds are present in amounts of 0.1–0.4%. They have fewer hydrocarbons (which are hydrophobic) and it would be expected that the smaller molecules, like the monoterpenes such as sabinene, α- and β-pinene and α- and β-phellandrene, would be more likely to occur with larger sesquiterpenes absent. However, caryophyllene has been shown to be present in hydrolats of melissa and clary sage and germacrene shown to be present in hydrolats of melissa and marjoram. The other groups of chemical compounds found in essential oils are also present in varying amounts. These include alcohols (e.g. linalool, geraniol), aldehydes (e.g. 3-Methyl-butanal), ketones (e.g. carvone, thujone), acetates (e.g. Linalyl acetate, lavendulyl acetate) and oxides (e.g. 1,8-cineole).

Rose Water/Hydrolat

The complexity of the aqueous products situation can be illustrated by Rose Water. It is a long established product with a history of applications in cosmetics, skincare and culinary preparations. Initially it may be produced from different botanical species e.g. typically Wild rose (*Rosa canina*), Damask rose (*Rosa damascena*) and Cabbage rose (*Rosa centifolia*).

Box 7.24 shows the analysis for a natural rose water.

AROMAFACT

Genuine, unadulterated rose hydrolat varies from commercially produced rose water that is formulated in the laboratory. Some regulations (including the BP) require ethanol to be added as a preservative and this can make up to 15% of the composition. It is important to check the origins, composition and production method of anything described as rose water.

There are many properties attributed to Rosa hydrolats. It has been suggested that their specific therapeutic properties may be linked to the % composition of functional group compounds present. This theory is unproved but finds favour with many aromatherapists.

- Aldehydes 5–6% – anti-infectious, antiviral, anti-inflammatory, hypotensive, calming, antipyretic, tonic.
- Esters 8–9% – antifungal, anti-inflammatory, antispasmodic, calming, uplifting, balancing (nervous system).
- Alcohols 32–66% – anti-infectious, bactericidal, antiviral, stimulating, decongestant.

Melissa Hydrolat

Melissa officialis or lemon balm has a hydrolat with a lemony scent with a wide variety of both internal and external uses. Its culinary applications are widespread and other uses include skincare, insect bites, digestive disorders and menstrual problems.

AROMAFACT

Melissa essential oil is expensive and difficult to distill as it contains many hydrophilic (water loving) molecules. This means that the correctly produced hydrolat has many of these molecules in its aqueous solution and its properties are similar to that of the essential oil.

Box 7.25 shows the analysis of two samples of melissa hydrolat. Both samples are from reputable producers and illustrate variations in composition. These can be due to a variety of factors including the nature of the plant material used, the distillation parameters and the operating systems of the analytical method.

Box 7.24   Analysis of a Natural Rose Water

Distillation water: Bulgarska Rosa Plovdiv
Appearance: Clear liquid
Colour: Colourless
Odour: Typical of roses

Physico–chemical indices
Essential oil content %:   Min 0.025
Ethanol content %:   Max 4
pH: 4–7.5
Composition: Contains the basic ingredients of rose oil: geraniol, citronellol, nerol, phenyl alcohol, ethyl alcohol
Packing: 200 dm^3 barrels with a protective inner coating
Storage: In dark and cool
Expiry term: One year

%	Compound
0.11	cis- and trans-Linalyl oxide
4.9	Linalool
0.2	Terpineol-4
0.05	Neral
1.8	α-Terpineol
0.18	Geranial
28.5	Citronellol
7.15	Nerol
0.52	β-phenylethyl acetate
27.9	Geraniol
7.4	β-phenylethyl alcohol
0.19	Methyl eugenol
0.2	Eudesmol
0.9	Eugenol
0.55*	Carvacrol
0.23	Citronellic acid
0.69	Neric acid
8.7	Geranic acid

* [possible contamination from thyme water] Essential oil/water ratio <0.02%.
Courtesy of Len Price, taken from Understanding Hydrolats: The specific Hydrosols for Aromatherapy. A Guide for Health Professionals (Churchill Livingstone)

Box 7.25   Analysis of melissa hydrolat

Melissa officinalis [LEMON BALM] Lamiaceae*

%	Compound
1.83	Acetone
4.98	Dimethyl sulphide
19.27	2-Methyl propanal
19.83	3-Methyl butanal
12.87	2-Methyl butanal
0.28	Dimethyl disulphide
1.11	Hexanal
4.36	2-Hexenal
0.82	2,5-Diethylterahydrofuran or isomer
5.31	6-Methyl-5-hepten-2-one
1.14	3-Octanone
0.71	3-Octanol
5.17	Linalool
0.46	cis-Rose oxide
0.28	trans-Rose oxide
0.66	2,2-Dimethylocta-3,4-dienal or isomer
1.34	Isomenthone
0.63	Isopinocamphone
5.38	Neral
4.06	Probably methyl 3,7-dimethyl-6-octenoate or isomer
8.54	Geranial
0.20	Neryl acetate
0.76	Geranyl acetate

* Source from Farming co-operative in Drome valley

Melissa officinalis [LEMON BALM] Lamiaceae**

%	Compound
4.19	Acetone
0.65	2-Methyl propanal
4.12	3-Methyl butanal
1.44	2-Methyl-butanal
0.54	2,5-diethyltetrahydro-furan or isomer
25.54	6-Methyl-5-hepten-2-one
0.80	3-Octanol
5.84	Linalool
0.28	cis-Rose oxide
0.24	trans-Rose oxide
0.79	2.2-Dimethylocta-3,4-dienal or isomer
27.09	Neral
28.48	Geranial

** Source from Herbes de Chevenoz

Courtesy of Len Price, taken from Understanding Hydrolats: The Specific Hydrosols for Aromatherapy. A Guide for
Health Professionals (Churchill Livingstone)

Again specific therapeutic properties have been linked to amounts of functional group compounds present:

- Ketones 3–10% – anti-inflammatory, analgesic, skin healing, calming, digestive, expectorant, sedative.
- Aldehydes 69–73% – anti-infectious, antiviral, anti-inflammatory, calming, hypotensive, tonic.

Widely available hydrolats include lavenders, chamomiles, orange flower, carrot, everlasting, juniper berry, marjoram, tea tree, melissa, peppermint, geranium, Scots pine, rosas, rosemary, sage, clary sage and sweet thyme. The types available are increasing as interest grows. As the use of hydrolats becomes more widespread, experience and shared knowledge should enhance their use as a valuable material for the aromatherapist.

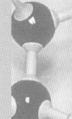

Chapter **8**

Handling, safety and practical applications for use of essential oils

INTRODUCTION AND BACKGROUND

A knowledge of the chemical and physical properties of the essential oils and materials used gives a logical background that can inform and guide in their applications in aromatherapy. The everyday storage, handling and use of oils with clients involve an underlying understanding of safety coupled with an awareness of the ever-increasing burden of legislation. The basics of anatomy and physiology appropriate to aromatherapy and the links to psychological well-being also need to be considered within this context. Topics in this chapter draw directly on the concepts previously covered in analysis and composition of oils. Important sources of information about properties and handling of essential oils can be found in established literature, in specialist journals and from the individual Safety Data Sheet for that oil. Safety Data Sheets cover areas including composition, health hazards, first aid procedures, dire and explosion hazard, procedures for accidental release, handling, storage, ecological implications, transport, labelling, regulations and other information. The oil supplier should have Safety Data Sheets for the materials they sell. An example for *Eucalyptus globulus* is shown in this chapter, and in the previous chapter we saw such sheets for rosemary and lemongrass, where they were linked with analytical data.

STORAGE OF OILS

Containers

It is important that the container is made of material that will not interact, either physically or chemically, with the essential oil. For the quantities handled by the aromatherapist, neutral glass is the best choice. Suppliers will use metal containers for larger quantities. Aluminium with an internally lacquered surface would be suitable for amounts up to 10 kg, while internally lacquered steel drums would be appropriate for amounts above 10 kg.

AROMAFACT

Plastic is usually avoided as it can absorb constituents from the oil, thus altering the composition of the oil. Also, this can cause the container walls to swell and weaken. Chemicals in the plastic may also be absorbed by the oil, thus altering its composition again. When components of the plastic become dissolved in the oil, detectable changes often occur in its odour.

Closures

The container must be sealed by a closure. If air is allowed to enter and interact with the essential oil, the chemical reaction of oxidation can occur. Oxidation in this case can be considered the addition of oxygen to an oil constituent to form a new compound. New compounds formed will alter the composition of the oil. Water vapour may also enter from the air. An open or incompletely sealed container will allow essential oil components to escape as vapours, and this will change the balance of constituents. The best choice of closure for a bottle is a screw cap fitted with a wad or washer. Ideally bottles are fitted with childproof tops and drop dispensers to control amounts dispensed.

 AROMAFACT

Essential oils like *Citrus limon* (lemon) and *Pinus sylvestris* (Scotch pine), which are high in terpenes such as limonene and pinene, are particularly prone to oxidation. The air provides oxygen, and oxidation is the chemical reaction in which oxygen adds onto another substance, to form a new compound. Small amounts of essential oil should not be kept in large bottles with a large amount of air above the oil. As the oil is used up, its level goes down and the amount of air above it increases. If an oil is stored in a large bottle, the number of times it is opened will also probably be more than for a smaller one, and this also exposes it to the air each time.

Protection from light

Essential oils should be protected from the light. Sunlight causes photocatalytic activity – that is, there are reactions that are speeded up by light. These reactions cause the essential oil to deteriorate. Artificial lights such as filament bulbs and fluorescent tubes are far less active than sunlight, but are still harmful.

AROMAFACT

Metal containers give complete protection against light, but amber glass will afford adequate protection for the majority of oils used by the aromatherapist.

Temperature

It is important to store essential oils under cool conditions. Woody oils such as *Cedrus atlantica* (cedarwood), *Santalum album* (sandalwood), *Pogostemon cablin* (patchouli) and *Vetiveria zizanioides* (vetivert) can be stored at a low room temperature, no higher than 15 °C. Resinoids can be kept at low temperatures, no higher than 10 °C, as may be found in a cellar. All other oils are best stored at temperatures found in a typical domestic refrigerator at around 5 °C. Rose otto and rose absolute and a few other oils may congeal or solidify at low temperatures, but re-melt at room temperature. It is important that they are allowed to do this gradually without application of artificial heat.

AROMAFACT

Citrus essential oils and many herbal essential oils that are rich in highly volatile, low boiling point monoterpenes will deteriorate very quickly if not kept cool. Ideally they should be used within six months of purchase, but if they are stored and handled carefully this can be extended for up to a year. Most other essential oils should be used within a year of purchase or first opening, but this may be extended to two years if they are handled carefully and stored in a refrigerator. These effects can be explained by the fact that the rate of deterioration *doubles* for every 10 °C rise in temperature.

In conclusion, the general storage rules for essential oils would be: store in tightly stoppered, small, dark glass bottles that will be used up quickly with minimal times of opening to prevent entry of air or loss of volatile components. They should be stored at cool temperatures and used within a year of purchase.

Flammability and spillages

Essential oils are flammable and must be kept away from naked flames. Small spillages can be wiped up with paper or a cloth which should then be placed in an external bin, as this waste can easily ignite. Large spillages should be absorbed onto a suitable inert material and then put into sealed containers. Under no circumstances should these be incinerated or discharged into drains or sewers.

AROMAFACT

Essential oils have a value called a flash point, which gives a measure of their flammability. It can be defined as the lowest temperature at which the vapour above a liquid can be ignited in air. Typical values for essential oils are in the range 33 °C to 77 °C. The lowest values are found in oils such as *Boswellia carteri* (frankincense) at 32 °C and citrus oils at around 43 °C, and the highest in woody oils, with *Santalum album* (sandalwood) having a flash point above 100 °C and *Cedrus atlantica* (Atlas cedarwood) one of 110 °C.

LABELLING

From practical considerations, the actual size of the label on a typical essential oil bottle is very small. This will limit the amount of information it can carry. There are a number of recommendations and guidelines for labelling from various regulatory and professional bodies, which need to be applied with certain legislative requirements in mind. These include guidance from AOC (Aromatherapy Organizations Council), IFRA (International Fragrance Association) and ISO (International Organization for Standardization). The EC regulations are explained in Chapter 7.

Details of labelling will be covered in the aspects of Professional Practice on an aromatherapy course. For practical purposes the label for an essential oil should indicate the following:

1. The botanical name and the part of the plant the oil is derived from, e.g. *Syzygium aromaticum* (clove) from bud, leaf or stem; *Juniperus communis* L. (juniper) from berry or needle.
2. The amount of the oil in the bottle.
3. The concentration of the oil. Many pre-blended oils are 5% in a carrier oil, and that carrier oil should also be named.
4. An indication of the useful shelf-life of the oil.
5. Storage precautions and temperature implications, usually stated as keep cool, tightly sealed, not in direct sunlight and out of reach of children.
6. Cautions: do not use neat, keep away from eyes, for external use only – do not ingest.
7. Name of supplier, with a contact point.

AROMAFACT

Oils that are bought directly from a supplier or through a retail outlet will probably carry most of the information listed above. However, you may supply an essential oil, or a blend of oils that is specifically formulated for use with an individual client. This will need additional labelling and must link to your therapists' record-keeping system. These oils will need to have additional information, including the client's name, date administered, directions for use and any special precautions or interactions. This is similar to the situation for drugs dispensed through a pharmacy. In terms of safety, the abbreviation GRAS on a label means Generally Recognized as Safe.

LEGISLATION AND REGULATORY BODIES

Aromatherapists need to be aware of a number of legislative regulations. These include The Medicines Act (1968); COSHH, Control of Substances Hazardous to Health; HSWA, Health and Safety at Work Act (1974); and CHIP, Chemicals (Hazard Information and Packaging for Supply) Regulations (CHIP 2 1994). The MCA (Medicines Control Agency) also has significant implications and constantly encroaches on the supply and use of products related to health.

HSWA – Health and Safety at Work Act   In 1974 the government passed the Health and Safety at Work Act. This enabling legislation allows regulations to control health and safety to be issued and revised as required, with new acts being passed. Such regulations cover working conditions, manual handling and, of particular relevance to aromatherapists, COSHH, CHIP and Safety Data Sheets.

COSHH – Control of Substances Hazardous to Health   This is a broad set of regulations designed to protect people from substances that are hazardous to health. When considering the implications of COSHH, an assessment is made based on a consideration of the risk to health resulting from work with potentially hazardous substances. It must include a justification for using the hazardous substance and a consideration of means of minimizing exposure to any substance identified as hazardous. The importance of this is highlighted by the Health and Safety Commission's Approved Code of Practice. It is useful to distinguish between hazards and risks. The term *hazard* means the inherent potential for danger to human health. A substance with a low hazard is one that is inherently safe, e.g. water. A substance with a high hazard is one that is dangerous even in low doses, e.g. potassium cyanide. A *risk* is the actual chance that danger to health results from use of a substance. A knowledge of the hazard of a substance and the circumstances under which it will be used are needed to assess the risk.

AROMAFACT

Essential oils should always be used in a controlled manner and this usually involves a low concentration reaching the metabolizing tissues. This is consistent with the reasoning behind COSHH. There is no such thing as a harmless substance, but there is such a thing as a harmless dose.

It is essential to understand the hazards of chemical products so that they can be used safely. Important sources of information for aromatherapists include guidelines from bodies such as RIFM (Research Institute for Fragrance Materials), IFRA (International Fragrance Association), product labels and MSDS (Material Safety Data Sheets).

CHIP – Chemicals (Hazard Information and Packaging for Supply Regulations)   The specific regulations applicable to aromatherapy are the CHIP 2 Regulations 1994; they are again related to whether a chemical is hazardous. The fundamental requirement of the CHIP regulations is to allocate what type of hazard a substance has: this is the category of danger and how the substance is classified. The hazard is then described by allocation of a risk phrase, hazard symbol and safety phrase. CHIP regulations may apply to essential oils and aromatherapy products. For example, the R65 risk phrase sets out criteria for classifying and labelling chemicals that could cause lung damage if swallowed, which is the 'aspiration hazard'. This is possible because essential oils have low viscosity. Chemicals that meet the R65 risk category are classified as Harmful: May Cause Lung Damage if Swallowed, and the regulations require the appropriate danger symbol (a black **X** on an orange square with the word 'hazardous' below; represented in shorthand as Xn in printed or written matter) to be displayed on the labels and in the text for safety phrases. The container or label should display the advice 'if swallowed, do not induce vomiting, seek medical advice immediately and show this container or label'.

AROMAFACT

The R65 risk category would apply to essential oils with more than 10% hydrocarbons, which includes many essential oils including lavender, tea tree, cypress and bergamot. The wording on essential oils and aromatherapy products is obligatory if they are sold to, or likely to be used by, the general public and it is recommended for those used in industry.

MSDS – Material Safety Data Sheets (now usually referred to as SDS, Safety Data Sheets)   Suppliers, manufacturers and importers who make up the chain of supply of essential oils to the aromatherapist, and ultimately the client, are responsible for drawing up the MSDS. Each time an oil is repackaged or relabelled, a MSDS should be prepared and relevant additional information provided before it is passed on to the next customer in the chain of supply. When a chemical is supplied to the general public in retail outlets, by mail order or as free samples and prizes, a MSDS is only needed if the purchaser intends to use that chemical at work, if the chemical preparation is classified as dangerous for supply (according to the CHIP 2 regulation) or if the purchaser asks for a safety data sheet. For most practical situations the packaging and labelling will supply sufficient information for safe use. The labelling of aromatherapy oils and blends is described in Chapter 7.

A typical MSDS is shown for *Eucalyptus globulus* in Figure 8.1 and gives a fairly comprehensive range of information about the oil. The example is one provided by a British oil supplier, and shows that a reputable supplier can provide high-quality relevant data. There are a number of features included that are explained elsewhere in this book, i.e. specific gravity, LD_{50}, GRAS, CHIP regulations, flash point, RIFM, hazard symbols, R phrase and S phrase. In addition there are a number of other acronyms that need to be identified.

- *CAS – Chemical Abstracts Service Number* is a US-based service that gives a summary of articles and papers in the scientific and chemical literature that relate to the chemical properties of a compound or substance. Each substance is given a code number and using that code a summary of information can be found.

- *FEMA – Federal Emergency Management Agency* is a US-based organization that offers plans, services and help in disaster management.

- *FDA – Food and Drug Administration Agency* is again a US-based government organization whose mission is to promote and protect the public health by helping safe and effective products reach the market in a timely way, and monitoring products for continued safety after they are in use. It provides a blend of law and science aimed at protecting consumers.

- *INCI – International Nomenclature of Cosmetic Ingredients* is a document drawn up in response to the Cosmetic Products Directive of the EC and produces an inventory of fragrance ingredients (perfume and aromatic raw materials). The lists are representative of the basic materials used in perfumes and aromatic compositions. The lists were compiled mainly on the basis of information provided by EFFA (European Flavour and Fragrance Association). They constitute the inventory of fragrance ingredients. Fragrance ingredients do not need a common nomenclature because the fragrance or their ingredients must be indicated on the labels using the words 'perfume' or 'flavour'. Hence the information on the identity of these substances consists of a chemical name identifying the substances in the clearest possible way. Such a system already exists in the 'acquis communautair', namely the EINECS Inventory (European Inventory of Existing Commercial Chemical Substances) and ELINCS (European List of Notified Chemical Substances). Chemical substances can be described in an unequivocal manner with a chemical name, CAS number and EINECS number.

SAFETY DATA SHEET

Supplied in accordance with the provisions of:
Directive 91/155/EEC
Article 10 of Directive 88/379/EEC

1.1 Identity of substance:	Essential oil of: **EUCALYPTUS GLOBULUS** *Eucalyptus globulus* **Labill. spp. and other species.** **INCI Name:** *Eucalyptus globulus* **CAS: 8000–48–4.6** **FEMA: 2466.2. 6**
1.2 Supplier:	[Name] [Address] [Telephone no.] [Emergency contact]
2.0 Composition:	The chemical composition of natural essential oils can be tremendously variable. A typical composition for this material may be: 1,8-cineole 70–90%, with α-pinene, *d*-limonene, *para*-cymene, α-phellandrene, camphene, α-terpinene.
2.1 Physical data	Appearance: Clear liquid, with a pungent familiar 'medicinal' smell. Solubility in **water**: INSOLUBLE Solubility in ethyl **alcohol**: Minimum 80% required Specific gravity: 0.9050–0.930 @ 25.00 °C
3.0 *Health hazard data*	The acute ORAL LD50 of **1,8-cineole** in rats was 2.48 g/kg. *Jenner P. et al. 1964. Fd. Cosmet. Toxicol. 2, 327.*
3.1 Toxicity	The Dermal LD50 in rabbits exceeded 5 g/kg. *Moreno O. 1972. Report to the RIFM.*[1]

Caution: There are several reports of poisoning caused by relatively small amounts of Eucalyptus oil. Death has occurred in adults after ingesting as little as 4–5 ml. of oil. *MacPherson L. 1925. Med. J. Aust 2: 108–110 also Patel S. 1980. Arch. Dis. Child. 55: 404–6*

This product must be stored out of the reach of children
Eucalyptus oil was given GRAS status by FEMA[2] (1965)
Approved by the FDA[3] for food use (§ 172.510).
Approved by the Council of Europe. CE: 185n

Figure 8.1 A typical material safety data sheet. Courtesy of Medical Aromatherapy Training Services. Supplied by Charles Wells, Essentially Oils and Analytical Intelligence Ltd.

3.2 Adverse skin reactions	Eucalyptus oil tested at 10% caused no irritation or sensitisation on humans. *Kligman A. 1966 & 1973. Reports to the RIFM.*[1]
3.3 Primary routes of exposure	Skin contact: YES. Inhalation: YES. Eye contact: YES. Skin absorption: NO. Ingestion: NO (unless consumed).
3.3 Medical conditions aggravated by overexposure	Any pre-existing allergies to fragrance or other materials may be aggravated following exposure to this oil.

3.4 Effects of overexposure

(a) Eye contact effects:	May be very irritating to the eyes.
(b) Skin contact effects:	May be mildly irritating to skin.
(c) Inhalation effects:	Will be irritating if the vapour is excessively inhaled.
(d) Aspiration effects:	May be harmful to the lungs if aspiration occurs.
(e) Ingestion effects:	May be harmful if swallowed.

Suggested classification under CHIP regulations as per The British Essential Oil Association member recommendations.

Hazard symbol	Risk hazard	Hydrocarbon content	Safety phase
Xn	R.10, R65	15%	S62

(See 9.6 for explanation of symbols)

4.0 *First aid procedures*

4.1 Eye contact:	Flush immediately with cold milk if available, then flush with clean water for at least 15 minutes. **Contact a doctor or take the person to a casualty unit if problems persist.**
4.2 Skin contact	Remove any contaminated clothing or shoes. Wash affected areas thoroughly with soap and water for at least 15 minutes. Flush continuously with cold water. Contact a doctor if necessary or take the person to a casualty unit.
4.3 Inhalation	Remove from the exposure to fresh air. If breathing has stopped administer artificial respiration and oxygen if available. **Contact a doctor or ring the emergency services.**

Figure 8.1 *Contd*

4.4 Ingestion Wash out the mouth with milk or water provided the person is conscious. *Do not induce vomiting.* **Ring the emergency services immediately.**

5.0 *Fire and explosion hazard*

5.1 Flash point: 42 °C. 107 F

5.2 Storage: Keep away from heat and open flames.

5.3 Extinguishing media: Carbon Dioxide; Dry Chemical; Universal-Type Foam. **Do not use: Water.**

5.4 Special fire-fighting procedures: Self-contained breathing apparatus and protective clothing should be worn when fighting fires involving essential oils or chemicals. Carbon monoxide and unidentified organic compounds may be formed during combustion.

6.0 *Accidental release measures*

6.1 Reactivity data: Chemically stable, but reduce oxygen exposure.

6.2 Conditions to avoid: This product presents no significant reactivity hazard. It is stable and will not react violently with water. Hazardous polymerization will not occur.

6.3 Incompatibility with other materials: Avoid contact or contamination with strong acids, alkalis, or oxidizing agents.

6.4 Hazardous combustion or decomposition products: Carbon monoxide and unidentified organic compounds may be formed during combustion.

6.5 Spill or leak procedures: Eliminate all ignition sources and ventilate the area. Contain spill and recover free product. Absorb remainder on vermiculite or other suitable absorbent material. Use of self-contained breathing apparatus is recommended for any major chemical spills. Prevent the liquid from entering the drains and sewers. Report spills to appropriate authorities if required.

6.6 Waste disposal methods: Place material and absorbent into sealed containers and dispose of in accordance with current applicable laws and regulation.
   Note: Empty containers can have residues, gases and mists and are subject to proper waste disposal. **Do not incinerate closed containers.**

7.0 *Handling, storage and special protection information*

7.1 Store in a cool, dry place, away from sources of heat and ignition. Be cautious when handling with lifting equipment that the containers are not punctured.

Figure 8.1   *Contd*

7.2 Protective gloves: The use of chemical resistant gloves is recommended, particularly when handling large volumes of this oil.

7.3 Respiratory protection: Not generally required.

7.4 Ventilation protection: Adequate ventilation is essential in confined spaces.

7.5 Protective clothing: Not generally required unless handling bulk oils in hot, humid conditions.

7.6 Eye protection: Goggles or a face shield are recommended for bulk handling.

7.7 Other protective measures: Avoid inhalation and contact with skin and eyes. Good personal hygiene practices should be used. Wash after any contact, before breaks and meals, and at the end of the work period.

8.0 *Environmental and ecological information*

8.1 Biodegradability: Pure essential oils are extracted from plants and therefore will biodegrade in the same manner as plants.

8.2 Water course contamination: Since essential oils and similar extracts float on water, any spillage should not cause problems to fish. Microorganisms such as plankton may be killed, but ecological recovery will be swift. Evaporation and dispersion of the lighter fractions will be swift. Heavier fractions may remain for an undetermined period of time. Crustacean and Invertebrate contamination is possible.

If a major spillage occurred into a watercourse, harm could be caused to aquatic birds and aquatic mammals. Therefore **immediate measures to contain the spill are necessary and removal of such creatures from the area.** Cleaning of these creatures would be the same as for humans, i.e. the use of detergents to remove the oil and flushing with clean water.

9.0 *Transport and Labelling information*

9.1 UN Number 1993: Flammable Liquid N.O.S.

9.2 Land. Road, Railway: ARD/RID Class 3.3 NO 31 d.c. Code 30 Ident: 1197 Label 3. Trem Card required with road transport of bulk oil.

9.3 Inland Waterways Mark with '**Flammable**' label, '**With Care**' and '**This way up**' labels.

9.4 Sea IMDG Page 3372 No 1197 Class 3.3 No: III Ident: 3-05 No GSMU 310, 313. U.K. IMO Mark with '**Flammable**' label. '**Stow away from heat**'. Flash point should be given.

Figure 8.1   *Contd*

9.5 Air No.: ONU 1197 Class 3.3 Passenger 309 Freighter 310 (220L)
Complete with 'hazard' labelling in accordance with IATA regulations.

9.6 Labelling Information:
In accordance with E.C. Directive, 4th Amendment, Art 6.
Hazard Symbol : Xn. Hazard and Caution conditions apply. Label Xn.
R phase: R65-Harmful. May cause lung damage if swallowed. R10 Flammable.
S Phrase: S62-If swallowed do not induce vomiting. Seek medical attention immediately and show this container or label.
EINECS: 283–406-2.[5]

10 *Regulatory and other Information*

10.1 EC Legislation: Council Directive of 27 July 1976 76/768/EEC Laws relating to Cosmetic Products. EC Directive, 4th Amendment, Art. 6: labelling. EC Directive on Packaging and Packaging Waste.

10.2 UK Legislation: Health and Safety at Work Act 1974 and relevant Statutory Provisions. Management of Health and Safety at Work Regulations 1992, Control of Substances Hazardous to Health (COSHH) Regulations 1999. Chemicals (Hazard Information and Packaging for Supply) (CHIP) Regulations 1994. The Cosmetics Products (Safety) Regulations 1996. Approved Guide to the Classification of substances and preparations dangerous for supply (2nd Ed. 1993). CHIP-2. CHIP 1999 Upgrade.

10.3 UK Further Information: The Weights and Measures (Cosmetic Products) Order 1994. General Code of Practice to COSHH Regulations, HSE.HS (G) 97 A Step By Step Guide to COSHH Regulations, HSE.HS(G)65, Successful Health and Safety Management, HSE. The General Product Safety Regulations 1994 U.K. Packaging Waste Regulations. 1996

References
1. RIFM is the Research Institute for Fragrance Materials: Two University Plaza Suite 406 Hackensack, New Jersey 07601, USA. Tel: 201–488–5527 Fax: 201–488–5594
2. FEMA is the The Federal Emergency Management Agency, 500 C Street, SW Washington, DC 20472
3. FDA is the Food and Drug Administration USA. http://www.fda.gov/fdahomepage.html
4. Set 4 Plant Aromatics Safety data manuals by Martin Watt. http://www.aromamedical.demon.co.uk
5. EINECS is the European Inventory of Existing Commercial Chemical Substances
6. Allured's Flavor and Fragrance Materials 1999. ISBN 0–93170-64-2

Figure 8.1 *Contd*

DISCLAIMER

The information contained in the Material Data Sheets has been compiled from data considered accurate. However, properties are known to vary depending on the source of raw materials, climatic and other variables applicable to materials of botanical origin. [Company Name] expressly disclaim any warranty expressed or implied as well as any liability for any injury or loss arising from the use of this information or the materials described. This data is not to be construed as absolutely complete since additional data may be desirable when particular conditions or circumstances exist. It is the responsibility of the user to determine the best precautions necessary for the safe handling and use of this product for their particular application. This data relates only to the specific material designated and **not when used in combination with any other material.**

PREPARED BY: [Company or Agency Name]

Figure 8.1   *Contd*

Restrictions on the use of a given ingredient are identified. Restrictions are set out in the Directive itself or in the IFRA (International Fragrance Association) code of practice. These restrictions may take the form of a quantitative limitation (expressed as a percentage of the final product or as a concentration for application to the skin), or the ingredient may have to meet certain specifications or may only be used in conjunction with certain specified ingredients. These substances are marked with one asterisk * for IFRA restrictions or with two asterisks ** for restrictions in the Cosmetic Products Directive.

AROMAFACT

In the fragrance inventory various qualities of a given ingredient, such as geraniol, have not been recorded separately; the same applies to different qualities of natural products with the same botanical origin. Orange oils from Brazil, Florida, California, etc., concentrated or otherwise, are all indicated under a single entry, i.e. 'sweet orange extracts CAS8028-48-6, EINECS 232–433-8'. This rubric is defined as 'Extractives and their physically modified derivatives such as tinctures, concretes, absolutes, essential oils, oleoresins, terpenes, terpene-free fractions, distillates, residues etc. obtained from *Citrus sinensis*, Rutaceae'.

- RIFM – Research Institute for Fragrance Materials is a US-based body with an ongoing programme for the testing of fragrance ingredients, including essential oils. The research follows strict scientific guidelines by independent experts. Information is collated and evaluated by a committee of specialists in all aspects of safety, composition and applications of fragrance chemicals. The reports are then transmitted to IFRA (International Fragrance Association) and these are passed on to their members in regular 'IFRA Updates'. RIFM reports the results of safety testing on both essential oils and chemicals used in fragrances, in Raw Materials Monographs. The monographs generally include data on acute oral and dermal toxicity, skin irritation and sensitization and phototoxicity. A new volume of these is published every few years by Elsevier Science. Their function is to provide international links and encourage adherence to a good code of practice within the perfume industry and ensure that issues of safety are regularly addressed.

- IFRA – International Fragrance Association is based in Geneva and was founded in 1973. It represents the collective interests of the fragrance industry worldwide. It has established, and seeks to preserve, self-regulatory practices through the development and implementation of a code of Practice and Safety Guidelines utilized internationally, with the final objective being to protect consumers and the environment. Usage guidelines for fragrance materials are established through the application of available scientific data and by policing compliance with those guidelines. IFRA analyses and reviews relevant pending legislations and regulations and disseminates information and recommendations to members and other international organizations. The monitoring of legislative trends worldwide is one of its main missions, along with the promotion of a consistent approach and understanding essential for global cooperation. Its guidelines, in addition to the Code of Practice, cover categories including quality control, storage, handling, labelling and packaging, usage and safety standards for fragrance materials. The link between the work of RIFM and IFRA has been described whereby IFRA distributes advisory updates for use of materials based on reports from RIFM.

AROMAFACT

Much of the work of IFRA is relevant to essential oils used in aromatherapy and it is a very respected organization. Although primarily targeting the fragrance industry, it also makes important safety points for aromatherapy. For example, in 1998 IFRA recommended that the compound methyleugenol should not be used as a fragrance ingredient, as research had shown it to be carcinogenic in mice. It stated that the restriction did not currently apply to essential oils containing methyleugenol. A formal statement is now due to be issued following further scientific research relating to naturally occurring methyleugenol. It is a major component of *Melaleuca bracteata* (a type of tea tree known as black tea tree). Methyleugenol chemotypes exist for *Ocimum sanctum* and *Cinnamomum longepaniculatum*, but these are not usually available commercially. However, it is sometimes present as a trace constituent in oils of basil, cinnamon bark, citronella, rose and ylang ylang.

A final regulatory body that has implications for aromatherapy is the MHRA.

- *MHRA – Medicines and healthcare products* Regulatory Agency (formerly MCA – Medicines Control Agency). A UK based regulatory body responsible for the Medicines Act. It has catagories for medicines and foods and is looking at herbal products (in the Traditional Herbal Products Directive introduced in 2005) and other materials used in complementary health.

The agency is part of the Department of Health and is responsible for safeguarding public health by ensuring that all medicines on the UK market meet acceptable standards. For a medicine to be sold it must have a Product Licence, which is granted when the MHRA has researched and taken advice from other bodies like the Medicines Committee, the Committee on Safety of Medicines and the Committee on Dental and Surgical Materials. When the medicine meets the standards of the Medicines Act or relevant EU legislation it is granted a licence. The licence stipulates format for administration (cream, lotion, tablet), specific diseases and conditions it can treat, type of person suitable for usage, dosage amounts and timing. Essential oils are not medicines in the context of the Medicines Act and have not been granted Product Licences.

AROMAFACT

Specific medical claims cannot be made for essential oils or aromatherapy products; if such were made, the products would need a product licence. The licence is only granted after an exhaustive series of laboratory and clinical trials to prove safety and efficacy. The issues surrounding research and trials on the use of essential oils in clinical situations are still contentious, but there are increasing numbers of scientific studies and papers in reputable journals.

GENERAL SAFETY AND FIRST AID

When essential oils are used following the correct guidelines taught in professional practice, they present very little or no risk. In terms of safety, most essential oils available to aromatherapists present no problems. Those used commonly and generally considered to be safe are the lavenders, *Matricaria chamomila* (German chamomile), *Anthemis nobilis* (Roman chamomile), *Salvia sclarea* (clary sage), *Pelargonium graveolens* (geranium), *Santalum album* (sandalwood), *Pogostemon cablin* (patchouli), *Melaleuca cajeputi* (cajeput), *Cupressus sempervirens* (cypress), *Citrus reticulata* (mandarin), *Citrus sinensis* (sweet orange) and *Thymus vulgaris* (thyme) CT linalool. These are also considered to be baby- and child-safe, but care must be taken with certain chemotypes as previously described.

AROMAFACT

Never use an undiluted essential oil on a child. A good dilution guideline would be one-third the adult dose, so for a massage the oil would be diluted to between 1% and 1.5% dilution as opposed to the average 3% dilution for an adult. Roman chamomile is a particularly useful oil for young children, suitable for problems including rashes, teething and colic and as a generally calming oil promoting natural sleep.

Generally essential oils are used in very dilute forms and the main safety concerns are skin irritations, sensitizations, breathing difficulties and oral toxicity. These are dealt with in the context of the physiology and metabolism of the essential oils in the body. Accidents may occur with spillage of essential oils. When dealing with these the basic principle is to take action to dilute the oil to safe levels and remove it from any situation where it might represent a hazard. As essential oils are lipophilic (lipid- or fat-loving), the initial choice of diluent would be a carrier oil or full-fat milk, which will help to dissolve the oil. This would be followed by washing with water and soap or detergent.

Essential oils can easily become absorbed by the skin and present a hazard if not removed from the fingers, which may transfer that oil to other parts of the body. It is essential that hands are thoroughly washed with warm water and a fat-dissolving cleanser such as soap or a detergent like washing up liquid. If the essential oils come into contact with the skin in delicate areas of the body, the affected areas should be washed with warm soapy water and carefully and thoroughly dried, and if necessary a gentle skin cream or medicated cream should be applied.

AROMAFACT

Peppermint and cinnamon essential oils are particularly likely to persist on the skin of the fingers for a prolonged time. This needs to be considered by the aromatherapist when using them in massage blends.

If essential oils are present on the fingers, care must be taken not to rub the eyes. The eyes are particularly sensitive and any accidental entry of oils must be dealt with quickly. A diluted oil, such as that in a bath, will cause stinging and may damage the delicate tissues if it gets into the eye. Flushing with copious amounts of clean, warm water should be done immediately. For neat oils, flush with full-fat milk, followed again by clean warm water. If the stinging and irritation persist, medical assistance should be sought.

The eyes, mouth, nose, vagina and rectum have mucous membranes. These are sheets of epithelial (lining) cells that are moist owing to the production of a slimy secretion called mucus. Additionally, they line the alimentary (digestive) tract, respiratory tract and genito-urinary tracts. The mucus has a protective role to prevent injury to underlying tissues and traps foreign particles in the respiratory system.

AROMAFACT

Essential oils that may cause irritation of mucous membranes include fennel, pine, spruce, clove, oregano and thyme.

Breathing difficulties can occur if excess essential oil is inhaled; oils can also be dangerous in much lower amounts for some individuals. The best treatment is to get the excess oil diluted by removing the patient to fresh air and to flush the oil by allowing the air to dilute it. If breathing has stopped, this represents a critical situation – artificial resuscitation should be started and medical assistance sought.

AROMAFACT

Inhalations should be carefully monitored if a person is known to suffer from conditions such as asthma or any allergies such as hay fever. The inhalation route for administration of conventional drugs is usually restricted to treatments of the respiratory tract such as cold remedies or asthma drugs. Owing to the low interest in the use of the nose as an administration route for substances into the body, few studies have been carried out. The use of illegal substances by this route, however, is well known and documented.

Consumption of an essential oil is probably the most hazardous and serious accident that can happen. If excessive quantities are taken this is particularly dangerous as inappropriately ingested oils act as poisons. Prompt action is essential and immediate medical assistance should be sought, either by ringing your general practitioner or going to a hospital accident and emergency department. Do not try to induce vomiting unless specifically advised to do so by a health professional. The bottle or container the oil came from should be taken with the patient and, if possible, the amount consumed should be noted so that appropriate treatment can be administered. Advice may be sought from one of the national poisons units, which should only be contacted by medical personnel.

An inquest in 1999 into the death of a baby who had suffered from colic showed the danger of inappropriately administered essential oil. It appears that a prescription for peppermint water was incorrectly dispensed and either the neat or a very concentrated form of the oil was used.

AROMAFACT

When using a particular oil, the individual safety data sheet can be consulted for specific first aid procedures. For example:

Eucalyptus globulus

- Eye contact: Flush immediately with cold milk if available, then flush with clean water for at least 15 minutes. Contact a doctor or take the person to a casualty unit if the problems persist.
- Skin contact: Remove any contaminated clothing or shoes. Wash affected areas thoroughly with soap and water for at least 15 minutes. Flush continuously with cold water. Contact a doctor if necessary or take the person to a casualty unit.
- Inhalation: Remove from the exposure to fresh air. If breathing has stopped, administer artificial respiration and oxygen if available. Consult a doctor or ring the emergency services.
- Ingestion: Wash out the mouth with milk or water provided the person is conscious. Do not induce vomiting. Ring the emergency services immediately.

THE ADMINISTRATION OF ESSENTIAL OILS TO THE BODY

Entry routes

The routes for entry of essential oils into the body are by absorption from vaporizers, baths and skin massage. Oral administration and ingestion of essential oils are the most potent and effective methods, while rectal and vaginal routes can be harmful if the mucous membranes are damaged. This is summarized in Fig. 8.2, which also shows their absorption and assimilation and their loss from the body by elimination or excretion.

AROMAFACT

The acceptable methods of administration for the aromatherapist to use are inhalation of vapours through the nose and by dermal application massage through the skin. Internal routes – oral, intravenous, rectal or vaginal – require specialist training and experience. This should be left to a qualified aromatologist. The internal administration of essential oils is practised in France but it is done by medical practitioners and physiotherapists using oral preparations, injections, pessaries and suppositories.

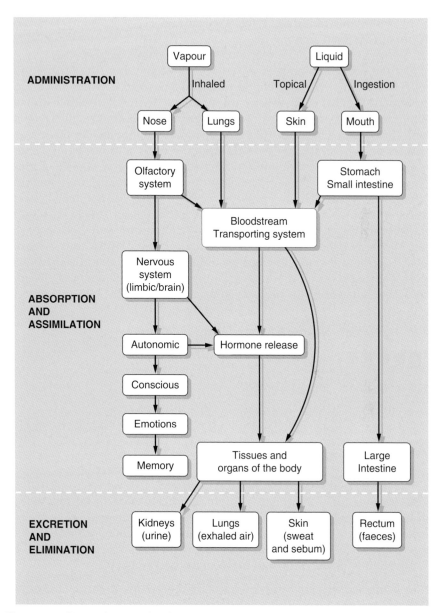

Figure 8.2   Routes for essential oils in the body.

However an oil enters the body, it must be taken up into the bloodstream to be transported around the body. The essential oils are lipophilic (fat soluble) and are carried to all organs of the body including the brain. It is believed that an essential oil does not stay in the circulation for a long period of time. Initially it goes to areas of high blood flow such as skeletal muscle and kidney. Eventually it may become absorbed into the fat (adipose) tissue. The blood flow to the liver is also high, and the liver itself holds a large volume of blood.

The liver is often referred to as 'the chemical factory' of the body and has an important role for regulating the amounts of substances in the blood, along with a large number of other reactions including detoxification.

Different components of essential oils will have differing biochemical properties and reactions affecting certain tissues and organs. The details of the physiological mechanisms are the subject of much research and are beyond the scope of this book. Substances produced after being involved in the chemical reactions of the body (metabolism) are lost by the process of excretion. Materials that pass through the body without being chemically changed are lost by elimination. The time a *drug* or substance stays in the body will vary from chemical to chemical. A quantitative measure of this is called the *biological half-life*: the time taken for the drug concentration in the blood to decrease to half its initial value. This is influenced by a number of factors, including transportation and metabolism of the drug by the body and its rate of elimination. Both drugs and essential oils are excreted through the kidneys in the urine, exhaled by the lungs, secreted through the skin or passed out in the faeces. The rate of elimination of a substance from the body is proportional to its concentration in the bloodstream.

AROMAFACT

It has been shown that most essential oils and their breakdown products are eliminated and excreted through the kidneys, with smaller amounts breathed out from the lungs. The skin and faeces account for the least loss.

Specific measures are used to quantify the effectiveness of the response to a drug or substance (ED_{50}) and its toxicity (LD_{50}). The ED_{50} and LD_{50} are often quoted in data, providing an indication of the effects of chemicals on the body. These values have been derived from animal studies, so variations will be found in human metabolism, but they can be used as a guide.

- ED_{50} is the *median effective dose*, a measure of response in the animal (other than death); the median effective dose is that at which 50% of the desired effect is achieved in 50% of the animals tested. Values for ED_{50} are known and quoted for acute oral values.
- The LD_{50} is the *median lethal dose*, which kills 50% of test animals.

Both values need to be related to the body weight of an animal, and are usually quoted in grams of substance to kilogram of animal weight. This means that the different weights of individuals must be taken into account when formulating dosages. If the LD_{50} of a substance is 10 g/kg, and an individual weighs 80 kg, the dose will be 800 g. The higher the LD_{50} value the safer a substance is, and values above 5 g/kg are considered nontoxic.

AROMAFACT

The LD$_{50}$ values are known for most essential oils, but they represent a measure of acute oral value. It is one of many measures quoted when describing properties of essential oils. Aromatherapists do not practise the use of oral administration but full tables of LD$_{50}$ values can be found in established texts and on safety data sheets. As essential oils are products of natural origin with variations in composition the values will also show some variations due to this. Also oils from different parts of a plant will have different chemical compositions and this will be reflected in the different LD$_{50}$ values. For example

- Clove (*Syzygium aromaticum*)
- Buds: LD$_{50}$ = 2.65 g/kg
- Stems: LD$_{50}$ = 2.03 g/kg
- Leaves: LD$_{50}$ = 1.37 g/kg

Wormwood is an oil for food flavouring at very low concentration (60 ppm (parts per million)); it is not suitable for aromatology or aromatherapy owing to its toxicity, with an LD$_{50}$ of 0.96 g/kg. Peppermint (*Mentha Piperata*) has an LD$_{50}$ of 4.4 g/kg; lemongrass (*Cymbopogon citratus*) has an LD$_{50}$ of 5 g/kg.

The amounts of essential oil entering the body in aromatherapy by inhalation or massage are very small. It has been estimated that an oral dose of an essential oil will have a ten times greater concentration than that from a massage.

Inhalation and respiratory system

The importance of scent molecules picked up in the olfactory epithelium and directly stimulating the brain has been described previously in Chapter 5 where the nose can be considered to be a valuable detector of an essential oil. However, the main stream of inhaled air will not reach this small sensitive area of olfactory cells. The tissues that cover the lining of the nasal passages are very thin and have an extensive blood capillary network. There is a high concentration of capillaries. A relatively high proportion of the molecules from the essential oil will enter the circulatory system here. Also, the inhaled air with essential oil passes along the pipes of the *trachea* (windpipe) and the *bronchi* (tubes that enter the lungs). The lungs are spongy structures made up of air spaces called *alveoli*. The alveoli also have an extensive blood capillary network that provides a high surface area for gas exchange between air in lungs and the bloodstream when breathing. Essential oil molecules can enter the bloodstream along with the other gases involved in breathing. Figure 8.3 shows the structure of the respiratory system.

AROMAFACT

An increased rate and depth of breathing will enhance the uptake of gases. When considering the needs of a client and administering essential oils to them, the aromatherapist should consider the effects of the oil on themselves. Giving a client a massage will be physically demanding for the therapist, causing them to breathe faster and deeper than the client. In this way they may absorb more of the oil by inhalation than the client. Conditions such as a warm room increase the vaporization of the oil. It is recommended that the therapist should follow basic precautions. Good ventilation is possibly the most significant factor for aromatherapists to consider. Simple guidelines to prevent overexposure would include the following practices.

- The treatment room should be adequately ventilated and thoroughly aired with a time break of at least five minutes between each client.
- The aromatherapist should store and dispense oils in a separate room and always wash hands after each treatment.

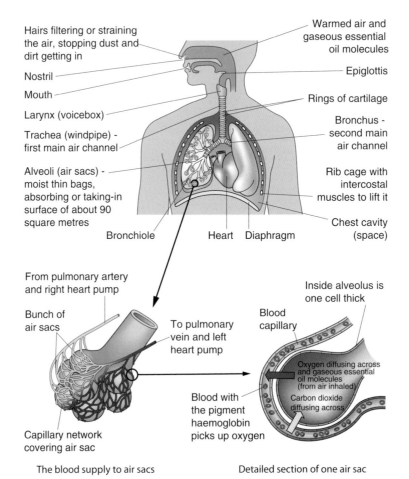

Figure 8.3   The respiratory system.

Massage and dermal application

Massage constitutes a topical or dermal application. A number of factors need to be considered when offering massage to a client. These include types and combinations of essential oils chosen, dosage or amounts of essential oil to use, choice of carrier oils, physiological properties of the oils, skin type and health of the client. A number of safety factors, including contraindications to essential oil used on the skin, must also be evaluated. Dermal application also covers the uses of creams, ointments and compresses – anything that brings the essential oil into contact with the skin.

Blending and dosage

When an essential oil is used for massage, it is diluted in a carrier or base oil. Carriers are vegetable oils such as sweet almond, grapeseed, wheatgerm, jojoba, etc. They have different compositions and properties and these are briefly described in Chapter 7. The resultant mixture of essential oil and carrier is called a blend. The amounts used or dosages are rather subjective and will vary according to a number of factors.

In general, for the commonly used essential oils the percentage dilution is within the range 1–5%. Most aromatherapy books will describe blend compositions in terms of 'drops' of oil, whereas a clearly defined measure such as a ml (millilitre) would be more scientific. However, this would not be very practical in practice.

assuming 20 drops		22 drops	25 drops	30 drops
1 drop =	0.05 ml	0.0454 ml	0.04 ml	0.0333 ml
2 drops =	0.1 ml	0.0908 ml	0.08 ml	0.0667 ml
5 drops =	0.25 ml	0.227 ml	0.2 ml	0.1668 ml
½ drop =	0.025 ml	0.0227 ml	0.02 ml	0.0167 ml

AROMAFACT

A typical blend for a massage would be 7 drops of essential oil in 20 ml of carrier oil. This would be a 1.75% dilution, calculated by 0.35 ml (amount of essential oil in 7 drops) divided by the amount of carrier (20 ml) and multiplied by 100:

$$(0.35 \div 20) \times 100 = 1.75$$

As a general rule for skin application, 30–60 drops in 100 ml of carrier would be used. This gives dilutions of 1.5–3%.

The choice of essential oils and quantities used for aromatherapy will vary according to a number of factors. These include method of use, size, age, state of health of the client and purpose of the treatment. In aromatherapy, dosages and dilutions are not strictly laid down or standardized and amounts administered are not always accurately measured. It is an important part of clinical practice to understand the properties and therapeutic strengths and limitations of individual oils and blends. These need to be viewed in a holistic manner and will vary in effects with different clients. It is outside the scope of this book, but amplifies the importance of thorough training and experience in practice. In terms of safety, it is reassuring to know that if essential oils are administered by a qualified aromatherapist following known guidelines for use of oils in correct dilutions, the amounts of pharmacologically active substances will be significantly lower than those found in the dosages of orthodox drugs.

AROMAFACT

Essential oils should always be diluted before application. Historically lavender and tea tree have been used with caution directly to the skin. This may represent a risk and this practice is no longer advised.

The time taken for an oil, or certain of its components, to become absorbed into the bloodstream will vary, but it is accepted that this will usually be slower for dermal application than for oral dosing. The concentrations are less likely to build up to high levels as the oil components are being continually metabolized and removed from the body.

Appreciation of the value of massage and the entry of oils into the body via the skin needs an understanding of the structure, functions and physiology of the skin.

The skin

The skin is considered to be an organ of the human body. It has a large surface area – for an adult this is approximately 2 square metres. The skin has a number of important functions.

- *Protection.* The skin acts as a barrier to prevent injury to underlying tissues and invasion by microbes. The skin itself houses a number of microorganisms including bacteria that are not harmful in that situation. They are called commensal organisms and live with us in a symbiotic relationship, that is one that is mutually beneficial. It can be dangerous to remove these helpful microbes as they have a defensive role in protecting the body from invasion by other pathogenic (disease-causing) microbes.

- *As a sensory structure.* The skin contains receptors providing information about our surroundings and changes in the environment. The receptors are part of the nervous system and those in the skin are sensitive to touch, pressure, pain and changes in temperature. The sensory receptors are made up of modified nerve endings in the dermis. When they are stimulated they generate nerve impulses that travel to the region of the brain called the cerebral cortex.

- *Regulation of body temperature.* The core temperature of the human body is kept fairly constant at around 37 °C. Heat gained or produced by the body must be balanced by the heat that is lost. Only the heat lost through the skin can be regulated; the other routes (urine, faeces, breathing out) cannot be controlled. The skin achieves regulation by altering the amounts of blood flowing through the blood vessels of the dermis and by varying the production of sweat.

- *As an excretory organ.* This is usually considered to be a minor function. Substances that are lost include salt (sodium chloride) and urea in the sweat, the amounts of which will vary according to internal bodily levels. Each individual will produce a characteristic odour, which can be detected by sniffer dogs that have a more acute sense of smell than humans.

AROMAFACT

Aromatic substances such as garlic and certain spices are lost through the skin and can be smelt on individuals who have eaten them. Certain essential oils are also lost in this way and may be detected.

Structure of skin

A knowledge of the structure of the skin is fundamental for understanding the benefits of massage and the dermal uptake of essential oils in aromatherapy. Skin contains hair, nails and glands and is arranged in two main layers: the outer *epidermis* and the underlying *dermis*.

Below the dermis and above the underlying structures is a layer of subcutaneous fat (or adipose tissue). Figure 8.4 shows the arrangement and names of these structures.

Epidermis

This outer layer is made up of other sublayers. The surface layer is the *stratum corneum*, or *horny layer*, and is made up of thin, flat cells high in the protein keratin. They are dead cells and are constantly shed from the body. Certain areas, such as the heels of the feet, have a thicker stratum corneum and have a protective function to prevent damage by friction to the underlying structures. The deepest layer is the *germinative layer*, where the living cells are actively dividing and growing and progress upwards to the stratum corneum. The epidermis is completely replaced about every 40 days.

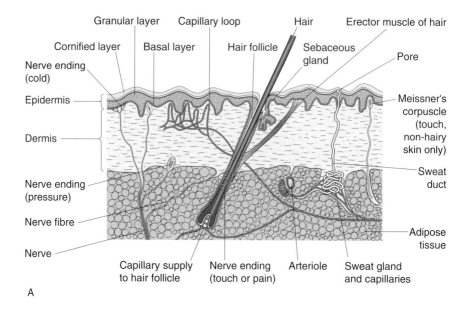

A

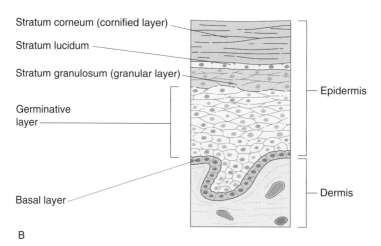

B

Figure 8.4   (A) The structure of the skin. (B) The main layers of the epidermis.

AROMAFACT

Some oil components are able to stay in the stratum corneum for several hours, so it may be thought of as a reservoir.

The substance *melanin* is found in the germinative layer, where it is formed by cells called *melanocytes*. The number of melanocytes is fairly constant and differences in skin colour are due to the amount of melanin produced. Exposure to sunlight promotes the synthesis of increased amounts of melanin. The function of melanin is to protect the skin from the harmful effects of some of the sun's rays.

AROMAFACT

Photosensitization is when the skin becomes abnormally sensitive to sunlight or ultraviolet radiation and tans very rapidly. It can follow contact with certain phototoxic substances found in essential oils. Citrus oils extracted by cold pressing or expression from the peel may contain large amounts of furanocoumarins (also called furocoumarins or psoralens), molecules that may cause phototoxicity problems. The presence of the furanocoumarin bergaptene (or 5-methyoxypsoralen) in bergamot at concentrations of 0.3–4% (explained previously in Chs 3 and 7), expressed lime (0.1–0.3%) and expressed lemon (0.15–0.25%) is well documented. Although the essential oils access the barrier of the skin quite quickly, it is better not to use an ultraviolet sunbed or sunbathe after using citrus oils.

Certain oils cause an *irritation* to the skin, which appears as itchiness or inflammation. These are often oils with a high proportion of phenolic or aldehyde compounds. For example, cassia (*Cinnamomum cassia*) has 78–88% aldehyde and 5–6% phenol. It is very caustic (burning) to the skin. This is also true of essential oils from cinnamon, lemongrass, oregano, clove and thyme. Considering the dilution of the essential oil in a massage blend and the large area of skin it is applied to, the likelihood of irritation is low. Skin sensitization differs from irritation. Sensitization occurs once the skin has reacted to a particular substance; then upon subsequent exposure to that substance it becomes even more sensitive very rapidly. A patch test prior to use of an essential oil or blend may be advisable and you will learn about this in your practical training.

AROMAFACT

A typical patch test is performed using the chosen essential oils at twice the concentration you intend to use in the massage. They are applied to the inside of the forearm and monitored over 48 hours for redness, itching or swelling. This is explored further later in this chapter under 'cautions and contraindications'.

Structures and substances that originate in the dermis such as hairs, sebaceous gland secretions and the ducts of the sweat glands pass through the epidermis to reach the surface of the body.

Dermis

The dermis is made up of collagen and elastic fibres overlying connective tissue. A number of important structures are located here.

Blood vessels   These comprise the *arterioles* (which are the smaller vessels branching from the *arteries* that carry blood from the heart to the tissues), *venules* (which are smaller vessels that join up into the *veins* and return blood from the tissues and back to the heart) and *capillaries*. Capillaries are the thin-walled vessels that exchange materials between the bloodstream and the cells. Together they form an extensive fine network to provide blood to the hair follicles, sebaceous glands and sweat glands. The blood provides nutrients and oxygen for the growth and healthy functioning of the tissues of the dermis. The high pressure of the blood in the arteries is responsible for the formation of tissue fluid, which directly bathes the cells. Blood, as such, does not leave the vessels. Tissue fluid containing waste products, including carbon dioxide from respiration, is returned to the bloodstream and returns to the heart in the veins. The veins contain valves to ensure the correct direction of flow back to the heart.

AROMAFACT

A massage will stimulate blood flow to the skin and this can be seen by a reddening effect or erythema. The increased blood flow, in turn, increases the surface temperature and a pleasant warming and relaxing effect is experienced.

Lymphatic system

Lymph vessels   These are part of the *lymphatic system*, made up of vessels, nodes and organs such as the spleen and tonsils. Important functions for the body include internal defensive mechanisms. The lymph vessels form a tubular network throughout the body carrying a fluid called *lymph*. Lymph is made up of a colourless fluid containing white blood cells that is collected from the tissues of the body. The lymph vessels pick up and regulate the tissue fluid formed by the bloodstream, which bathes and nourishes the cells. The lymph is circulated through the lymphatic vessels and is eventually returned to the bloodstream.

Figure 8.5 shows the lymphatic system and vessels.

AROMAFACT

A good massage will increase the blood flow to the skin and promote the uptake of nutrients and the respiratory gas oxygen. The waste products, including carbon dioxide produced by the chemistry of respiration in the cells, must not be allowed to build up, so their removal by the bloodstream and lymphatic system is equally important. The contentious issue of cellulite is often attributed to the build-up of waste products and toxins around the cells of the skin and associated tissues. A good massage technique will enhance the lymphatic drainage of the tissues and removal of harmful toxins. The lymph flows within lymph vessels in one direction and there are valves present to ensure this. When doing a massage, the strokes must be in the direction of the flow of blood and lymph, that is towards the heart and proximal lymph nodes.

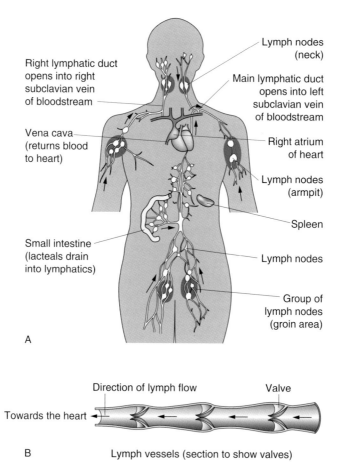

Right lymphatic duct opens into right subclavian vein of bloodstream

Lymph nodes (neck)

Main lymphatic duct opens into left subclavian vein of bloodstream

Vena cava (returns blood to heart)

Right atrium of heart

Lymph nodes (armpit)

Spleen

Small intestine (lacteals drain into lymphatics)

Lymph nodes

Group of lymph nodes (groin area)

A

Direction of lymph flow   Valve

Towards the heart ←

B   Lymph vessels (section to show valves)

Figure 8.5   (A) The lymphatic system. (B) Section of a lymph vessel to show valves.

Sweat glands   Sweat glands are found throughout the skin but are more numerous in areas such as the soles of the feet, palms of the hand, armpits and groin. The body of the gland is made up of a coiled tube, surrounded by a good blood supply, and a duct, which opens onto the skin surface through a pore. Other glands open into the hair follicles after puberty. The important function of the sweat glands is to form the fluid sweat. The sweat is formed from the bloodstream, so in times of high sweat production the body's water intake and balance must be regulated. When liquid sweat changes to a vapour and evaporates from the skin surface, it takes heat away from the body. If the body is cold, the sweating mechanism is inhibited. Temperature regulation is controlled by a part of the brain called the hypothalamus responding to the core temperature of the blood.

AROMAFACT

Essential oils enter the body through the skin by the ducts of the sweat glands and the hair follicles. The permeability of the skin at various locations in the body can be linked to the number of available ducts acting as entry points. Sites such as the palms of the hands, soles of the feet, armpits, genitals, forehead and scalp are quite permeable to absorption of essential oils, while the limbs, buttocks, abdomen and trunk are relatively impermeable.

Sebaceous glands   Sebaceous glands are present in all areas of the skin except the palms of the hands and soles of the feet. They produce an oily secretion called *sebum*. The function of sebum is to keep the hair soft and lubricated and it gives the skin some waterproofing properties and acts as an antibacterial/ antifungal agent preventing invasion by some microbes. It is important to prevent the skin drying out.

AROMAFACT

Sebum can act as a barrier to the passage of essential oils through the skin, so a greasy skin may inhibit the absorption of the oil. Similarly, greasy ointments or cosmetics that promote skin hydration by slowing water evaporation will also act as an obstructive layer. It is always desirable to perform a massage on clean skin.

Hairs   That part of the hair that shows above the skin is called the shaft and the remainder is the root. The hair follicle in the dermis has a cluster of cells called the bulb, which is the site of the cell division responsible for hair formation. Nutrition for growth comes from the bloodstream; the new cells are pushed upwards and as they die they become keratinized. Keratin is the strong fibrous protein found in both hair and skin. Hairs have associated muscles called *arrector* muscles, which make the hair stand up when they contract. These muscles are stimulated by the nervous system in response to cold and fear.

Sensory nerve endings and receptors   The skin is an important sensory organ, providing us with information about conditions in our surrounding environment. The range of nerve endings and sensory receptors are sensitive to touch, pressure, pain and changes in temperature. The nerve endings and receptors generate nerve impulses when stimulated, and these impulses are then conveyed to the central nervous system (CNS), which is the brain and spinal cord. It is in the CNS that the impulses are interpreted and initiate appropriate action by the muscles or glands.

AROMAFACT

We are all aware of the importance of tactile stimulation or touch. Babies and young animals do not thrive unless cuddled by their mothers, and individuals so deprived often go on to develop behavioural problems in adult life. When something hurts we instinctively 'rub it better', and the comforting hug directly conveys sympathy in times of crisis.

The importance and implications of the massage process are multifaceted. The significance of a good rapport between masseur and client should never be underestimated. A skilful masseur will stimulate both physiological and psychological benefits in the client. A number of body systems are involved, including the circulatory, lymphatic, musculo-skeletal and nervous systems. The oils, with their varying chemical compositions and properties, have differing effects on the individual systems, the body as a whole and each client. The aromatherapist needs to establish a rapport with the client, discussing choice of oils and inspiring cooperation and confidence in the chosen treatment. The manual touch to the skin is not only comforting but is highly sensuous, stimulating receptors that send impulses to the brain that are interpreted as pleasurable. A massage is relaxing when it helps the muscles to relax and reduces tightness and tension.

Subdermal fat or subcutaneous fat needs to be mentioned as this underlying adipose tissue can also act as a reservoir for oils. The lipophilic or fat-/lipid-loving molecules can be retained on a temporary basis, and will not undergo rapid diffusion. As subcutaneous fat has a poor blood supply, the oil does not enter the circulation very easily and a person with a high amount of fat will retain more oil in this way.

General considerations and other factors influencing dermal absorption

The efficiency of a massage, in terms of amounts of essential oil absorbed into the body, will be affected by a number of factors. These include the choice of essential oils and carrier, the concentration of the blend, the part of the body being massaged and the total area that the blend is applied to. A more viscous oil will be absorbed more slowly than a thinner one. The skin is highly permeable to essential oils, which are fat-soluble but are also partially water-soluble.

The skin should be clean and grease-free, and warmer skin will absorb oils more quickly owing to increased capillary circulation.

AROMAFACT

It is usual practice to cover the skin with a nonpermeable material after completing a massage. This helps to increase the absorption of the oil into the bloodstream, and works by increasing the temperature and hydration of the skin. This covering of the skin is referred to as *occlusion*.

The essential oils move by a passive process called diffusion, whereby molecules move from a region of high concentration to one of lower concentration, along a concentration gradient. Small molecules move faster than large ones, and substances with a molecular weight greater than 500 are unlikely to pass through the skin and into the bloodstream.

CAUTIONS AND CONTRAINDICATIONS

When used sensibly following correct professional guidelines, essential oils present little risk. Good-quality oils from a reputable supplier, made to careful formulations and dilutions in appropriate blends, should always be used. The main safety considerations are skin irritation and sensitization and oral toxicity. Other predisposing factors specific to each client must be assessed upon their individual merits, referring to professional practice and established guidelines. A number of situations and conditions may make it inappropriate to carry out a massage on a client. When initially assessing the client, any existing medical problems should be noted. Those that need particular caution are heart and circulatory conditions such as high (hypertension) or low (hypotension) blood pressure, clotting disorders and varicose veins. Also diabetes, epilepsy, fractures and infectious diseases must be carefully considered. The use of aromatherapy for cancer patients needs to be assessed in terms of the condition of the individual patient and in conjunction with their mainstream treatment. High temperatures or fevers and recent vaccinations (within the previous 48 hours) would also be contraindications for a massage. Medications being taken should also be noted and any possible interactions assessed.

Before performing a massage it is also important to assess the condition of the skin of each client. Any localized damage should be noted and avoided. Very small cuts, bruises and boils can be covered with thin transparent tape.

Any openings to the body can provide direct access to the bloodstream and this must be avoided. Recent scar tissue may benefit from use of a diluted essential oil, but it should not be rubbed in and the area should not be over-stimulated. Inoculation sites should be avoided for at least 24 hours. Existing skin conditions such as acne, eczema and psoriasis can often be helped by aromatherapy, but the choice of oils, both essential and carrier, is crucial. Certain allergies can be triggered and this should also be considered. Dermatitis is a common condition in which the skin becomes irritated and inflamed with characteristic redness and itching. It is triggered by many chemicals or substances and often has other predisposing factors such as stress. Conditions such as eczema are thought to be examples of allergic reaction.

Reactions to essential oils can affect both the client and the aromatherapist. Sensitization is an allergic reaction to a particular or specific substance, which causes an interaction with the body's immune system. The sensitizing substance is called the antigen and it triggers the type of white blood cells called lymphocytes to make antibodies. The antibodies function to neutralize or eliminate the harmful effects of the antigen. The antibodies are specific and act only on the antigen that stimulated their formation. Typical allergies are triggered by proteins found in foods such as cheese, milk, gluten in flour, pollen, airborne moulds and biological washing powders containing enzymes. They can cause a full-scale immune reaction and once the body has been exposed to the antigen and has produced the antibody it is said to be sensitized, when it can quickly produce antibody on future exposure to that antigen. When this occurs on the skin, itching, rashes and blistering are typical signs.

AROMAFACT

A small number of essential oils have been shown to cause sensitization of the skin. These include cinnamon bark (containing cinnamic aldehyde), clove bud (containing the alcohol eugenol) and, surprisingly, ylang ylang. It is advisable for people with sensitive skin or a history of dermatitis to avoid the use of essential oils of geranium, ginger, pine, citronella and cassia. Wheatgerm carrier oil, owing to its protein origin, is often contraindicated for those with certain allergies. The use of the patch test is always advised, as previously described.

On a more general note, it is better not to give a massage to a client under the following conditions:

- If he or she has just engaged in vigorous sport.
- If he or she is very hungry or has had a heavy meal or has been drinking alcohol.
- For women it is better to avoid the first three days of the menstrual cycle, as blood loss may be increased.

- Pregnancy and aromatherapy can be a controversial issue: caution is always advised for the first three months, but careful choice and use of essential oils can be very helpful.
- Clients with any existing medical conditions or course of drugs that may be adversely affected.

Again, professional practice training and reference to specialist safety guides coupled with common sense should ensure a safe approach. If in doubt, err on the side of caution and consult an experienced practitioner.

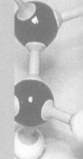

Bibliography and sources of information

Further reading: books

Battaglia S 1997 The complete guide to aromatherapy, 2nd edn. Watson Ferguson, Brisbane

British Herbal Pharmacopoeia 1996 British Herbal Medicine Association, PO Box 304, Bournemouth, Dorset BH7 6JX

Buckle J 2004 Clinical aromatherapy, essential oils in practice. Churchill Livingstone, Edinburgh

Crowe J, Bradshaw T, Monk P 2006 Chemistry for the biosciences. Oxford University Press, Oxford

Davies P 1999 Aromatherapy: an A to Z, 3rd edn. CW Daniel, London

Devon T K, Scott A I 1972 Handbook of naturally occurring compounds: terpenes, volume 2. Academic Press Inc, New York

Doty R L 2003 Handbook of olfaction and gustation. Marcel Dekker, New York

Ernst E 2006 The desktop guide to complementary and alternative medicine: an evidence based approach. Mosby, London

Franchomme P, Penoel D 1990 L'aromatherapie exactment. Jollois, Limoges, France

Fullick A 1998 Human health and disease. Heinemann, Oxford

Gadd K, Gurr S 1994 Chemistry (University of Bath Sciences 16–19). Thomas Nelson, Walton-on-Thames

Gunther E 1972 The essential oils. Kneger, Flanders

Hine R S, Martin E 2005 Dictionary of biology. Magpie Books, London

Isaacs A, Daintith J, Martin E 2005 Dictionary of science. Magpie Books, London

Lawless J 1999 Complete essential oils. Mustard/Parragon, London

Lewith G, Jonas W B Walach H 2003 Clinical research in complementary therapies. Churchill Livingstone, Edinburgh

Lis-Balchin M 1995 Aroma science. The chemistry and bioactivity of essential oils. Amberwood Publishing, East Horsley

Lowrie R, Ferguson H 1975 Chemistry: an integrated approach. Pergamon, London

Mackean DG 1988 Human life John Murray, London

McGuiness H 2001 Aromatherapy therapy basics. Hodder and Stoughton, London

Miall L, Sharp D 1986 A new dictionary of chemistry, 4th edn. Longman, Harlow

Onions C 1986 The shorter Oxford English dictionary. Clarendon Press, Oxford

Open University 1996 S102: a science foundation course, units 17–18. The chemistry of carbon compounds. Open University Press, Milton Keynes

Price L, Price S 2004 Understanding hydrolats: the specific hydrosols for aromatherapy. Churchill Livingstone, Edinburgh

Price L, Smith I, Price S 2006 Carrier oils for aromatherapy and massage. Riverhead, Stratford-upon-Avon

Price S 1995 Aromatherapy workbook. HarperCollins, London

Price S, Price L 1995 Aromatherapy for health professionals. Churchill Livingstone, Edinburgh

Roberts D 2002 Signals and perception; the fundamental of human sensation. Open University Press and Palgrave Macmillan

Rockett B, Sutton R 1996 Chemistry for biologists. John Murray, London

Rounce J 1988 Science for the beauty therapist. Stanley Thornes, Cheltenham

Sell C S, 2006 Chemistry of Fragrances, from Perfumer to Consumer. RSC, London

Sellar W 1997 The directory of essential oils, 5th edn. CW Daniel, London

Simonsen J, Barton D H R 1952 The terpenes; the sesquiterpenes, diterpenes and their derivatives. Cambridge University Press, Cambridge

Temay A 1979 Contemporary organic chemistry. Saunders, Philadelphia

Tisserand R, Balacs T 1995 Essential oil safety. Churchill Livingstone, Edinburgh

Towards safe medicines. Available from the MCA, Market Towers, Nine Elms Lane, London SW8 5NQ

Turin L 2006 The secret of scent. Faber and Faber, London

Williams D 1989 Lecture notes on essential oils. Eve Taylor, London

Williams D 1996 The chemistry of essential oils. Michelle Press, Weymouth

Wilson J, Waugh A 1999 Anatomy and physiology, 8th edn. Churchill Livingstone, Edinburgh

Further reading: journals

Albone E 1996 Web of scent. *Chemistry Review* Jan: 18–23

Ali Z, O'Hare L 1997 Analysing food flavours. *Chemistry Review* May: 2–7

Anon 1994 Gas chromatography in pictures *Chemistry Review* Nov: 16–17

Barnes J 1998 Complementary medicine – aromatherapy. *The Pharmaceutical Journal* 260: 862–867

Barnes J, Williamson EM 2000 Aromatherapy and essential oils – useful information for pharmacists. Information sheet commissioned by the Royal Pharmaceutical Society of Great Britain

Fowler P, Wall M 1997 COSHH and CHIPS: ensuring the safety of aromatherapy. *Complementary and Therapeutic Medicine* 5: 112–115

Kingston R 2001 It's only natural. *Chemistry in Britain* Jan: 18–20

Mills G, Ottewill G 1997 Chromatography. *Catalyst* Nov: 7–9

Useful journals and publications

Aromatherapy Times (Journal of the IFA) 2–4 Chiswick High Road, London W4 1TH

Aromatherapy Today (Australian publication) PO Box 273, Zillmere Qld 4034, Australia. (distributed by Essentially Oils)

International Journal of Essential Oil Therapeutics (formerly International Journal of Aromatherapy) Published by Essential Oil Resource Consultants, Au Village 83840 La Matre, province, France

NAHA Aromatherapy Journal (formerly Scentsitivity) 3327 W.Indian Trail road, PMB 144, Spokane WA 99208, USA

In Essence the Journal of the *International Federation of professional Aromatherapists* (formerly Aromatherapy World) IFPA House, 82 Ashby Road, Hinckley, Leics, UK

Chemistry World, Monthly Journal of the Royal Society of Chemistry (RSC)

Complementary Therapies in Clinical Practice, Elsevier Health

Complementary Therapies in Medicine, Elsevier Health

Essential Oil Monographs, detailing the composition of oils, edited by Brian Lawrence and published by Allured Publishing Corporation, 362 S. Schmale Road, Carol Stream, IL 60188, USA

Fragrance Raw Materials Monographs, published by Elsevier Science, The Boulevard, Langford Lane, Kidlington, Oxford OX5 1 GB

International Therapist, The Journal of the Federation of Holistic Therapists, Southampton

Journal of Essential Oil Research, edited by Brian Lawrence, published by Allured Publishing Corporation, 362 S. Schmale Road, Carol Stream, IL 60188, USA

Raw Materials Monographs, volumes published every few years by RIFM (Research Institute for Fragrance Materials). Available in the UK through Elsevier Science Ltd, The Boulevard, Longford Lane, Kidlington, Oxford, OX5 1 GB

Websites

AFNOR – Association Française de Normalisation – Safety and composition of oils
http://www.afnor.fr/bas_gb.htm

Aromatherapy Book Store, books only about aromatherapy and related topics in association with Amazon.com
http://www.angelfire.com/hi/oasisbydesign/bookstore.htm/

Aromatherapy Consortium (Aromatherapy Consortium)
http://www.aromatherapy-regulation.org.uk

Aromatherapy Council (AC)
http://www.aromatherapycouncil.co.uk

ATC (Aromatherapy Trade Council)
http://www.a-t-c.org.uk

Atlantic Institute of Aromatherapy
http://atlanticinstitute.com/oils.html

BACIS Archives – Wealth of information listing published papers relating to essential oils
http://www.xs4all.org/~bacis/pom9804l.html

B and R Harris, Essential Oil Resource Consultants, information on education and research in essential oils and aromatherapy
http://www.essentialorc.com

Essentially Oils Limited – Suppliers of oils, books and associated aromatherapy materials. Excellent monthly newsletter
http://www.essentiallyoils.com

FACT – Focus on Alternative and Complementary Therapies. A review journal aiming to present evidence about complementary medicine in an analytic and impartial manner. Written by research staff within the Department of Complementary Medicine, University of Exeter
http://www.exeter.ac.uk/FACT/aboutFACT.htm

FDA – US Food and Drug Administration
http://www.fda.gov/opacom/hpview.html

Federation of Holistic Therapists (FHT)
http://www.fht.org.uk

Green, environmental issues, official government information *http://direct.gov. uk/en/Environmentandgreenliving/Greenershopping*

Guardian Unlimited:

health and well-being – *http://www.lifeandhealth.guardian.co.uk* and

science – *http://www.guardian.co.uk/science*

House of Lords Report on Complementary and Alternative Medicine
www.publications.parliament.uk/pa/ld/ldsctech.htm
IFRA – International Fragrance Association
http://www.infraorg/About/Ifra.asp
INCI – International Nomenclature of Cosmetic Ingredients
http://dg3.eudra.org/inci/index.htm
International Journal of Aromatherapy (IJA)
http://www.elsevierhealth.com/journals/ija
International Journal of Clinical Aromatherapy (IJCA)
http://www.ijca.net/information.htm
ISO – International Standards Association
http://www.iso.ch/infoe/intro.htm
IFPA (International Federation of Professional Aromatherapists (IFPA)
http://www.ifparoma.org
International Journal of Clinical aromatherapy
http://www.ijca.net
Kew Gardens (Royal Botanic Gardens)
http://kew.org
The Complementary and Natural Healthcare council (CNHC)
http://www.cnhc.org.uk
General Regulatory Council for Complementary therapists (GRCCT)
http://www.grcct.org
MHRA (Medicines and Healthcare Regulatory Agency)
http://mhra.gov.uk
Details of NOS (National Occupational Standards)
http://www.skillsforhealth.org.uk
Plant Aromatics Safety Data Manuals by Martin Watt
http://www.aromamedical.demon.co.uk
Phytobotanica Centre – Covers the Phytobotanica Centre, organic farm and oil producer, education centre (Hygeia school). Useful information.
http://www.phytobotanica.com
Quinessence Aromatherapy oils supplier with good product information and current issues
http://www.quinessence.co.uk
RIFM – Research Institute for Fragrance Materials
http://pwl.netcom.com/~bcb56/RIFM.htm
Royal Horticultural Society
http://www.rhs.org.uk
Sabia's future<nature forum – information about wide range of aromatherapy issues
http://www.sabia.com
Soil Association
http://www.soilassociation.org
Statistics and Research Methods link on British Medical Journal (BMJ) site
http://www.bmj.com/allshtml
Telegraph
health issues – *http://www.telegraph.co.uk/health* and
science – *http://www.telegraph.co.uk/earth*
Times Online Health
http://www.timesonline.co.uk/tol/life_and_style/health

Molecular models

The Molymod System as used in this book. Supplied by Spiring Enterprises Ltd, Beke Hall, Billingshurst, West Sussex RH14 9HF – *http://www.molymod.com*

Analytical services

Analytical Intelligence, 10 Mount Farm, Junction Road, Churchill, Chipping Norton, Oxfordshire, OX7 6NP – *www.essentiallyoils.com*

Essential Analyses, Dr William Morden, Elm Cottage, Old Road, Whaley Bridge, High Peak. SK23 7HS – *www.essentialanalyses.co.uk*

Glossary

Absolute Materials obtained from a plant using enfleurage or solvent extraction. Enfleurage produces a pomade, which is a mixture of fat and essential oil, while solvent extraction gives a concrete made up of fats, waxes, essential oils and other plant materials. The absolute is then extracted by use of ethanol as a solvent.

Acid A compound that can form hydrogen ions (H^+); when dissolved in water gives the hydroxonium ion H_3O^+. Inorganic acids include sulphuric and nitric acid; organic acids contain the –COOH group (carboxylic acid) and include a large number of compounds such as ethanoic acid (formerly known as acetic acid). They are usually water soluble.

Absorption In biological items, movement of a fluid or dissolved substance across a cell membrane.

Adsorption A process where a substance, usually a gas, accumulates on the surface of a solid forming a thin film.

Adulteration The introduction of an impurity that is either accidentally or more normally deliberately introduced into a product and that alters its composition and properties, making it of an inferior quality.

Alcohol An organic compound containing one or more hydroxyl groups (–OH) attached directly to hydrocarbon structures other than benzene rings.

Aldehyde An organic compound containing the carbonyl group positioned at the end of the carbon chain, with a general formula

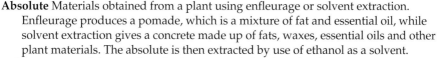

for example formaldehyde

Alkali A compound which when dissolved in water gives rise to any increase in hydroxyl ion (OH⁻) concentration. An alkali is a substance that, when in aqueous solution, gives a pH greater than 7.

Alkanes Saturated hydrocarbon compounds with the general formula C_nH_{2n+2}. Found in natural gas and petroleum, e.g. methane (CH_4), or natural gas. The larger molecules (e.g. $C_{16}H_{34}$) are waxy solids. Hexane (C_6H_{14}) is used as a solvent for extraction of plant materials. Alkanes are insoluble in water but dissolve easily in organic solvents such as chloroform.

Alkenes Unsaturated hydrocarbon compounds with the general formula C_nH_{2n} in the simplest cases. They contain double covalent bonds. Terpenes, an important constituent of essential oils, are alkenes.

Alkynes Unsaturated hydrocarbon compounds with the general formula C_nH_{2n-2} in the simplest cases. They contain triple covalent bonds. Uncommon in essential oil components.

Allergy An abnormal reaction by the body in response to a substance called an allergen (or antigen), e.g. 'foreign' proteins such as found in pollen. The body produces antibodies that are specific to that antigen and that cause a reaction on exposure to that antigen again. This allergic reaction is due to the presence of these previously formed antibodies and is called sensitization. This can take many forms, but on the skin it typically shows irritation and reddening.

Alpha (α) *See* Greek letters.

Amino acids The basic units that join together to make proteins. They contain functional groups amines ($-NH_2$) and carboxylic acids ($-COOH$), hence their name. The chemical bonds formed between amino acids when joining together to form proteins are called *peptide* links.

Analysis The identification of the composition of a substance. Physical methods used for essential oil mixtures include GC-MS. The identification of substances is called qualitative analysis, while the estimation of the amounts of components present is quantitative analysis.

Anion *See* Ion.

AOC Aromatherapy Organizations Council.

Aqueous Involving water: for example, an aqueous solution is a solution in water.

Aroma chemical A chemical that has a useful odour and is safe and legal for use as a fragrance or flavour.

Aromatherapy The use of essential oils in a controlled manner for the benefit of other living organisms. It does not usually involve internal application of essential oils.

Aromatic A term originally used to categorize organic compounds that were fragrant, though this now has little significance. In the chemical sense it describes the property of *aromaticity* as illustrated by benzene. For many years the structure of benzene presented a problem, and was shown with alternating single and double bonds in a hexagonal ring

It did not show properties of typical unsaturated compounds, suggesting that ordinary $-C=C-$ double bonds were not present. The bond lengths determined by X-ray analysis showed that all the carbon-to-carbon bonds in the ring were the same length. The chemical reactions normally undergone by double-bonded compounds were not shown by benzene. This was explained by assuming that six of the electrons in the benzene, one from each carbon atom, are able to move freely around the ring. They form new orbitals where electrons circulate freely, not attached to any particular carbon atom. The electrons are said to be *delocalized*, and are spread out, resulting in a more stable configuration.

The delocalized structure is often described as a hybrid or blend of two nominal structures:

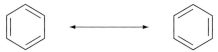

These structures are called *canonical* forms, and the actual resulting blended structure is called a *resonance hybrid*. They are usually represented as an aromatic sextet of *delocalized* electrons, represented by a circle within the benzene ring:

Delocalized structure

In derivatives of benzene, a hydrogen atom is replaced by a functional group. The group C_6H_5- is called a *phenyl* group, and the general name for substituted derivatives of the phenyl group is *aryl*.

Aromatology Use of essential oils for their pharmacological properties.

Artefact A product that may appear in analysis as a result of conditions of the analytical method is termed an artefact.

Asymmetric carbon atom A carbon atom with four different atoms or groups of atoms attached. This gives rise to optical activity. See isomerism.

Atom The smallest portion of an element that can enter into chemical change, and cannot be further subdivided without destroying its identity. The modern view of an atom is of a positively charged nucleus (made up of electrically neutral neutrons and positive protons) surrounded by a 'cloud' of negatively charged electrons.

Atomic number The number of protons in the nucleus of an atom.

Atomic weight Originally, and still useful as a close approximation, the atomic weight of an element was defined as the ratio of the weight (mass) of one atom of the element to that of one atom of hydrogen (hence, the atomic weight of hydrogen). Now atomic weight is defined as the ratio of the mass of one atom of the element to $\frac{1}{12}$ of the mass of the carbon-12 isotope ^{12}C.

Base (1) In simple chemical terms, a substance that in aqueous solution reacts with an acid to form a salt and water; considered to be hydrogen ion acceptors. (2) In perfumery, it refers to an ingredient specially formulated to represent a natural source or a blend of natural sources of fragrance, or an abstract fragrance concept.

Baseline The horizontal line on a graph (such as a spectrogram or chromatogram) drawn by the pen recorder when no signal is coming from the instrument.

Base note Shown by aromatic materials of low volatility, giving an extended persistence of fragrances.

Benzene ring The molecular structure of the cyclic, unsaturated, aromatic hydrocarbon benzene, C_6H_6:

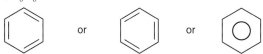

(*See* Aromatic) Compounds that contain one or more benzene rings in their molecules are called *benzenoid compounds*.

Beta (β) *See* Greek letters.

Body note *See* Middle note.

Boiling point The temperature at which a liquid boils; it is the temperature at which a liquid changes to a gas at atmospheric pressure.

Bond The means by which the atoms in a molecule are attached to each other giving them their positions in space (*see also* Covalent bond, Ionic bonding, Valency).

B.P. British Pharmacopoeia.

Carbonyl group Name given to the C=O group (carbon atom joined to an oxygen atom by a double bond) found in compounds such as aldehydes and ketones.

Carboxyl group
(a carbon atom joined to an oxygen atom with a double bond and to a hydroxy

$$-C\overset{OH}{\underset{O}{<}} \quad \text{group}$$

group by a single bond) found in organic acids.

Carboxylic acids Organic compounds containing one or more carboxyl groups. They are weaker acids than the mineral acids such as hydrochloric acid.

Carrier gas A chemically inert gas, e.g. nitrogen or helium, used to transport vapour through the column of a GLC/GC (gas–liquid chromatograph). Called the moving or mobile phase of the system.

Carrier oil Also called Fixed Oil, in which the essential oil is diluted, always coming from vegetable origins, e.g. sweet almond, grapeseed, jojoba. Unlike the essential oil they do not evaporate readily at room temperature.

Cation *See* Ion.

Centrifugation The separation of substances by use of a centrifuge, which is a machine using centrifugal force to obtain high rates of sedimentation or filtration in order to separate a solid and liquid or two immiscible liquids.

Chemical bond *See* Bond.

Chemical properties Properties shown by a substance when it undergoes a change in composition or reacts with another substance, e.g. in oxidation.

Chemical purity The extent to which a substance is made up of that substance only, usually expressed as a percentage.

Chemical reactions A rearrangement of atoms or ions with accompanying energy change.

Chemotype Plants from a given botanical species whose chemical composition varies from the average due to environmental growing conditions.

Chemovar Same as chemotype, meaning a chemical variety.

CHIP Chemicals Hazard Information and Packaging for Supply.

Chromatography A process for the separation of the constituents of a mixture of chemicals by passing a solution of the mixture or its vapour through a column of adsorbent material. The constituents of the mixture are adsorbed at different rates, more or less strongly, on the column and layers or bands of individual chemicals build up. *See also* GLC/GC. The instrument is termed a chromatograph and the trace produced a chromatogram.

cis/trans **isomers** *See* Isomerism.

Column The tube containing the stationary phase, through which the carrier gas takes the vaporized sample of material to be separated in the GLC/GC.

Compound A substance made up of specific numbers of atoms of two or more elements that are chemically bonded together.

Concentration The amount of a substance dissolved in a given amount of another substance. It may be expressed as a percentage (%), grams per litre or as mole fraction. For percentages these may be mass/mass, e.g. grams/100grams, or mass/volume, e.g. grams/100ml, or volume/volume, e.g. ml/100ml. Mole fraction is a fraction of the gram molecular weight of the compound in question.

Concrete The aromatic, waxy or fatty extract from plant material obtained by washing with a hydrocarbon solvent (such as hexane). Concretes are usually solid or semi-solid and contain essential oil, wax and soluble plant materials like pigments.

Condensation (1) Physically, the change of state of a substance from a gas or vapour phase to a liquid or solid. (2) Chemically, the addition of one molecule to another with the elimination of a simple molecule such as water.

Condenser A cooling device, in a distillation apparatus, that enables the vapour to change to a liquid (condense).

COSHH Control of Substances Hazardous to Health.

Covalent bond A type of bond joining together either atoms of the same element to give a molecule of that element (e.g. oxygen) or atoms of two or more elements to give a molecule of a compound (e.g. carbon dioxide). The component atoms share outer electrons to gain overall stability. When one electron from each atom is used in the bond, this represents a *single* bond; two electrons from each participating atom form a *double* bond; and three electrons from each participating atom form a *triple* bond. Covalent bonds are typically found in nonmetallic elements, and covalent bonding is the predominant form of bonding in organic chemistry.

Cutting A dilution or weakening of a substance. Essential oils may have additions to increase their volume such as alcohols, terpenes from other oils, and DPG (dipropylglycol) used for bulking up lavender.

Cyclic A molecule with atoms arranged in one or more rings, e.g. benzene, cyclohexane.

Delta (Δ and δ) *See* Greek letters.

Dermatitis An irritation or inflammation of the skin characterized by a redness and itching. The most common cause is due to contact with certain substances.

Detector Something that will react to a change and generate a measurable signal in response. Changes such as temperature, humidity or pressure are commonly encountered. In GC analyzers electrical conductivity changes are picked up by a flame ionization detector. Electrical signals from detectors in analytical instruments are then amplified and transmitted to a computer and chart recorder or monitor to give a visual display and record of the analytical results.

Dextrorotatory A molecule or material capable of rotating the plane of polarized light in a clockwise direction. *See* Optical isomers/Polarimeter.

Diffusion The inherent spreading out of a gas, or a solute in a solution, until it becomes evenly distributed throughout the system. It is movement of particles from a region of high concentration to that of low concentration, i.e. along a concentration gradient. It is explained on the basis of the kinetic theory whereby molecular motion leads to a uniform distribution of the molecules. Diffusion is an important mechanism for movement of materials in living systems.

Dilution Making something less concentrated; a solution is said to be dilute when it contains a small proportion of the dissolved solute. Essential oils are diluted in carrier oils.

Distillation The process of separating a liquid from a solid, or other liquids, by vaporizing it and then condensing the vapour. Fractional distillation separates mixtures into series of fractions of different volatilities (boiling points) by means of distillation. *See also* Steam distillation.

Diterpenes Unsaturated hydrocarbons with the empirical formula $C_{20}H_{32}$, considered to be dimers of monoterpenes $C_{10}H_{16}$.

Double bond (*See also* Covalent bond) A bond between two bonds involving four electrons, two from each atom.

Electromagnetic spectrum The complete range of electromagnetic radiation from the longest radio waves to the shortest gamma radiation. Those used in chemical analysis include ultraviolet (UV) and infrared (IR).

Electron The negatively charged particle of very small mass (1/2000 that of a proton) that orbits around the nucleus in the atom.

Electrovalency A numerical value used for combining power of an atom equal to the number of electrons it can either lose or gain when forming ions. (*See* Ionic bonding)

Element A substance that cannot be broken down to yield other simpler substances by chemical methods. An element is made up wholly of atoms having the same nuclear charge, that is their nuclei all contain the same number of protons, and consequently the same number of electrons. Elements are basic substances from which all others are built up by chemical combination.

Empirical formula Simplest whole-number formula expressing the composition of a chemical compound. For example, the empirical formula for the sesquiterpene bisabolene is C_5H_8, while its molecular formula is three times that, giving $C_{15}H_{24}$.

Enantiomers or enantiomorphs Optical isomers. The dextrorotary and laevorotatory forms of an optically active substance are said to be enantiomorphic. (*See* Isomerism (3))

Enfleurage The method of absorbing essential oils, from living flowers into preserved fat over a period of time. Now obsolete.

Essential oil Many definitions exist, referring to the odoriferous and volatile products from natural sources. Usually extracted by expression or steam distillation from a single species, producing an essential oil that corresponds to that species in chemical composition and odour.

Esters The product of the reaction between an alcohol or phenol (with the –OH functional group) and a carboxylic acid (with the –COOH functional group). The ester formed has the functional group

$$(R)-\overset{\displaystyle \overset{O}{\|}}{C}\underset{\displaystyle O-(R)}{}$$

and water is lost in the reaction. Considered to be gentle and safe components of essential oils, e.g. geranyl acetate, linalyl acetate.

Ether Organic compounds with molecules containing an oxygen atom bonded to two hydrocarbon chains or ring structures. Insoluble in water but soluble in organic solvents and alcohol, e.g. diethyl ether ($C_2H_5OC_2H_5$), a colourless, sweet, characteristically smelling, highly volatile and flammable liquid. Used as an early anaesthetic administered by inhalation.

Evaporation The change of a liquid or solid to a gas or vapour phase.

Expression A mechanical method using compression and pressure for removing essential oils from the skins of citrus fruits, e.g. lemon, orange, bergamot.

Extraction The removal of a soluble material from a solid mixture by means of a solvent, or removal of one or more components from a liquid mixture by use of a solvent with which the liquid is immiscible. An extract is the soluble matter from a natural source washed with solvent, followed by removal of the solvent to give products such as concretes, absolutes and resinoids.

Fixed oil A vegetable oil that does not evaporate at normal room temperature and pressure, e.g. olive, sweet almond.

Flash point The temperature, under standardized conditions, at which a liquid begins to evolve flammable vapours.

Floral oil *See* Infused oil.

Floral water *See* Hydrosol.

Formulation A systematic description of components from the process of composing a formula for a product such as a cream or massage blend.

Fractional distillation A distillation process that separates a mixture into portions of different volatilities/boiling points, which may be collected in separate receivers. A *fraction* is one of these separately collected distillate portions. The *fractionating column* is the vertical column, made of inert material such as glass or stainless steel, used to separate the different fractions from the vapours coming from the distillation vessel.

Functional group That group of atoms or atom within a molecule that is the most chemically reactive and gives the molecule its chemical characteristics. Compounds are classified and named accordingly, e.g. –OH functional groups in alcohols, named -ol as in linalool.

Furanocoumarins Also called furocoumarins, methoxypsoralens or bergaptenes. Found in cold-pressed citrus oils, e.g. bergamot. An oxygen-containing cyclic structure associated with phototoxicity on exposure to ultraviolet light.

Gamma (γ) *See* Greek letters.

GC/GLC (Gas–liquid chromatography) Now usually called GC. A technique for separating volatile samples of mixtures into their components. The sample is vaporized and constituents separate owing to differential solubilities in the nonvolatile absorbent column coating of the chromatography column through which they pass. The vaporized sample is carried by the inert carrier gas and all the constituents are maintained in the vapour phase by the apparatus. Results of the analysis are recorded on a chromatogram made up of a series of peaks, drawn by the pen recorder or recording device. Each peak corresponds to a particular constituent and has a characteristic position. [The abbreviation GC is also often applied to the apparatus (gas chromatograph) as well as to the technique (gas chromatography).]

Geometric isomerism *See* Isomerism.

GLA (Gamma linoleic acid) An essential fatty acid that the body requires to be provided in the diet for the manufacture of important bodily chemicals such as hormones and participation in other beneficial reactions. Found in evening primrose, starflower, borage, blackcurrant seed and rosehip seed.

Greek letters Greek letters are used to symbolize objects and phenomena in science. In chemistry they are used to describe configurations in isomers of molecules, e.g. α- and β-pinenes to describe the position of the double bonds. The most commonly encountered are the first few letters of the Greek alphabet, which are

Alpha (α)

Beta (β)

Gamma (γ)

Delta (upper case Δ, lower case δ)

Hazardous oils Those considered too dangerous to use at all, or that need to be handled with extreme caution.

Homologous series A series or family of compounds whose molecules vary only in the length of the hydrocarbon portion by the number of methylene ($-CH_2$) groups.

Hydrocarbon A compound whose molecules are made up of only atoms of hydrogen and carbon.

Hydrogen bond A weak, electrostatic bond between oppositely charged parts of molecules; for example an oxygen atom in an alcohol is slightly negatively charged ($\delta-$) and will be attracted to the hydrogen atom, slightly positively charged ($\delta+$), of another molecule of alcohol.

Hydrolysis In general a reaction between a substance and water; for example, esters can be hydrolysed to form alcohols and carboxylic acids.

Hydrosol (or Hydrolat) Also known as floral waters. The water collected when plants are distilled to extract essential oils. Considered gentle and therapeutically useful, especially for skin conditions, as they can be applied without dilution: e.g. lavender water, orangeflower water, chamomile hydrolats.

Hydroxyl group The $-OH$ functional group found in molecules of alcohols and water. NB: Do not confuse it with the hydroxide ion, which has a negative charge $OH-$.

IFRA International Fragrance Association. An advisory body for safety of materials.

Inflammation The production of redness, swelling, heat and pain in a tissue in response to chemical or physical injury, or to infection. When the body tissues are damaged, the chemical histamine is released, which increases blood flow, causing the redness and heat.

Infrared (IR) Electromagnetic radiation of longer wavelength than red light, in the range 730 billionths of a metre (730 nm) to about 1 mm.

Infrared (IR) spectroscopy A spectroscopic instrumental technique measuring the absorption of infrared radiation over a range of frequencies by molecules of a substance. The infrared spectrogram (or 'spectrum') is produced as an analytical record of this absorption; it is unique to each compound (when performed under standard conditions) and can be useful as a 'fingerprint' for comparative identifications.

Infused oil Produced by immersion of plant material in vegetable oil, often gently heated to release aromatic products from the plant into the oil. Also called macerated oils or herbal oils.

Inhalation The entry of gases into the body through the nasal tract.

Injection point The site for introduction of small quantities of material to be analyzed into a gas–liquid chromatograph.

Inorganic chemistry The chemistry of the elements other than carbon.

Instrumental analysis The analysis of material using an analytical instrument such as a GC (gas chromatograph) or MS (mass spectrometer).

Integrator A computer that processes results produced by an analytical machine such as a gas chromatograph.

Ion An atom or molecule that has either lost or gained one or more electrons to give a charged particle, called an ion. Typically metal atoms lose electrons to give positive (+) ions termed cations, while nonmetals gain electrons to give negative (−) ions called anions.

Ionic bonding (Sometimes called electrovalent bonding.) A bond formed between + ions (cations) and − ions (anions). The oppositely charged ions exert an attractive force to give aggregate structures or lattices that are typically high melting point solids soluble in water. Found predominantly in inorganic chemistry.

Ionization The process whereby an ion is formed (i.e. gain or loss of electrons by atoms or molecules).

Isolate The term for a single constituent that has been separated from a mixture of volatiles such as an essential oil, e.g. citral from lemongrass, limonene from citrus oils.

Isomerism The existence of a compound in the form of molecules with the same molecular formula but a different structural arrangement of the atoms. Different types of isomerism exist.

(1) *Structural isomerism*, where atoms are arranged in different configurations; for example the molecular formula C_2H_6O can be either C_2H_5OH (ethanol) or CH_3OCH_3 (dimethyl ether).

(2) *Geometric isomerism*, found in compounds with double bonds where there is no free rotation of the attached atoms or groups of atoms about the bond. This gives rise to two isomers, denominated *cis* and *trans*; for example for but-2-ene (C_4H_8) the *cis* isomer has the methyl groups ($-CH_3$) on the same side of the bond, while the *trans* form has them on opposite sides:

cis   trans

(3) *Optical isomerism* occurs in molecules with an asymmetric carbon atom – that is one that is attached to four different atoms or functional groups. The two different optical isomers are called optical isomers or enantiomers and rotate polarized light in opposite directions. The *d*-isomer rotates it clockwise and is called *dextrorotatory*; the *l*-isomer rotates it anticlockwise and is called *laevorotatory*. Despite their structural similarity, optical isomers exhibit significantly different physiological properties. In the case of essential oils their smells can be very dissimilar. When a compound is made up of equal amounts of the *d*- and *l*-isomers it will be optically inactive and is called a *racemic mixture*, or *racemate*.

ISO The International Organization for Standardization. Relates to criteria for composition of essential oils, among a vast range of other products and services.

Isoprene The basic building unit of the group of chemicals called the terpenes (2-methylbuta-1,3-diene), molecular formula C_5H_8.

Ketones Organic compounds containing the carbonyl C=O functional group. Present in essential oils and often considered very powerful and potentially toxic; thujone is an example.

Lactone An organic compound that contains an ester group incorporated into a carbon ring structure. Lactones include the coumarins, e.g. umbelliferone or 7-hydroxycoumarin. Lactones and furocoumarins, e.g. bergaptene, exist in small quantities in essential oils and should be used with care. Lactones can be neuro-toxic (poisonous to the nervous system) and cause skin allergies. Bergaptene is well known for its phototoxicity on the skin.

LD$_{50}$ Lethal dose 50%. A traditional method for determining toxicity of a substance. The value is the dosage required to kill 50% of the animals used in the test sample. The animals used are usually rats or mice; the LD$_{50}$ value is expressed in terms of the ratio of grams of test substance to kilograms of the animals' body weight. The experimental value is then extrapolated from test animal values to humans.

Litre Originally described as the volume occupied by 1 kg of pure water. Now defined as 1 cubic decimetre, written as dm^3.

Maceration A method of extracting materials, such as herbs, by soaking the plant material in water or alcohol for several days. The resulting material is called a *tincture* when ethanol is used. Tinctures were traditionally used in pharmaceuticals and perfumes but are practically obsolete now (*see also* Infused oil).

Mass number The sum of the numbers of protons and neutrons in the nucleus of an atom.

Mass spectrometer (MS) The instrument used to perform mass spectrometry. The abbreviation MS is often used for the instrument as well as the technique. The record made is termed a mass spectrum.

Mass spectrometry (MS) An analytical technique for determining the composition of a compound. The molecule breaks into separate fragments as a result of bombardment by high-energy electrons and these fragments are sorted by mass. The mass and abundance of each fragment are displayed as a fragmentation pattern, which is characteristic of the original molecule.

Melting point The temperature at which a solid turns into a liquid.

Metabolism The sum total of the chemical processes that occur in living organisms, divided into *anabolism*, which consumes energy (e.g. synthesis of proteins) and *catabolism*, which releases energy (e.g. breakdown of complex molecules in respiration).

Microlitre One millionth of a litre; written as μl (Greek prefix 'mu').

Middle note A fragrance note of intermediate volatility and lasting power.

Millilitre One thousandth of a litre, written as ml.

Miscibility Describing the ability of two liquids to disperse fully and uniformly in one another. Two *miscible* liquids are liquid substances that are fully dispersed together, e.g. essential oils in alcohol. *Immiscible* when they are incapable of mixing together, e.g. oil and water.

Molarity A *molar* solution contains one *mole* of a substance (element or compound) dissolved in a litre of solution.

Mole A *mole* is a measure of amount of substance. One mole is the formula weight of the substance expressed in grams. For example, for limonene, formula $C_{10}H_{16}$, the formula weight is $(C = 12) (10 \times 12) + (16 \times 1) (H = 1) = 136$ so that one mole of limonene is 136 grams of the compound. One mole of any substance contains the same number of 'units' (atoms, molecules or ions). This is termed the Avogadro number, 6.022×10^{23} in scientific notation.

Molecular formula The formula that expresses the numbers of each constituent element atom present in one molecule of a compound. For example, geraniol has 10 carbon atoms, 18 hydrogens and 1 oxygen, so its molecular formula is $C_{10}H_{18}O$.

Molecular structure A description of the position, type, direction and arrangement of bonds holding the atoms of a molecule together.

Molecular weight (or mass) The sum of all the atomic weights (masses) of the atoms in the molecule.

Molecule The smallest particle of compound that can exist in the free state.

Monomer An individual chemical compound whose molecule is capable of joining to others of the same type to form a polymer. The *polymer* is a large molecule made up of many repeated monomer units linked together by chemical bonds.

Monoterpene A terpene with the molecular formula $C_{10}H_{16}$ (two isoprene units). Present in almost all essential oils depending on the distillation conditions, e.g. pinene and limonene.

Moving phase The carrier gas in gas chromatography, also known as the *mobile phase*.

Nanometre (nm) A unit of measure for length frequently used for measuring very small structures. It is 10^{-9} metre, or one billionth of a metre.

Nature identical oils A combination of synthetically produced chemicals, or chemicals extracted from cheap oils, made to imitate a genuine essential oil. Owing to the complex and variable nature of natural essential oils, synthetics cannot hope to replicate their properties and are not suitable for aromatherapy.

Neutron The electrically neutral particle, designated one unit mass, found in the nuclei of an atom.

Nose Essential for aromatherapy, as it is where the volatile molecules of the oil are inhaled and can reach the bloodstream. The olfactory system links into the nervous system for interpretation and appreciation of smell.

Note A classification of aromatic components of essential oils and perfumes. Top notes are sharp, penetrating and highly volatile (e.g. citrus oils, peppermint). Middle note characteristics are used to give body to blends (e.g. geranium, lavender). Base notes are the least volatile and used as fixatives to give more permanence (e.g. sandalwood, vetivert).

Nucleus (1) In chemistry, the central body of an atom, made up of positively charged protons and electrically neutral neutrons. Virtually all of the mass of an atom is in the nucleus. (2) In biology, in living cells the nucleus is a dense area, within a membrane, containing the genetic material (DNA).

Odorant Any substance with an odour.

Odour The property of a substance that gives a characteristic scent or smell.

Olfactory Term relating to the sense of smell. The olfactory system is made up of a pair of small patches of epithelial tissue at the top of the nose called the *olfactory organs*. Microscopic threads called *olfactory hairs* detect the presence of odorous molecules and send impulses along the *olfactory nerve* to the brain for interpretation.

Optical isomers *See* Isomerism (3).

Optical rotation *See* Isomerism (3).

Orbitals The region in space, around the nucleus of an atom, where electrons circulate.

Organic acid *See* Carboxylic acid.

Organic chemistry The study of the chemistry of carbon compounds, other than those involving ionic bonding such as carbonates; i.e. the study of carbon compounds with covalent bonds.

Oxidation A type of chemical reaction in which oxygen combines with another element or compound, or in which hydrogen is removed from a compound. It is also used as a generalized term for the loss of one or more electrons from an atom, ion or molecule.

Oxide A compound of oxygen with another element. The most commonly occurring oxide in aromatherapy is 1,8-cineole, or eucalyptol, where the oxygen atom is included in a ring structure.

Oxygenated constituent A general term relating to constituents of essential oils that contain combined oxygen, e.g. monoterpene alcohols.

Partition The partitioning (distribution) of an essential oil between different solvents, utilizing the different solubilities of the oil components. Usually the distribution of a solute between two immiscible solvents in contact with each other; for example an essential oil in solvents pentane (a hydrocarbon) and aqueous methanol will separate into their constituents. Oxygenated compounds and terpenes will dissolve in both solvents, but terpenes mainly in the pentane and oxygenated compounds mainly in the alcohol.

Pathogenic Causing disease.

Peak area *Peaks* in a chromatogram represent the various constituents that have been separated. The area of the peak is approximately proportional to the amount of that substance. *Peak height* is the vertical distance from the baseline to the peak apex.

Percolation An extraction method for getting essential oils from plants. It is similar to distillation, but the steam is produced in a generator above the plant material and percolates downwards through it.

Perfume A fragrant material, traditionally a mixture of alcohol and fragrant essential oils extracted from plants but now more likely to be a blend of synthetic chemicals.

Periodic table An arrangement of the chemical elements in order of their atomic numbers. Arranged as horizontal *periods* and vertical *groups* or families of elements with similar properties. Its initiation is attributed to the nineteenth century Russian chemist Mendeleyev. A modern periodic table, which differs significantly from early ones, is shown on page **283**.

The *periodic law* states that the properties of the elements are a periodic (i.e. regularly repeating after an interval) function of their atomic numbers.

pH A measure of acidity or alkalinity of an aqueous solution expressed as a numerical value calculated from the concentration of hydrogen ions present. A pH less than 7 is acidic, pH 7 is neutral, and pH above 7 is alkaline. NB: The lower the number the more acidic the solution.

Phenol(s) Aromatic molecules in which one or more hydroxyl groups (–OH) are directly attached to a benzene ring. Phenols are powerful antibacterial compounds and essential oils containing phenols need to be used with caution. Examples of phenols in essential oils include thymol, carvacrol and eugenol. Phenol is the name for the parent compound, the simplest of the phenols (C_6H_5OH).

Phenylpropane derivatives The name given to compounds of phenol that have a three-carbon-atom (propyl) chain attached; those most commonly found in essential oils are thymol, carvacrol, chavicol (*see* Phenols).

Photosynthesis The metabolic reactions of green plants (and some other organisms such as certain bacteria) that produce sugars and ultimately other vital components for the plant. Photosynthesis requires sunlight as an energy source and carbon dioxide and produces oxygen as a by-product.

Phototoxicity An excessive reaction to sunlight (or UV light) caused by chemicals such as the furanocoumarins (e.g. bergaptene in bergamot oil) when applied to the skin. The phototoxic substances are able to absorb the UV light and cause it to produce abnormally dark pigmentation and reddening and burning of the surrounding skin. The darkened skin may remain for years and the burns can be slow to heal. Dilution is an important factor here. It is recommended that skin that has been treated with oils such as bergamot or expressed lime should not be exposed to sunlight or UV lamps for at least 12 hours if the oils are used in concentrations in excess of 0.4% and 0.7%, respectively. Even expressed oils of bitter orange, grapefruit and lemon should be used carefully, and again treated skin should not be exposed to sunlight or UV lamps for at least 12 hours if these oils were used at concentrations of more than 1.4%, 4.0% and 2.0%, respectively. This should be taken into account when formulating blends of such oils.

Periodic table

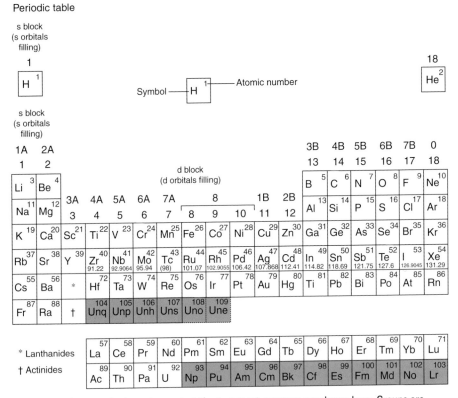

There are various numbering schemes but the two most common are shown here. Groups are traditionally numbered 1 (or I) to 8 (or VIII), with the left-hand groups designated A and the right-hand groups B, with the noble gases being Group 0. In a more recent scheme, the groups are numbered straight across, 1 to 18. (Hence the noble gases are variously described as Group 0 or Group 18.)

After period (row) 3, the order of filling of the subshells (designated s, p, d, f) within each main shell shows less regularity than in the first three periods. The 4s subshell starts to fill before the 3d and because the f subshells in periods 6 and 7 fill up 'inside' already filled outer subshells, the blocks of elements labelled lanthanides and actinides are each shown occupying a single position. This partly reflects their very great chemical similarity to one another (so that each block effectively forms a single group), but is also a practical device to avoid expanding the table to an unwieldy length and having 32 groups.

The elements above atomic number 92 (shown shaded) are not found in nature but can be created in 'atom smashers'; the atoms break up in radioactive decay processes very quickly.

Physical properties Those properties of a substance that do not involve any chemical change, e.g. melting point, boiling point, specific gravity and optical rotation. The tests used to measure physical properties are called *physical tests*.

Placebo An inactive substance administered to a patient, usually to compare its effects with those of the real drug. *The placebo effect* is a positive therapeutic effect claimed by patients after receiving a placebo believed by them to be an active drug.

Polarimeter Instrument that measures the optical rotation of a transparent liquid or solid.

Polarization Describes a state of a light ray in which the vibration is in a single plane as the light propagates. The separation of light rays with vibrations in all planes into light vibrating in a single plane is achieved by an instrument called a polarizer. The *plane of polarization* is the plane in which light vibrates following polarization.

Polarized light Light (electromagnetic radiation) with a specific plane of polarization.

Polymer A large molecule made up of many smaller repeating units called *monomers*.

Pomade The product formed by enfleurage, made up of fat containing fragrance materials.

Positional isomer *See* Isomerism.

Proton The positively charged particle in the nucleus of the atom, designated one unit mass; the number of protons present in the element is its atomic number.

Psoriasis A skin condition characterized by formation of reddish spots and patches covered with silvery scales.

Qualitative analysis Identification of the components of a substance, e.g. compounds present in an essential oil, without measuring their amounts or concentrations.

Quantitative analysis Measurement of the amounts or concentrations of components in a substance, e.g. percentage amounts of compounds in an essential oil.

Reaction *See* Chemical reaction.

Reagent A substance used in, and undergoing, chemical reactions.

RCO Reconstituted oils. Created in the laboratory and unlike natural and genuine oils with their complexity of trace amounts of unidentified components and slightly variable composition. Not suitable for aromatherapy.

Rectification The process whereby an essential oil is processed to remove unwanted components, e.g. by redistilling.

Refractive index (RI) The measure of the bending of the path of a light ray when passing from a less dense into a more dense medium, e.g. air to water, or vice versa. It is measured by an instrument called a *refractometer*. May be used as an analytical technique for examining essential oils.

Resinoid The purified, viscous, highly scented material produced by extraction of plant material with hydrocarbon solvents, e.g. benzoin.

Retention time The time a vaporized compound takes to pass through the column in gas–liquid chromatography (i.e. the time it is 'retained' in the column).

RIFM Research Institute for Fragrance Materials. Important for testing and advising on safety of perfumery ingredients and relevant to essential oils.

Saturated compound An organic compound with no multiple (double or triple) bonds, i.e. with only single bonds.

Sensory Related to the senses and sensory system. Provides information about changes in the environment and sends them to the central nervous system (CNS) for interpretation, e.g. in response to the smell of an oil.

Sesquiterpene A terpene with the molecular formula $C_{15}H_{24}$, literally 1½ monoterpenes, e.g. farnesene.

Sesquiterpenoid Derived from a sesquiterpene but containing a functional group such as an alcohol; e.g. bisabolol, called a sesquiterpenol.

Shelf life That period of time during which a product is considered fit for use.

Skeletal formula The representation of an organic compound's carbon-to-carbon bonds by lines. A single line represents a single bond with double and triple lines for double and triple bonds, respectively. The carbon-to-hydrogen bonds are assumed but not shown apart from the outline, but other functional groups or elements use their conventional representation.

Skin irritation A reaction to an irritant that produces itchiness and inflammation. The reactions of different individuals to a given potential irritant can vary, as there is a wide tolerance range. The majority of essential oils in aromatherapy used in the correct dilutions are perfectly safe, but potential irritants are usually used at a strength of 1% or less.

Skin sensitization This differs from skin irritation in that, once the skin has reacted to the substance, upon subsequent exposure it will be even more sensitive. This is an example of an allergic response (*see* Allergy) as the immune system has reacted to produce antibodies. Upon subsequent exposure, antibodies can be rapidly released again. Essential oils used by aromatherapists that may cause this effect are cinnamon bark and ylang ylang.

Smell (verb) To perceive the scent of a substance by means of the olfactory apparatus (*see* Odour, Olfactory).

Smell (noun) The odour emitted from a substance and perceived by the olfactory apparatus.

Solvent A liquid or substance capable of dissolving another. The substance dissolved is the *solute* and the resulting homogeneous mixture of molecules is called a *solution*.

Specific gravity (SG) The ratio of the weight of a given volume of a substance to the weight of an equal volume of water measured at a stated temperature and pressure.

Spectrogram A diagram or graph of a spectrum resulting from the spectroscopic examination of a substance; e.g. a graph of the absorption of infrared (IR) radiation by a substance, plotted over a range of wavelengths.

Spectroscopy Spectroscopy is the practice of using spectrometers and spectroscopes and analysing spectra. The spectrometer is the instrument that produces a spectrum (usually where wavelengths, energy or intensity can be measured). The spectroscope is the instrument that uses the electromagnetic radiation of a material to form the recording or spectrum or spectrogram.

Standard sample A sample of a product that conforms to a given specification for that product. It is kept for purposes of comparison for evaluating other samples.

Standard solution A solution containing a known weight of a solute in a known volume of solution, i.e. of precisely known concentration. Molar solutions are commonly used in chemistry (*see* Molarity).

Stationary phase In GC (GLC) the term used for the nonvolatile adsorbent material lining the column.

Steam distillation A type of distillation in which steam under pressure heats and releases the volatile components from the sample of material. For essential oils, the material is the plant tissue.

Stereoisomer *See* Isomerism, Optical isomerism.

Still The name given to distillation equipment.

Straight chain The series of carbon atoms joined together in an unbranched succession in noncyclic organic compounds.

Synergy The increased effect achieved by two or more substances working together over and above the simple additive effect. Synergy is important in genuine essential oils, where components are synergistic and the effect of the whole is greater than the sum of its separate parts.

Synthesis The building up of more complex compounds from simpler compounds or elements.

Synthetic oil An aroma chemical made up of synthetic chemicals.

Terpeneless essential oil An essential oil with all or part of the terpene content removed by solvent extraction or vacuum fractionation.

Terpenes A significant family of naturally occurring unsaturated hydrocarbon compounds. They, and the compounds derived from them called the terpenoids, are widespread in nature. They constitute a large number of compounds present in plants including the essential oils. They have the empirical formula $(C_5H_8)_n$. When $n = 2$, the compound is a monoterpene; $n = 3$ corresponds to sesquiterpenes; $n = 4$ to diterpenes; $n = 5$ to sesterterpenes; and $n = 6$ to triterpenes. Terpenes up to $n = 4$ are found in distilled essential oils.

Terpenoids Components of essential oils based on the hydrocarbon skeleton of terpene plus a functional group such as an aldehyde, alcohol or ketone.

Tincture The alcoholic solution of extractable matter from suitable material, prepared by maceration.

Top notes The most volatile ingredients of an essential oil or perfume. The first smells perceived by the olfactory apparatus.

Toxin A poisonous substance of plant or animal origin.

Triple bond A covalent bond between two atoms, made up of three pairs of electrons.

Unsaturated compound A compound with molecules containing one or more double or triple bonds.

Ultraviolet (UV) Electromagnetic radiation with wavelengths shorter than visible light but longer than X-rays (13 to 400 billionths of a metre; 13–400 nm). Used in analytical chemical techniques. Reacts with components of the skin.

Ultraviolet (UV) spectroscopy Measurement of the absorption of UV light in a range of wavelengths as a means of identifying compounds.

Valency The combining power of an atom or ion: e.g., the valency of C is 4, of H is 1 and of O is 2.

Viscosity The extent to which a fluid resists a tendency to flow.

Volatile A volatile substance is capable of readily changing from a solid or liquid to a vapour or gas. Gives a basis for the concept of classification of aromatic components into top (most volatile), middle (intermediate volatility) and base (least volatile) notes. Used as a noun to denote a volatile compound or substance.

Virus Smallest microorganism, consisting of nucleic acid surrounded by protein and only able to reproduce within another living organism. Responsible for diseases such as influenza, common cold.

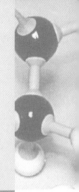

Index

NB: Page numbers in **bold** refer to boxed, figures and tables. Page numbers in *italics* refer to glossary entries.

A

Absolutes, 53, 83–84, 86, 156, 189
    definition, 130, *271*
    resin, 200
    'true', 201
Absorption, *271*
    molecular weight and, 22
    spectrum, IR spectroscopy and, 103
Acetic acid, 80
Acids, 69, **70**, *271*
    aromatic, **70**
    carboxylic, **40**, 65, 209, *274*
    in essential oils, **70**
    polyacids, 41
'Acquis communautair', 237
Acupuncture, 5
Acyclic chain structure, 42
Additions, 92–93
Adenosine monophosphate, cyclic (cAMP), 111
Adenosine triphosphate (ATP), 111
Adsorption, *271*
Adulterated oils, **90**
Adulteration, 23, 87, 88, 131, *271*
    acceptable, 159
    detecting, 106, 133
Advisory bodies, 130–132
Affinity, GC and, 97
Alcohols, 16, **39**, **42**, 54–58, **55**
    aromatic, 58
    chemotypes, 148–149, **149**
    clary sage and, 141
    definition, *271*

    functional groups, 54, 103
    monoterpene, in essential oils, 54, **55**
    noncyclic, 128
    non-terpene-derived aliphatic, 58
    phenylethyl (PEA), 82, 92
    removal, 83
    santanol, 195
    sesquiterpene, in essential oils, 56, **57**
    as solvents, 92
Aldehydes, 38, **40**, **42**, 63–66, **63**
    definition, *271*
    in essential oils, **65**
    functional groups, 53
    properties of, 65
    synthetic fatty, 65
Aliphatic alcohols, non-terpene-derived, 58
Aliphatic chain structure, 42
Aliphatic hydrocarbons *see* Hydrocarbons
Alkali, *271*
Alkanes, **29**, 38–39, **39**, *271–272*
    bonds, IR spectroscopy and, 103
Alkenes, **29**, **39**, 42, *272*
    bonds, IR spectroscopy and, 103
Alkyl groups, 60
Alkynes, **29**, *272*
Allergy, 217, 218, 247, 263, *272*
Allopathic medicine, 1, 116, 117, 119
Alternative medicine *see* Complementary and alternative medicine (CAM)
Aluminium atom, 18
Aluminium ion, 18
Alveoli, 251
Amber glass, containers, 232
Amino acids, *272*
Ammonaceae, 190–195
Amygdala, 113

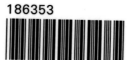